PPE PREPARTICIPATION EVALUATION

6TH EDITION

Editors
Joel S. Brenner, MD, MPH, FAAP, FAMSSM
Cynthia R. LaBella, MD, FAAP, FAMSSM

American Academy of Family Physicians

American Academy of Pediatrics

American College of Sports Medicine

American Medical Society for Sports Medicine

American Orthopaedic Society for Sports Medicine

American Osteopathic Academy of Sports Medicine

With endorsement and contributions by
American Heart Association
National Athletic Trainers' Association
National Federation of State High School Associations

American Academy of Pediatrics

DEDICATED TO THE HEALTH OF ALL CHILDREN®

American Academy of Pediatrics Publishing Staff
Jeff Mahony, *Senior Director, Professional and Consumer Publishing*
Chris Wiberg, *Senior Editor, Professional/Clinical Publishing*
Carrie Peters, *Editor, Professional/Clinical Publishing*
Annika Hawkinson, *Editorial Assistant*
Shannan Martin, *Production Manager, Consumer Publications*
Theresa Wiener, *Production Manager, Clinical and Professional Publications*
Soraya Alem, *Manager, Digital Publishing*
Emily Slayden, *Marketing Manager, Professional Resources*

Published by the American Academy of Pediatrics
345 Park Blvd
Itasca, IL 60143
630/626-6000
www.aap.org

The American Academy of Pediatrics is an organization of 67,000 primary care pediatricians, pediatric medical subspecialists, and pediatric surgical specialists dedicated to the health, safety, and well-being of all infants, children, adolescents, and young adults.

While every effort has been made to ensure the accuracy of this publication, the American Academy of Pediatrics does not guarantee that it is accurate, complete, or without error.

The recommendations in this publication do not indicate an exclusive course of treatment or serve as a standard of medical care. Variations, taking into account individual circumstances, may be appropriate.

Statements and opinions expressed are those of the authors and not necessarily those of the American Academy of Pediatrics.

Any websites, brand names, products, or manufacturers are mentioned for informational and identification purposes only and do not imply an endorsement by the American Academy of Pediatrics (AAP). The AAP is not responsible for the content of external resources. Information was current at the time of publication.

The publishers have made every effort to trace the copyright holders for borrowed materials. If they have inadvertently overlooked any, they will be pleased to make the necessary arrangements at the first opportunity.

This publication has been developed by the American Academy of Pediatrics. The contributors are expert authorities in the field of pediatrics. No commercial involvement of any kind has been solicited or accepted in the development of the content of this publication. Financial and conflict of interest disclosures for the authors of this book can be found at https://publications.aap.org/aapbooks/pages/MA1231.

Every effort has been made to ensure that the drug selection and dosages set forth in this publication are in accordance with the current recommendations and practice at the time of publication. It is the responsibility of the health care professional to check the package insert of each drug for any change in indications or dosage and for added warnings and precautions.

Every effort is made to keep *PPE: Preparticipation Evaluation* consistent with the most recent advice and information available from the American Academy of Pediatrics.

Please visit www.aap.org/errata for an up-to-date list of any applicable errata for this publication.

Special discounts are available for bulk purchases of this publication. Email Special Sales at nationalaccounts@aap.org for more information.

Printed in the United States of America

9-543/0926 1 2 3 4 5 6 7 8 9 10
MA1231
ISBN: 978-1-61002-906-3
eBook: 978-1-61002-907-0
Cover and publication design by Peg Mulcahy
Library of Congress Control Number: 2026934321

PREPARTICIPATION EVALUATION WORKING GROUP AND AUTHORS

Author Societies

American Academy of Family Physicians
American Academy of Pediatrics
American College of Sports Medicine
American Medical Society for Sports Medicine
American Orthopaedic Society for Sports Medicine
American Osteopathic Academy of Sports Medicine

Endorsing and Contributing Societies

American Heart Association
National Athletic Trainers' Association
National Federation of State High School Associations

Editors

Joel S. Brenner, MD, MPH, FAAP, FAMSSM
Cynthia R. LaBella, MD, FAAP, FAMSSM

Organization Representatives

Stephanie Aldret, DO, CAQSM, FAOASM
Holly Benjamin, MD, FACSM, FAAP
Bonnie P. Gregory, MD, FAAOS
Sarah E. Henson, MD, FAAP
Jason M. Matuszak, MD, FAAFP, FAMSSM
Teri McCambridge, MD, FAAP
Alex McDonald, MD, CAQSM, FAAFP
Kody Moffatt, MD, MS, FAAP, FACSM
Stephen Paul, MD, MA, CAQSM, FAMSSM
Amy Powell, MD, FACP, FAMSSM
Francisco Silva, MD, MPH, FAAP
Mary Solomon, DO, FACOP, FAOASM
Siobhan M. Statuta, MD, FACSM, FAMSSM
Ciara Taylor, EdD, LAT, ATC
Edwin Tingstad, MD
Andrew Watson, MD, MS, FAMSSM, FAAP

With grateful acknowledgment of Mark Price, MD, PhD

Additional Contributors (Staff)

American Academy of Family Physicians
Michael Monroe

American Academy of Pediatrics
Anjie Emanuel, MPH
Heather Stob

American College of Sports Medicine
Angela Chastain

American Heart Association
Laurie Whitsel, PhD

American Medical Society for Sports Medicine
Jim Griffith, MBA, CAE

American Orthopaedic Society for Sports Medicine
Lynette Craft, PhD, FACSM

American Osteopathic Academy of Sports Medicine
Mary Solomon, DO, FACOP, FAOASM

National Athletic Trainers' Association
A.J. Duffy III, MS, ATC, PT

National Federation of State High School Associations
Bob Colgate

Contents

Preface

The authoring societies (American Academy of Family Physicians, American Academy of Pediatrics, American College of Sports Medicine, American Medical Society for Sports Medicine, American Orthopaedic Society for Sports Medicine, and American Osteopathic Academy of Sports Medicine) along with the consulting societies (American Heart Association, National Athletic Trainers' Association, and National Federation of State High School Associations), recognize the important role the preparticipation evaluation (PPE) plays in the health care of individuals, particularly the adolescent population. The societies believe the ideal physical activity screening evaluation is done in the medical home as an individual encounter incorporated into the annual health supervision visit. A PPE that is completed in the medical home by a provider who knows the individual and has access to their medical record has the greatest chance of integrating full past medical and family history into the medical eligibility determination.

PPE: Preparticipation Evaluation, 6th Edition, reflects a rigorous effort by the writing group to identify and outline evidence-based and expert opinion principles and practices in the evaluation and medical eligibility decision. We have added new content on nutrition, cancer survivors, preventing and addressing abuse and sexual violence, and implementation of the PPE in clinical practice. In addition, we have expanded content on mental health, individuals with disabilities, and the medical clearance form. We also created more streamlined history and physical examination forms. One major change from the previous edition is that the title has been changed from *Preparticipation Physical Evaluation* to *Preparticipation Evaluation* to reflect the fact that the screening encompasses much more than a physical examination. It involves a comprehensive history, family history, and medical record review. In addition, the sixth edition is no longer called a monograph. This term was appropriate when the first edition was published in 1992; however, the current work is more properly called a book, as it includes hundreds of pages of critical information and resources. The writing process included

- Definition of the issues surrounding the PPE
- An extensive review of the current literature
- Use of position, policy, and consensus statements from major organizations
- Review of expert opinion
- Peer review by other experts from all the authoring societies (assisting in content revisions)

This edition of *PPE: Preparticipation Evaluation* has been reviewed extensively, and we greatly appreciate the excellent recommendations of the many professionals from the societies who have reviewed the document. These individuals include experts in primary care and multiple specialties, in both private practice settings and academic settings.

The authoring societies are confident this book will be a valuable resource for health care providers performing PPEs and will enhance the health and safety of all physically active individuals. We recommend a standardized approach to the PPE, as this will set the stage for data collection, which can be used to evaluate the PPE process, as well as immediate and long-term health outcomes. Incorporating the PPE into the electronic health record would promote standardization and establish a platform for data collection.

We acknowledge that the PPE is used in a variety of settings to determine medical eligibility for youth, high school, and college sports. Because of continued barriers to performing research on the PPE, there is a lack of data demonstrating its overall effectiveness in preventing adverse outcomes, even after more than 3 decades of use. Since publication of the first edition of *PPE* in 1992, debate has continued about its effectiveness as a screening tool for an individual's safety and medical eligibility for sport participation. For some adolescents, the PPE is their only contact with a medical provider. Performing the PPE in the medical home provides a good opportunity for health supervision, including evaluating mental health and risk-taking behaviors. For children and adolescents who do not participate in organized sports, incorporating the PPE into the health supervision visit is still beneficial, as it provides an opportunity for health care providers to promote exercise as a path to long-term health and screen for any conditions that may affect physical activity.

CHAPTER 1

Vision and Goals of the PPE

A medical home is an approach to providing comprehensive primary care that facilitates partnerships between patients, clinicians, medical staff, and families. A medical home extends beyond the 4 walls of a clinical practice. It includes specialty care, educational services, family support, and more.[1]

The preparticipation evaluation (PPE) is considered a best practice for the care of participants by many sports organizations and governing bodies around the world. However, the content and conduct of these evaluations is not standardized across organizations or countries and the evidence for their efficacy is limited.[2] For this 6th edition, the PPE authoring societies redefined and updated the 5 goals of the PPE (Box 1-1). The primary goal of the PPE is to consistently promote optimal health and safety during physical activity, training, and competition. The main way the PPE accomplishes this goal is by identifying conditions that predispose the individual to injury, illness, or even disabling and life-threatening conditions that could occur during physical activity. The PPE also includes a discussion of general emotional and physical well-being, psychological health, and lifestyle issues. There is stronger emphasis on having the evaluation take place in the individual's medical home, ideally in conjunction with their annual health supervision visit.

Box 1-1. Goals of the Preparticipation Evaluation

1. Promote optimal and safe physical activity
2. Provide a framework to assess, promote, and discuss physical and psychological health related to physical activity in conjunction with the annual health supervision visit
3. Encourage use and/or establishment of a medical home for continuity-based health care
4. Identify conditions that may be life-threatening or disabling, or those that may predispose to injury or illness related to physical activity
5. Provide an opportunity for discussion of health and lifestyle issues

In the United States, over 60 million children and adolescents, including over 8 million high school students, participate in sports activities, and these numbers have consistently increased over the past 4 decades.[3] The PPE is currently used to determine medical eligibility for youth athletics, yet it is *not* meant to exclude individuals from participation. The active role a health care provider plays in the determination of clearance for physical activity and sports participation is based on the foundational principle of "do no harm." The practice of medicine has evolved from an authoritarian approach of unilateral decision-making and absolute exclusion to that of education, guidance, individualization, risk stratification, activity modification, and optimization of injury- and disease-specific treatments.[4] Historically, only 1% to 2% of individuals screened will ultimately be restricted from a specific type or level of sports participation.[5–14] One large systematic review[15] of the PPE (> 20,000 evaluations) identified only 3 athletes (0.01%) who were completely excluded. A larger percentage, typically ranging from 3.1% to 13.9%, is referred for additional evaluation before ultimately being cleared for participation.[5–14,16] The PPE is a screening tool for conditions that may predispose the individual and/or others to injury or illness during participation; these range from minor to disabling or even life threatening. The information obtained is the basis for shared decision-making regarding medical eligibility and clearance status among the involved parties, such as the individual, their family, their personal physician, the team physician, subspecialty consultants, and any nonphysician clinicians who are involved in longitudinal care. It is recommended that associated medical staff such as a school-certified athletic trainer and a member of the athletic department and any third-party stakeholders be involved in the postdecision implementation phase as this is a critical component that is often overlooked.[4] Because the history and physical examination forms may contain sensitive information or information regarding genetic screening (eg, sickle cell trait), it is important for health care providers performing PPEs to be aware of applicable Health Insurance Portability and Accountability Act (HIPAA) and Family Educational Rights and Privacy Act (FERPA) laws and inform the individual and their parent/guardian how their protected health information will be handled (see Chapter 3).

The intention of the PPE authoring societies (American Academy of Family Physicians [AAFP], American Academy of Pediatrics [AAP], American College of Sports Medicine [ACSM], American Medical Society for Sports Medicine [AMSSM], American Orthopaedic Society for Sports Medicine [AOSSM], and American Osteopathic Academy of Sports Medicine [AOASM]) is that this resource will enhance the health of active individuals and increase safety, regardless of the type or level of sport or physical activity in which they are engaged. The PPE provides a framework to assess, promote, and discuss physical and psychological health related to physical activity, ideally in conjunction with the annual health supervision visit. It is also an opportunity to discuss health and lifestyle issues and is intended to be a useful experience for both the examiner and the individual participants.

The PPE authoring societies strongly recommend that the PPE be part of continuity-based health care that occurs in the individual's medical home. The AAP defines a medical home as an approach to providing comprehensive primary care that facilitates partnerships between patients, clinicians, medical staff, and families. A medical home extends beyond the 4 walls of a clinical practice. It includes specialty care, educational services, family support, and more.[1] PPEs occurring outside the medical home are discouraged for a variety of reasons. For example, when performed in an urgent care setting or a retail clinic, there can be poor communication with schools and primary care physicians; in addition, these settings are not conducive to proper follow-up. There can be a lack of privacy and confidentiality in certain settings. Also, there is often a lack of access to relevant medical records, prior test or imaging results, vaccination status, allergies, and/or a current list of medications prescribed. Unfortunately, however, sometimes there are significant barriers to medical home access for PPEs, including a lack of medical insurance, inability to schedule appointments, transportation issues, limited financial resources, and communication or language barriers.

HISTORY OF THE PPE

The origins of the PPE have been traced back to 600 BC in India.[17] In fact, Hippocrates himself assisted with the ancient Olympic games, and even the Roman gladiators of Pergamum were screened by Galen, a great philosopher and physician to Marcus Aurelius.[18,19]

The origins of the modern PPE date back to a movement in the 1890s to bring routine physical education into schools in Britain. Prominent physicians recommended obtaining "a much more detailed account of a child's physical background and conditions at the time of entering school."[20] This information was intended to ensure appropriate physical activity (but also was used to separate the social classes),[20] and it was considered important for keeping the learning environment healthy.[21]

During the mass screenings of World War II draftees, the US Selective Service deemed 1 in 4 young men unfit for military service,[22] and an integrated effort to prepare students for military service was started in US high schools.[23] This led to supplementing the established health examination for school entry with a standardized preparticipation evaluation. The examination included provisions for prevention and modification of "correctable defects" patterned after the military evaluation to put more adolescent boys onto a path to successful integration into the military.[22–24] In the mid-1960s, the American Medical Association (AMA) called for youth-athlete screening, and the PPE process for young athletes was initiated in the United States.[25]

EVIDENCE FOR THE PPE

The PPE was not developed as an evidence-based process, and there is a notable lack of outcomes data to demonstrate the overall effectiveness even after several decades of use.[26] Furthermore, as few as 37% of physicians surveyed after publication of the 4th edition of *PPE: Preparticipation Physical Evaluation* reported being aware of it.[27] Despite over 30 years and 4 revisions to the original guidelines, PPEs remain challenging for physicians and nonphysician providers.[26] Logistical barriers to effective performance of the PPE include uncertainty or unfamiliarity with how to perform the PPE, unclear significance of each component, and lack of both time and a standardized approach to completion.[26,27] One cross-sectional survey of 616 AAFP and AMSSM members showed only one-half performed the 90-second musculoskeletal screen, and there have been no additional data to support the process.[26] Effective PPE screening also depends on truthful and accurate documentation by the athlete, their parent/guardian (if a minor and/or present), and the examiner. Clear communication with all stakeholders involved and adherence to the clearance recommendations are essential components of the evaluation.[4,28] Despite the lack of efficacy data, the examinations are widely performed, with every US state requiring some level of PPE for high school scholastic athletes. Some authors express skepticism,[29,30] including that "the PPE as currently practiced is ineffective and illogical" and "a research agenda that would provide data to more effectively promote adolescent health both on and off the playing field" is sorely needed.[30]

CURRENT USE OF THE PPE

Content

The National Federation of State High School Associations (NFHS) recommends referring to the 6th edition PPE book to perform a PPE on every student-athlete before participation. However, the NFHS has neither the authority nor the ability to mandate the PPE or standardize it across its member state associations.[31] As a result, organizations at the state level have made a variety of modifications to the PPE form published in previous editions of this book, with each state having the ability to create its own version. An increasing number of states have incorporated into their PPE forms the recommendations of the American Heart Association (AHA) or the 5th edition of this book regarding the cardiac screening questions and cardiopulmonary physical examination (see Chapter 5A); however, this is not yet universal.[7,32–35] The current state-to-state variability may be an avenue to judge the efficacy of the PPE if a database can be developed to evaluate the outcomes of the PPE at the high school level when a standardized approach is used.

Frequency

The interval between examinations is not standardized and varies across states, ranging from annual to every 3 years.[31] There are no data suggesting a difference in participant outcomes based on the frequency of the examinations.

Examiners

Providers with varying levels of training and expertise are permitted to administer the PPE to high school athletes in most states.[34] Equally wide variation exists in physician knowledge and understanding of the process and how the examinations are conducted and documented.[27] One goal of this book is to improve knowledge of the key questions that are most likely to identify at-risk individuals who plan to participate in physical activities or sports.

At the collegiate level, the National Collegiate Athletic Association (NCAA) recommends, and most institutions require, a PPE at entrance to the program, but the content of the evaluation, including who obtains, reviews, and performs the history and physical examination, is not standardized. Follow-up for those participants who are not cleared, choose to terminate, or drop out on matriculation is at the discretion of each institution, with no national oversight.[36,37] Outside of scholastic-based competition, some youth sports programs and organizations, such as the Special Olympics, require a PPE for participants (see Chapter 7). Similarly, other niche activities or crafts that require significant physical and mental effort may benefit from a PPE that can assess any unique risks affecting participation. Notably, the movement to expand the use of the PPE outside of organized sports has extended to the performing arts community. In 2022, The DIVA (Dancers, Instrumentalists, Vocalists and Actors) Screening Protocol was created through a special initiative between the ACSM and the Performing Arts Medicine Association (PAMA).[38] The DIVA is a 30-minute consensus best-practice screening PPE tool that focuses on musculoskeletal injuries and mental health conditions. It includes vocal health survey and audiological screening questions, all identified by members of the performing arts community as frequently encountered problems. It is important for physicians and nonphysician providers to understand that performing artists benefit from PPE screening as much as a traditional sport athlete.

RATIONALE FOR INCORPORATING THE PPE INTO THE ANNUAL HEALTH SUPERVISION VISIT

Youth sport governing bodies and clubs do not have uniform or consistent requirements for a PPE. Thus, young individuals have little or no formal screening before participating in sports activity other than routine health supervision examinations. This leaves many with no structured PPE except for those individuals who eventually decide to start scholastic-based sports activity. However, there are no data to compare outcomes between the individuals screened with a PPE and those who were not. In addition, every child should be active for health reasons, and many children and adolescents participate in vigorous exercise or activities that are not organized, and they do not undergo any formal PPE screening. With the large number of young individuals participating in physical activity outside the scholastic or organized sports arena, it makes sense to incorporate the PPE into routine health supervision visits. Doing so also sends the implied public health message that all children and adolescents should be active. The PPE guidelines in this book, as well as the forms (eg, history, examination, and clearance), can be used for physical activity screening at virtually any age.

Therefore, the second major goal of the PPE is to provide a framework to assess, promote, and discuss physical and psychological health related to physical activity in conjunction with the annual health supervision visit. The third goal is to encourage use and/or establishment of a medical home for continuity-based health care as a best practice strategy. It is well recognized that adolescents benefit from routine health care from a provider in a medical home. The Society for Adolescent Health and Medicine (SAHM) recommends that health care for adolescents be readily available, visible, confidential, affordable, and flexible.[39,40] SAHM estimates that 5% to 10% of adolescents have a chronic condition that requires ongoing care, and up to half of adolescents will have less severe medical problems.[41] For some adolescents, the PPE is their only contact with a medical provider and the health care system in any given year.[8,15] Preventive services are better delivered when associated with an annual health supervision visit, but the number of adolescents receiving preventive care remains low.[22,42] However, the health care landscape is changing in the United States. In 2012, 74% of insured and 46% of uninsured adolescents (approximately 5% of the US population is uninsured) had an annual health supervision examination, suggesting there may be a good opportunity to perform PPE screening simultaneously if pertinent PPE questions are included.[9] Such increased adolescent exposure to the health care system reinforces the need for the examination to be performed by an individual's primary care physician in the medical home, but it also requires that nonphysician providers at all levels understand the PPE process and rationale. Integrating the PPE into an individual's regular health supervision visits would provide the opportunity to facilitate general health care and update immunizations, emphasize the importance of regular vigorous exercise beyond the confines of organized sport, enable providers to assess mental health and risk-taking behaviors,[8] and reduce duplication of services.[9] With the emphasis on preventive care and the medical home, the PPE needs to be in the toolbox of every pediatrician, family physician, and nonphysician provider, as the key components of the PPE encourage regular moderately strenuous physical activity for the long-term health of every child, adolescent, and young adult. Ideally, the PPE findings will be used by physicians, nonphysician providers, and various ancillary health care team members (athletic trainers, sports physical therapists, and others) as part of an overall health care program that focuses on the prevention, assessment, treatment, and rehabilitation of athletic injuries and promotes the clear health benefits of exercise and sport participation.

ACCESSIBILITY OF THE PPE

The Affordable Care Act (ACA) has increased the number of children with medical benefits, particularly in low-income households. A comparison of preventive services before and after implementation of the ACA shows a small increase in the use of preventive care.[30,42] The greatest impact has been on minority and socioeconomically disadvantaged adolescents.[30] The AAP recommends including in the PPE several identifying characteristics to encompass minority status such as race, ethnicity, gender identity, sexual orientation, and physical or mental disability that predispose to health care inequities. Individuals with minority status have a higher incidence of health problems, mental health issues, and at-risk behaviors; therefore, arguably, this group has the greatest need for a medical home where consistent efforts can be made to address social drivers of health and overcome systemic inequalities. Regardless of whether the PPE is initially performed in the medical office, an urgent care setting, or a group setting, it offers an opportunity to establish or refer to a medical home.

It is in the medical home setting that all the PPE objectives can reasonably be achieved and integrated into the medical record. When the PPE is viewed as a point of entry to the health care system, there are clear benefits to having the medical home as the site for the PPE. When station-based group examinations are used, follow-up becomes much more difficult. A careful and deliberate process for follow-up visits and referrals is critical for group model PPEs not performed one-on-one in the medical home.

HISTORY IS THE MOST IMPORTANT COMPONENT OF THE PPE

The fourth goal of the PPE focuses on history as the most relevant aspect, and obtaining an accurate history is the highest-yield component of the PPE. It is well known that at least 75% of relevant medical and orthopedic conditions are detected by history.[14,20,34,43–45] Additionally, over one-half of disqualifying conditions—many of which are musculoskeletal—are identified by history alone.[5,46] However, the history has a low sensitivity and a high false-positive rate. It is problematic that the history questions are based primarily on expert opinion and have not been validated. In addition, there are wide variations in the skill level and thoroughness of the examiners, and the evaluation depends on honest and accurate reporting by the individual. An accurate personal and family history to search for red flags, coupled with appropriate follow-up to investigate potentially life-threatening or disabling medical or musculoskeletal conditions, is most likely to occur when the PPE takes place in a medical home.[28] There are no outcome-based data to show that a screening PPE will reliably identify important, but clinically silent, conditions (such as many of the cardiac conditions associated with sudden cardiac death),[19,33,47] yet the authoring societies believe that a comprehensive, uniformly applied approach to the PPE offers the best opportunity to meet this objective. Controversy exists related to augmenting the history and physical examination with electrocardiography for the general athlete population versus selective use for higher-risk populations. Details related to this controversy are highlighted in Chapter 5A.

The PPE encounter is most likely to identify the following:
- **Acute, recurrent, chronic, or untreated injuries or illnesses**
- **Inadequately rehabilitated prior injuries**
- **Inadequate neuromuscular control predisposing to injury**
- **Congenital or developmental problems**

Prior injury or illness is a leading risk factor for many sports-related problems. Identification and treatment of certain conditions prior to participation in sport may minimize lost participation time and reduce the risk of persistent injury or reinjury.[48–51] Lastly, regular follow-up examinations are recommended for all individuals, even if the initial screen yields entirely normal results.[52] For anyone found to have abnormalities on history, physical examination, or diagnostic testing, follow-up needs to be individualized according to current guidelines.

PPE AS AN OPPORTUNITY TO DISCUSS HEALTH AND LIFESTYLE ISSUES

The last goal of the PPE is to provide an opportunity to discuss health and lifestyle issues. Discussion of sensitive topics, like mental health, is best performed in a familiar environment. There is little solid evidence that supports brief counseling interventions for adolescent lifestyle choices (eg, tobacco and alcohol consumption), but the AAP, SAHM, AAFP, AMA, and others recommend such counseling for preventive health visits.[24,53,54] The PPE provides an opportunity to begin this dialogue and to screen for mental health conditions. Most adolescents relate that they are not comfortable with questions related to risky behaviors, substance use, sexuality, or weight and diet in the context of a station-based examination,[25,44,45,55] further supporting PPE integration into the medical home. The opportunity for counseling an individual and answering health-related questions requires patient comfort and confidentiality, which are difficult to provide during group examinations or in urgent care settings. However, it is feasible when done in an office-based setting or perhaps in a less optimal, modified, one-on-one coordinated medical team examination (see Chapter 2).

In addition to an explanation of any abnormal findings from the PPE, topics such as proper training techniques, weight-control behaviors, nutrition, sleep, social media influence, tobacco use, alcohol or drug use, driving while impaired or distracted, seat belt use, prevention of sexually transmitted infections, and birth control, along with immunization education, may be discussed or introduced for discussion at a later visit. This objective may be difficult to achieve, but it may be the most important part of the encounter. The AAP, AAFP, and SAHM have resources that address many of the risks faced by an adolescent (www.adolescenthealth.org/Resources/Clinical-Care-Resources.aspx). The information obtained during the PPE can provide a means to initiate discussion with an individual or to make referrals for health-related and lifestyle issues.

ROUTINE SCREENING TESTS

Routine laboratory, cardiac, and pulmonary screening tests for PPEs remain controversial. Evidence-based studies indicate that the utility of adding screening tests is lacking. The PPE authoring societies concur that no routine screening tests are required during the PPE for determining medical eligibility of asymptomatic individuals. A good screening test should influence a disease or health outcome that has a significant impact on public health. On the basis of the current World Health Organization criteria, screening works best when applied to a population with a justifiably high disease prevalence to make a difference in outcomes. Key to effective screening is detecting an asymptomatic problem and demonstrating improved long-term outcomes. There is a difference between finding a potentially hazardous condition and changing the outcome of the condition. This judgment hinges on the difference between screening tests and diagnostic tests. The value of a screening test or procedure depends on 2 variables: (1) the predictive value of the proposed screening test, which is in turn affected by the prevalence of the condition in the population being screened, and (2) the ability to reduce morbidity and mortality by identifying the condition with the screening method. The screening test also needs to be acceptable in cost and potential side effects. The questions used in the PPE are based on time-honored expert opinions and are intended to draw out red flag conditions and direct a focused case finding evaluation. The AAP recognizes the tragic nature of sudden cardiac arrest (SCA) and sudden cardiac death (SCD) in youths and proposes that all children, not just athletes, undergo a set of questions so that health care providers can identify and focus on those who may be at risk.[33] The PPE authoring societies recommend that all examiners who perform PPEs have a strategy for screening, evaluating, and managing those at risk of SCA and SCD.

The value of a diagnostic test, as compared with a screening test, is the ability to confirm a condition for which suspicion already exists based on history or physical examination findings. When evaluating screening tests for the PPE, studies have not supported the use of urinalysis, complete blood cell count, chemistry profile, lipid profile, ferritin level monitoring, or screening for sickle cell trait.[56–59] Since the institution of sickle cell trait screening at the college level as required by a legal settlement with the NCAA, exercise-associated sickle cell deaths have decreased in number, but it is difficult to determine whether that is a product of the screening or the associated educational component of the requirement.[60] Similarly, cardiopulmonary screening with electrocardiography, echocardiography, exercise stress testing, or spirometry lacks research to demonstrate that the tests clearly meet screening criteria in asymptomatic individuals across the 12- to 18- and 19- to 24-year-old age groups generally assessed in the PPE process.[61–67] The current literature and expert opinion recommendations for cardiovascular screening tests are addressed in Chapter 5A.

CASE-FINDING DIAGNOSTIC TESTS

Findings from the PPE medical history or physical examination may indicate a need to arrange specific case-finding diagnostic tests. The examiner may elect to defer the final medical eligibility decision for sports participation while awaiting completion of diagnostic testing. Additional diagnostic tests are recommended to evaluate for specific conditions in some cases but are not part of the standardized screening examination. For example, a complete hematologic profile may be recommended to check for anemia or nutritional deficiency in an individual who has fatigue, pallor, performance decline, heavy menstrual bleeding, low caloric intake, or a diet lacking red meat. A lipid profile to test for familial dyslipidemia is recommended for a student who has a family history of premature atherosclerotic heart disease or dyslipidemia. Urinalysis may be indicated for an individual with dysuria, hematuria, or a family history of certain types of kidney disease. Urine screening, not as a part of the PPE but as part of a drug-testing program for performance-enhancing drugs, is common among elite-level and professional athletes and is becoming more common for intercollegiate athletes.

Mandatory HIV screening for sports participation is not recommended because of the low risk of transmission, although certain boxing organizations require it.[68,69] However, voluntary testing is encouraged for all teenagers because the AAP, Centers for Disease Control and Prevention, and US Preventive Services Task Force recommend that all youth 13 years and older be routinely screened for HIV. Therefore, if there is an opportunity or a need to perform HIV screening, it can be completed during the PPE or ordered as a future test. The current literature and expert opinion regarding testing for certain blood-borne diseases are reviewed in Chapter 5C.

SUMMARY

This 6th edition of the PPE book provides a state-of-the-art, practical, and effective evaluation tool for health care providers who perform PPEs for individuals participating in physical activity in elementary school, middle school, high school, and college. It can be broadly and easily used to screen any individual who is engaging in regular physical activity in virtually any setting or environment. The PPE can be performed as a stand-alone evaluation or incorporated into health supervision visits within the medical home. The process and forms are designed to be easily adaptable to suit individual or institutional needs.

The 6th edition of the publication:

- Describes the goals, process, timing, setting, and frequency of the evaluation
- Details the history, physical examination, and medical eligibility considerations
- Provides guidelines for determining medical eligibility and return to play
- Addresses medicolegal and ethical concerns
- Includes practical tips for implementation in practice

This book reviews the rationale for primary and secondary history questions as well as the examination maneuvers. While most of the content is based on the expert opinion level of evidence, whenever there is higher-level evidence for the content, it is noted in the text (Table 1-1), and numerous up-to-date references are provided.

Table 1-1. Strength of Recommendation Taxonomy (SORT)

In general, only key recommendations for readers require a grade of the "Strength of Recommendation." Recommendations should be based on the highest quality evidence available. For example, vitamin E was found in some cohort studies (Level 2 study quality) to have a benefit for cardiovascular protection, but good quality randomized trials (Level 1) have not confirmed this effect. Therefore, it is preferable to base clinical recommendations on the Level 1 studies.

Strength of Recommendation	Definition
A	Recommendation based on consistent and good-quality patient-oriented evidence[a]
B	Recommendation based on inconsistent or limited-quality patient-oriented evidence[a]
C	Recommendation based on consensus, usual practice, opinion, disease-oriented evidence,[a] and case series for studies of diagnosis, treatment, prevention, or screening

Use the table below to determine whether a study measuring patient-oriented outcomes is of good or limited quality, and whether the results are consistent or inconsistent between studies.

Study Quality	Diagnosis	Treatment/Prevention/Screening	Prognosis
Level 1			
Good-quality patient-oriented evidence	Validated clinical decision rule Systematic review (SR)/meta-analysis of high-quality studies High-quality diagnostic cohort study[b]	SR/meta-analysis of randomized controlled trials (RCTs) with consistent findings High-quality individual RCT[c] All-or-none study[d]	SR/meta-analysis of good-quality cohort studies Prospective cohort study with good follow-up
Level 2			
Limited-quality patient-oriented evidence	Unvalidated clinical decision rule SR/meta-analysis of lower-quality studies or studies with inconsistent findings Lower-quality diagnostic cohort study or diagnostic case-control study[b]	SR/meta-analysis of lower-quality clinical trials or of studies with inconsistent findings Lower-quality clinical trial[c] Cohort study Case-control study	SR/meta-analysis of lower-quality cohort studies or studies with inconsistent results Retrospective cohort study or prospective cohort study with poor follow-up Case-control study Case series

Table 1-1. Strength of Recommendation Taxonomy (SORT) *(continued)*

Level 3	
Other evidence	Consensus guidelines, extrapolations from bench research, usual practice, opinion, disease-oriented evidence (intermediate or physiologic outcomes only), and case series for studies of diagnosis, treatment, prevention, or screening
Consistency Across Studies	
Consistent	Most studies found similar or at least coherent conclusions (coherence means that differences are explainable) *or* If high-quality and up-to-date systematic review or meta-analyses exist, they support the recommendation.
Inconsistent	Considerable variation among study findings and lack of coherence *or* If high-quality and up-to-date systematic reviews or meta-analyses exist, they do not find consistent evidence in favor of the recommendation.

[a] Patient-oriented evidence measures outcomes that matter to patients: morbidity, mortality, symptom improvement, cost reduction, quality of life. Disease-oriented evidence measures intermediate, physiologic, or surrogate end points that may or may not reflect improvements in patient outcomes (ie, blood pressure, blood chemistry, physiologic function, pathologic findings).

[b] High-quality diagnostic cohort study: cohort design, adequate size, adequate spectrum of patients, blinding, and a consistent, well-defined reference standard.

[c] High-quality RCT: allocation concealed, blinding if possible, intention-to-treat analysis, adequate statistical power, adequate follow-up (> 80%).

[d] An all-or-none study is one where the treatment causes a dramatic change in outcomes, such as antibiotics for meningitis or surgery for appendicitis, which precludes study in a controlled trial.

Reprinted with permission from Ebell MH, Siwek J, Weiss BD, et al. Strength of Recommendation Taxonomy (SORT): a patient-centered approach to grading evidence in medical literature. *Am Fam Physician.* 2004;69(3):548–556. https://www.aafp.org/afp/2004/0201/p548.

NEW CONTENT IN THE 6TH EDITION

New to the 6th edition are resources in each chapter with links to make them more user-friendly. Based on feedback from the previous editions, the 6th edition includes system-based history, examination, medical eligibility content, return to play, when to refer, particulars for athletes with disabilities, information pertinent to different populations (ie, middle and high school athletes, college athletes, and nonorganized sport participants), administrative concerns, research gaps, and updated future directions. The information on mental health is also expanded, and a chapter has been added on preventing and addressing abuse and sexual violence.

The 6th edition has prioritized inclusiveness for all individuals, as the benefits of physical activity are universal. In 2021, the AAP published a clinical report promoting the participation of children and adolescents with disabilities and cancer survivors in sports, recreation, and physical activity. The PPE for these individuals may occur more frequently, with input from a multidisciplinary team (physicians, coaches, physical education teachers, school nurses, adaptive recreation specialists, physical and occupational therapists, and others). Child, family, societal, and financial barriers to participation need to be addressed by examiners to help reach the goal of inclusion in either sports (including competitive, adaptive, or therapeutic) or recreational activities.[70] Succinct, comprehensive, and easily used forms (pp 293–304) are supplied for participants, parents or guardians, and clinicians. The PPE authoring societies advocate for and support future research to create evidence-based history questionnaires; identify the optimal timing and frequency of evaluations; optimize screening criteria for high-risk diseases, injuries, and illnesses; and support the implementation of a universal form and process.

REFERENCES

1. American Academy of Pediatrics. Medical home. Accessed May 9, 2025. https://www.aap.org/en/practice-management/medical-home/
2. Roberts WO, Löllgen H, Matheson GO, et al; American College of Sports Medicine (ACSM); Fédération Internationale du Médicine du Sport (FIMS). Advancing the preparticipation physical evaluation: an ACSM and FIMS joint consensus statement. *Clin J Sport Med.* 2014;24(6):442–447. PMID: 25347259 doi:10.1097/JSM.0000000000000168
3. National Federation of State High School Associations. High School Athletics Participation Survey (2024–2025 School Year). Accessed March 5, 2026. https://a-us.storyblok.com/f/1022696/x/85a6414d04/2024-25-nfhs-high-school-athletics-participation-survey.pdf
4. Baggish AL, Ackerman MJ, Lampert R. Competitive sport participation among athletes with heart disease: a call for a paradigm shift in decision making. *Circulation.* 2017;136(17):1569–1571. PMID: 29061571
5. Rifat SF, Ruffin MT IV, Gorenflo DW. Disqualifying criteria in a preparticipation sports evaluation. *J Fam Pract.* 1995;41(1):42–50. PMID: 7798065
6. Smith J, Laskowski ER. The preparticipation physical examination: Mayo Clinic experience with 2,739 examinations. *Mayo Clin Proc.* 1998;73(5):419–429. PMID: 9581581
7. Glover DW, Maron BJ. Profile of preparticipation cardiovascular screening for high school athletes. *JAMA.* 1998;279(22):1817–1819. PMID: 9628714
8. Park MJ, Brindis CD, Vaughn B, Barry M, Guzman L, Berger A. Child Trends and the National Adolescent and Young Adult Health Information Center at the University of California, San Francisco. Adolescent Health Highlight. Health care services. October 2013. Publication 2013-10. Accessed May 9, 2025. https://pub-35cb1528455e4a46bbd4371582c4df39.r2.dev/media/2013-10HealthCareServices.pdf
9. National Center for Health Statistics. Health insurance coverage. Centers for Disease Control and Prevention website. Updated September 17, 2025. Accessed December 26, 2025. https://www.cdc.gov/nchs/fastats/health-insurance.htm
10. Klein JD, Slap GB, Elster AB, Schonberg SK. Access to health care for adolescents. A position paper of the Society for Adolescent Medicine. *J Adolesc Health.* 1992;13(2):162–170. PMID: 1627584
11. Rosen DS, Elster A, Hedberg V, Paperny D. Clinical preventive services for adolescents: position paper of the Society for Adolescent Medicine. *J Adolesc Health.* 1997;21(3):203–214. PMID: 9283943
12. Fuller CM, McNulty CM, Spring DA, et al. Prospective screening of 5,615 high school athletes for risk of sudden cardiac death. *Med Sci Sports Exerc.* 1997;29(9):1131–1138. PMID: 9309622
13. Lyznicki JM, Nielsen NH, Schneider JF. Cardiovascular screening of student athletes. *Am Fam Physician.* 2000;62(4):765–774. PMID: 10969856
14. Koester MC, Amundson CL. Preparticipation screening of high school athletes: are recommendations enough? *Phys Sportsmed.* 2003;31(8):35–38. PMID: 20086484
15. Stickler GB. Are yearly physical examinations in adolescents necessary? *J Am Board Fam Pract.* 2000;13(3):172–177. PMID: 10826864
16. Mayer F, Bonaventura K, Cassel M, et al. Medical results of preparticipation examination in adolescent athletes. *Br J Sports Med.* 2012;46(7):524–530. PMID: 22576783 doi:10.1136/bjsports-2011-090966
17. Tipton CM. The history of "Exercise Is Medicine" in ancient civilizations. *Adv Physiol Educ.* 2014;38(2):109–117. PMID: 25039081

18. Gwathmey FW, Hart J, Miller M. Principles of sports medicine. In: Wiesel BB, Sankar WN, Delahay JN, Wiesel SW, eds. *Orthopaedic Surgery: Principles of Diagnosis and Treatment.* Lippincott Williams and Wilkins; 2011:165–192
19. Andujo VD, Fletcher IE, McGrew C. Musculoskeletal preparticipation physical evaluation—does it lead to decreased musculoskeletal morbidity? *Curr Sports Med Rep.* 2020;19(2):58–69. PMID: 32028350
20. Carter AH. A discussion on the claims and limitations of physical education in school. *Br Med J.* 1890;2(1557):995–1001. PMID: 20753163
21. Neve M, Turner T. What the doctor thought and did: Sir James Crichton-Browne (1840-1938). *Med Hist.* 1995;39(4):399–432. PMID: 8558991
22. Gallagher J, Brouha L. Physical fitness: its evaluation and significance. *JAMA.* 1944;125(12):834–838.
23. Kleinschmidt EE. The schools contribute to national defense. *J Sch Health.* 2001;71(8):378–382. PMID: 11794280
24. Rowntree LG. A movement for improvement in health and physical fitness; what role should we play in Pennsylvania? *Pa Med J.* 1945;49(49):31–33. PMID: 21010225
25. American Medical Association Subcommittee on Classification of Sports Injuries and Committee on the Medical Aspects of Sports. *Standard Nomenclature of Athletic Injuries.* American Medical Association; 1966
26. LaBotz M, Bernhardt DT. Preparticipation physical examination: is it time to stop doing the sports physical? *Br J Sports Med.* 2017;51(3):151–152. PMID: 27935485
27. Madsen NL, Drezner JA, Salerno JC. The preparticipation physical evaluation: an analysis of clinical practice. *Clin J Sport Med.* 2014;24(2):142–149. PMID: 24231928
28. Kennedy M, Comer F, Young JA, Valasek AE. Increasing primary care follow-up after preparticipation physical evaluations. *Pediatr Qual Saf.* 2020;5(6):e358. PMID: 33134760
29. Best TM. The preparticipation evaluation: an opportunity for change and consensus. *Clin J Sport Med.* 2004;14(3):107–108. PMID: 15166897
30. Bundy DG, Feudtner C. Preparticipation physical evaluations for high school athletes: time for a new game plan. *Ambul Pediatr.* 2004;4(3):260–263. PMID: 15153048
31. National Federation of State High School Associations. Update on 2017 NFHS survey results on preparticipation physical evaluation. Presented at: Sports Medicine Advisory Committee; April 2017; Indianapolis, IN
32. Caswell SV, Cortes N, Chabolla M, Ambegaonkar JP, Caswell AM, Brenner JS. State-specific differences in school sports preparticipation physical evaluation policies. *Pediatrics.* 2015;135(1):26–32. PMID: 25535257 doi:10.1542/peds.2014-1451
33. Erickson CC, Salerno JC, Berger S, et al; American Academy of Pediatrics Section on Cardiology and Cardiac Surgery, Pediatric and Congenital Electrophysiology Society (Paces) Task Force on Prevention of Sudden Death in the Young. Sudden death in the young: information for the primary care provider. *Pediatrics.* 2021;148(1):e2021052044. PMID: 34155130 doi:10.1542/peds.2021-052044
34. Krowchuk DP, Krowchuk HV, Hunter DM, et al. Parents' knowledge of the purposes and content of preparticipation physical examinations. *Arch Pediatr Adolesc Med.* 1995;149(6):653–657. PMID: 7767421
35. Fuller CM. Cost effectiveness analysis of screening of high school athletes for risk of sudden cardiac death. *Med Sci Sports Exerc.* 2000;32(5):887–890. PMID: 10795776
36. MacAuley D. Does preseason screening for cardiac disease really work? The British perspective. *Med Sci Sports Exerc.* 1998;30(10 suppl):S345–S350. PMID: 9789860
37. Montalto NJ. Implementing the guidelines for adolescent preventive services. *Am Fam Physician.* 1998;57(9):2181–2188, 2189–2190. PMID: 9606308
38. Ackermann BJ, Guptill C, Miller C, Dick R, McCrary JM. Assessing performing artists in medical and health practice–the dancers, instrumentalists, vocalists, and actors screening protocol. *Curr Sports Med Rep.* 2022;21(12):460–462. PMID: 36508603
39. Copperman S. GAPS (AMA Guidelines for Adolescent Preventive Services). *Arch Pediatr Adolesc Med.* 1997;151(9):957–958. PMID: 9308879 doi:10.1001/archpedi.1997.02170460095019
40. Society for Adolescent Health and Medicine. Clinical Care Resources. Adolescent and young adult clinical care resources by topic. Accessed May 8, 2025. https://adolescenthealth.org/resources/clinical-care-resources/
41. Hulkower S, Fagan B, Watts J, Ketterman E, Fox BA. Clinical inquiries: do preparticipation clinical exams reduce morbidity and mortality for athletes? *J Fam Pract.* 2005;54(7):628–632. PMID: 16009094
42. Adams SH, Park MJ, Twietmeyer L, Brindis CD, Irwin CE Jr. Increasing delivery of preventive services to adolescents and young adults: does the preventive visit help? *J Adolesc Health.* 2018;63(2):166–171. PMID: 29929838 doi:10.1016/j.jadohealth.2018.03.013

43. Joy EA, Pescatello LS. Pre-exercise screening: role of the primary care physician. *Isr J Health Policy Res.* 2016;5:29. PMID: 27358724
44. Riebe D, Franklin BA, Thompson PD, et al. Updating ACSM's recommendations for exercise preparticipation health screening. *Med Sci Sports Exerc.* 2015;47(11):2473–2479. PMID: 26473759
45. Carek PJ, Futrell M. Athletes' view of the preparticipation physical examination. Attitudes toward certain health screening questions. *Arch Fam Med.* 1999;8(4):307–312. PMID: 10418536 doi:10.1001/archfami.8.4.307
46. Bakken A, Targett S, Bere T, et al. Health conditions detected in a comprehensive periodic health evaluation of 558 professional football players. *Br J Sports Med.* 2016;50(18):1142–1150. PMID: 27012663
47. Wingfield K, Matheson GO, Meeuwisse WH. Preparticipation evaluation: an evidence-based review. *Clin J Sport Med.* 2004;14(3):109–122. PMID: 15166898 doi:10.1097/00042752-200405000-00002
48. Corrente C, Silvis M, Murphy J, Gallo R, Onks C. Musculoskeletal practices for the preparticipation physical examination. *BMC Sports Sci Med Rehabil.* 2021;13(1):84. PMID: 34348781
49. Brunner R, Friesenbichler B, Casartelli NC, Bizzini M, Maffiuletti NA, Niedermann K. Effectiveness of multicomponent lower extremity injury prevention programmes in team-sport athletes: an umbrella review. *Br J Sports Med.* 2019;53(5):282–288. PMID: 30201793
50. Thorborg K, Krommes KK, Esteve E, Clausen MB, Bartels EM, Rathleff MS. Effect of specific exercise-based football injury prevention programmes on the overall injury rate in football: a systematic review and meta-analysis of the FIFA 11 and 11+ programmes. *Br J Sports Med.* 2017;51(7):562–571. PMID: 28087568
51. Mandelbaum BR, Silvers HJ, Watanabe DS, et al. Effectiveness of a neuromuscular and proprioceptive training program in preventing anterior cruciate ligament injuries in female athletes: 2-year follow-up. *Am J Sports Med.* 2005;33(7):1003–1010. PMID: 15888716
52. Albiński M, Balmer C, Wilhelm M, et al. Paediatric and adolescent athletes in Switzerland: age-adapted proposals for pre-participation cardiovascular evaluation. *Swiss Med Wkly.* 2022;152:w30128. PMID: 35195978
53. Moyer VA, Butler M. Gaps in the evidence for well-child care: a challenge to our profession. *Pediatrics.* 2004;114(6):1511–1521. PMID: 15574609 doi:10.1542/peds.2004-1076
54. Chang C, Putukian M, Aerni G, et al. Mental health issues and psychological factors in athletes: detection, management, effect on performance and prevention: American Medical Society for Sports Medicine Position Statement-Executive Summary. *Br J Sports Med.* 2020;54(4):216–220. PMID: 31810972
55. Society for Adolescent Medicine. Access to health care for adolescents and young adults. *J Adolesc Health.* 2004;35(4):342–344. PMID: 15481116
56. Dodge WF, West EF, Smith EH, Bunce H III. Proteinuria and hematuria in schoolchildren: epidemiology and early natural history. *J Pediatr.* 1976;88(2):327–347. PMID: 1249701
57. Peggs JF, Reinhardt RW, O'Brien JM. Proteinuria in adolescent sports physical examinations. *J Fam Pract.* 1986;22(1):80–81. PMID: 3941303
58. Taylor WC, Lombardo JA. Preparticipation screening of college athletes: value of the complete blood cell count. *Phys Sportsmed.* 1990;18(6):106–118. PMID: 27452100
59. Vehaskari VM, Rapola J. Isolated proteinuria: analysis of a school-age population. *J Pediatr.* 1982;101(5):661–668. PMID: 7131137
60. Tarini BA, Brooks MA, Bundy DG. A policy impact analysis of the mandatory NCAA sickle cell trait screening program. *Health Serv Res.* 2012;47(1 Pt 2):446–461 PMID: 22150647 doi:10.1111/j.1475-6773.2011.01357.x
61. Ades PA. Preventing sudden death: cardiovascular screening of young athletes. *Phys Sportsmed.* 1992;20(9):75–89. PMID: 29281438
62. Epstein SE, Maron BJ. Sudden death and the competitive athlete: perspectives on preparticipation screening studies. *J Am Coll Cardiol.* 1986;7(1):220–230. PMID: 3079780
63. Feinstein RA, Colvin ED, Kimoh M. Echocardiographic screening as part of a preparticipation examination. *Clin J Sport Med.* 1993;3(3):149–152
64. Lewis JF, Maron BJ, Diggs JA, Spencer JE, Mehrotra PP, Curry CL. Preparticipation echocardiographic screening for cardiovascular disease in a large, predominantly black population of collegiate athletes. *Am J Cardiol.* 1989;64(16):1029–1033. PMID: 2816733
65. Maron BJ, Bodison SA, Wesley YE, Tucker E, Green KJ. Results of screening a large group of intercollegiate competitive athletes for cardiovascular disease. *J Am Coll Cardiol.* 1987;10(6):1214–1221. PMID: 2960727
66. Rupp NT, Brudno DS, Guill MF. The value of screening for risk of exercise-induced asthma in high school athletes. *Ann Allergy.* 1993;70(4):339–342. PMID: 8466100

67. Rupp NT, Guill MF, Brudno DS. Unrecognized exercise-induced bronchospasm in adolescent athletes. *Am J Dis Child*. 1992;146(8):941–944. PMID: 1636661
68. Mast EE, Goodman RA, Bond WW, Favero MS, Drotman DP. Transmission of blood-borne pathogens during sports: risk and prevention. *Ann Intern Med*. 1995;122(4):283–285. PMID: 7825765
69. Drotman DP. Professional boxing, bleeding, and HIV testing. *JAMA*. 1996;276(3):193. PMID: 8667554
70. Carbone PS, Smith PJ, Lewis C, LeBlanc C. Promoting the participation of children and adolescents with disabilities in sports, recreation and physical activity. *Pediatrics*. 2021;148(6):e2021054664. PMID: 34851421

CHAPTER 2

Timing, Setting, and Frequency

The timing, setting, and structure of the preparticipation evaluation (PPE) depends on many factors, including the age of the participants, the presence of a team physician, the availability of qualified health care professionals who are trained and willing to do the examinations, and the health insurance available to the individual. For individuals in high school and younger, the PPE authoring societies recommend that the PPE be embedded into the annual health supervision visit at their medical home, around the time of the individual's birthday, to distribute the health care provider's evaluations throughout the calendar year.

QUALIFICATIONS OF THE EXAMINERS

Physicians with a doctor of medicine (MD) or doctor of osteopathic medicine (DO) degree and advanced practice providers (nurse practitioners [NPs] and physician assistants [PAs]) with the clinical training to address the broad range of problems that may be encountered during the PPE are allowed to complete the evaluation on the basis of individual state regulations. The PPE authoring societies concur that conducting and determining medical eligibility should be the responsibility of a physician (MD or DO), an NP, or a PA.[1–3] It is essential that whoever performs the PPE has the clinical training, knowledge, and expertise to conduct the evaluation and determine medical eligibility. Providers performing PPEs need to be able to fulfill the goals and objectives outlined in the previous chapter and should seek consultation with an appropriate specialist to address problems beyond their expertise.[1]

Regardless of their training, it is important that providers performing PPEs be competent to screen individuals for problems that would affect participation or place them at undue risk (greater than the inherent risk of the sport). Use of standardized history forms in paper or electronic format or more comprehensive electronic history forms establishes consistency of the evaluation across the various providers permitted to complete the PPE by their state regulations. At the collegiate, professional, national, and international competition levels, the respective athletic governing bodies determine who may perform the PPE, and standardized formats would likewise benefit those providers and athletes.[4]

TIMING OF THE EVALUATION

The PPE authoring societies recommend individuals have their PPE performed every 1 to 2 years during the annual health supervision visit with their primary care provider (PCP), who has access to medical records, can adjust treatment for chronic medical conditions, and can incorporate the examination into routine health supervision examinations. Both the American Academy of Family Physicians (AAFP) and the American Academy of Pediatrics (AAP) endorse the concept of the medical home as a patient-centered model to provide timely, well-organized, and regular care; eliminate barriers to care; and create greater access to preventive care services, including the PPE. In the medical home, these annual health supervision visits are typically performed around the individual's birthday, which evenly distributes the evaluations across the calendar year for PCPs. The authoring societies strongly oppose rules and regulations that require PPEs to be done after an arbitrary date during the year. Further, many health care insurance companies pay for one health supervision visit per year, so if there are separate dates for the annual health supervision visit and the PPE, only one of these would be an insurance-covered benefit. If performed during the same visit, both would be covered. However, for individuals with complex medical histories and needs, there may not be enough time to address everything related to health supervision and PPE in a single visit. Thus, more than one visit may be needed in these cases.

Whether the PPE is completed by a PCP or, when necessary, in a group examination format, individuals should schedule the examinations at least 6 weeks before the start of preseason practice. This approach allows the individual to complete any needed evaluations or consultations with less impact on school attendance and sports practice. Individuals examined at the end of the school year for the next fall sports season are asked to report any unresolved injuries or medical problems from summer activities to the PCP, team physician, athletic trainer, or school nurse before fall practice to allow for reevaluation. Many collegiate sports programs do not have athletes on campus 6 weeks prior to the fall season and therefore coordinate the PPE screening process as soon as they arrive on campus. The examinations then can be completed before the individuals begin practice in their respective sports. Students and parents or guardians need to assume responsibility for scheduling an appointment in the medical home before the start of the sport season (at least 6 weeks is preferable) and for accurately completing the health history section.

SETTING OF THE EVALUATION

The appropriate method and setting of the PPE (individual evaluation vs group-based assessment) depends on the age and competitive level of the individual, and the resources available at the possible settings. **For individuals who are high school aged and younger,** the PPE authoring societies recommend that the PPE be embedded into the annual health supervision visit at their medical home.

For individuals who are high school aged and younger, the PPE authoring societies recommend that the PPE be embedded into the annual health supervision visit at their medical home.

Having the PPE performed in the PCP's office allows for continuity of care. The PCP has an established relationship with the individual, is likely to know the personal history, and usually has a complete set of medical records, including family history, immunizations, and previous laboratory and imaging studies. Access to the complete medical record during the PPE reduces the possibility that a previously detected abnormality or family risk factor that would predispose the individual to unnecessary risk will be missed or omitted. The PCP may be less likely to overlook health issues inadvertently or consciously omitted from the PPE History Form by the individual. In addition, the PCP has a better appreciation of the individual's known medical problems, a sense of the individual's current health status, and knowledge of potential changes in treatment that would optimize participation. For example, an asymptomatic individual with a heart murmur and an echocardiogram showing benign findings can be readily cleared for participation. If needed, the PCP can easily coordinate care with consultants in a timely manner and arrange for proper follow-up for medical conditions considered a risk for sport participation before determining medical eligibility.

The office setting offers privacy, which supports discussion of confidential issues. Familiarity also provides an opportunity to counsel an individual on sensitive issues such as mental health, abuse in any form, gender identity, birth control, and prevention of sexually transmitted infections, in addition to a variety of risk-taking behaviors such as tobacco use, alcohol and recreational drug use, appearance- and performance-enhancing drug and supplement use, and unsafe nutritional practices. When appropriate, chaperones should be present. Adolescents can be seen apart from their parents or guardians for at least part of the evaluation so that the provider can inquire about risk-taking behaviors. Adolescents are often more willing to discuss these issues with someone they know and trust, rather than with a stranger in a group-based PPE assessment or at a retail or urgent care clinic. Additionally, if the screening identifies any concerning risk-taking behaviors, the PCP can promptly connect the individual with appropriate resources. Given the time constraints of a typical health supervision visit, it is important to focus screening and counseling on evidence-based interventions that have an impact on long-term morbidity such as depression and obesity along with risk-taking behaviors. Understanding the risk of exercise in relation to each question or physical examination finding is essential to improve the outcomes of the PPE encounter. One purpose of this book is to advance the quality of the PPE by closing that knowledge gap for PCPs. For a summary of the PPE administration process, see Box 2-1.

For individuals who are high school aged and younger, performing a PPE outside the medical home is ineffective and presents a barrier to both health supervision care and participation in sports and other activities.[5,6] These PPE encounters are unlikely to address all health and anticipatory guidance issues in a comprehensive manner. The PPE authoring societies consider group-based examinations (eg, performed in a gymnasium or locker room) inappropriate to accomplish the goals and objectives of the PPE process. Likewise, examinations done in an urgent care or a retail clinic lack access to an individual's medical record and are considered unsuitable. The most appropriate setting for a PPE is one with adequate resources and access to full medical records. Using the PPE to accrue market share

Box 2-1. The Preparticipation Evaluation Administration Summary

1. The preparticipation evaluation (PPE) authoring societies recommend the PPE be performed as part of the periodic health supervision visit at a minimum every 2 years, with updated interval histories at intervening health supervision visits yearly.
2. The PPE is best performed in the setting of the primary medical home, by a provider who knows the individual well or who has access to a comprehensive medical and injury history of the individual.
3. The PPE authoring societies do not recommend that these examinations be performed in a station-based or group setting or by providers who do not have access to the individual's comprehensive medical and injury history. The PPE authoring societies recommend that this approach be limited to those who do not have health insurance, a primary care provider, or a medical home.
4. If a station-based or group examination is used, it is important that review of the history and physical examination be performed by the same provider assessing medical eligibility and participation status.
5. The PPE authoring societies strongly oppose restricting the timing of the PPE to an arbitrary date; scheduling around the time of the individual's birthday is easy for families and reduces the burden on the provider.
6. Individuals and their parents or guardians are responsible for timely scheduling of PPEs, as problems that require additional testing may delay the completion of the evaluation in time for the start of season practices.
7. The final responsibility for a PPE lies with the provider who signs the Medical Eligibility Form and assumes the medical liability.
8. Individuals with problems discovered during the PPE that are beyond the scope and expertise of the examining provider are best managed by referring to an appropriate specialist for consultation regarding medical eligibility.
9. The standardized PPE History Form is the preferred format for documentation in either paper format or electronic format.
10. It is important for adolescents to be seen apart from their parents or guardians for at least part of the evaluation so that the provider can inquire about risk-taking behaviors.
11. Defined sections of the PPE are personal (and protected) health information and require confidential, secure handling and permission of the individual and/or parent or guardian to be shared beyond the individual's health care personnel.

in a community or as a fundraiser for the school or athletic department is also **inappropriate.** Individuals often arrive at group-based examinations with forms either partially completed or not completed at all and without a parent or guardian, so the data are inadequate for the health care provider's assessment and decision-making. Group-based examinations away from the medical home should be a last resort for high school students and younger individuals, such as for those who do not have health insurance, a PCP, or a medical home. Coordinated examinations for high school students are sometimes done as a community service for individuals in these categories. Part of this community service includes having a process in place to help individuals without a medical home establish one.

The PPE authoring societies consider group-based examinations (eg, performed in a gymnasium or locker room) inappropriate to accomplish the goals and objectives of the PPE process.

In sports settings with formal medical teams, group-based examinations may be preferred when full access to past medical history is available. This is common for college sports settings and rare for high schools. Coordinated medical team evaluations, where the athletes are evaluated and treated by a team of health care professionals, are common in this setting.

At both the high school and college levels, the group-based evaluations depend even more on individuals and their parents or guardians accurately and honestly completing the health history section. Coordinated medical teams are typically organized by the school team physician or a local clinic, and they often involve both primary care specialists and other sports medicine specialists. On-site medical specialists and other professionals may allow consultation for a wide range of problems.

When a coordinated medical team works together to complete the PPE, the PPE authoring societies recommend that the history review, physical examination, and sports medical eligibility process be done in a one-on-one examination with a single provider for all aspects of the evaluation. A quiet examination room is required to auscultate the heart. Private areas are needed for discussion of sensitive topics and to maintain confidentiality. It is important to carve out time for adolescents to be seen apart from their parents or guardians for at least part of the evaluation so that the provider can inquire about risk-taking behaviors.

When PPEs are done in a group setting, the team or lead physician coordinates the process and supervises the team of health care professionals such that all appropriate components of the assessment take place as outlined in Table 2-1. Insufficient provider recruitment and attendance can lead to more individuals being screened than the providers can manage in the session. It is better to be overstaffed to allow providers to spend appropriate time with each individual.

In the coordinated medical team approach with multiple providers (Box 2-2), the PPE authoring societies recommend that a single provider review the history and perform the examination for the individual. Individuals with known ongoing medical concerns can then be redirected to the appropriate medical consultant based on the condition's nature. Colleges typically use a coordinated medical team and may institute special evaluations uniquely useful for a given sport.

The team or lead sports physician is responsible for assembling an interdisciplinary group with the combined expertise to evaluate each athlete. On-site specialists in orthopedics and cardiology can help with difficult medical eligibility assessments related to those systems and can expedite the evaluation of athletes with medical eligibility concerns. Physical therapists, athletic trainers, nurses, and dietitians can help with check-in, check-out, "traffic control," vital sign measurements, patient education, musculoskeletal screening, and rehabilitation exercise instruction. Coaches and school administrators can be enlisted to help maintain order and discipline in what can be a chaotic group environment.

The team physician needs to choose a location that has adequate space for the substantial number of participants and one that has a private and quiet space for individual examinations. Many providers use their medical offices after hours to conduct these examinations so that examiners and athletes have privacy. The rooms can be arranged to allow an orderly flow of athletes and specific consultations.

Table 2-1. Elements of a Coordinated Medical Evaluation

Stage	Purpose
Waiting area	Sign-in, registration, and review, including careful instruction about completing required forms
Vitals station (private setting)	Height, weight, body mass index,[a] blood pressure, heart rate, and visual acuity may be measured by qualified personnel such as medical assistants, student athletic trainers, and medical students.
General medical examination station	History review and physical examination performed by a single health care provider for a given individual. Medical eligibility status or referral plan determined.
Specialty examination stations	Orthopedic assessment, cardiac evaluation, pulmonary function testing, or other systems-based examination
Optional stations	Education and immunization areas

[a] Body mass index can be calculated from height and weight (www.cdc.gov/growthcharts).

Box 2-2. Tips to Improve the Coordinated Medical Team Approach to Preparticipation Evaluations

Preparation
- Provide the individual with information in advance about the detailed nature of the evaluation.

Privacy
- Provide separate and private areas for examining male, female, and transgender individuals.
  - Require appropriate examination attire (eg, shorts and t-shirt or tank top).
  - Provide a private counseling room for discussion of sensitive issues.

Referrals
- Establish a clear protocol for return to the medical home or referral to specialists for more extensive evaluation or rehabilitation for individuals who are not medically eligible for sport participation.
- Aid individuals who need help arranging follow-up evaluations (ie, low-income, uninsured, and those without primary care providers).

Medically Ineligible or Limited Student-Athletes
- Keep a record of individuals who are not medically eligible or who require further evaluation before final medical eligibility is determined (see the Medical Eligibility for Participation content in each system section of Chapter 5). A process needs to be in place for following up with these individuals to establish the final disposition. Typically, this is done by the team physician or PPE site coordinator.
- Counsel any individual who is not medically eligible for the desired sport regarding modified participation or other possible activities.
- Filling out the history (p 293), physical examination (p 297), and medical eligibility (p 301) forms carefully before the evaluation can improve the entire process. Therefore, at the start of a coordinated medical team evaluation, explaining to the individuals and their parents or guardians how to correctly complete the forms will result in more useful final forms. Appropriate privacy, storage, and handling of forms can give an individual greater confidence in the confidentiality of the process.

When an individual does not meet medical eligibility requirements, effective communication among the evaluating provider, the individual, and their parents or guardians is essential. Communicating the medical details of the activity restriction to coaches and possibly the team athletic trainer requires permission of the athlete and parents/guardians (see Chapter 3). In a medical team setting, the team physician will often lead this discussion. The decision to restrict activity is often not finalized on the day of the evaluation. Rather, it occurs after consulting with medical subspecialists, reviewing risks of participation with the consultant, and then meeting with the individual (and family) in a private setting to discuss the specific issue limiting medical eligibility.

FREQUENCY OF THE EVALUATION

There are no outcomes-based data to guide the recommendations for frequency of the PPE, and following the initial PPE, one might consider the examination to be a periodic athlete health evaluation rather than a PPE.[7] The current PPE intervals for high school athletes are arbitrary and based on state or organization requirements. The American Heart Association recommends a cardiac evaluation every 2 years, but this is also an arbitrary recommendation based on the assumption that cardiac changes are detectable at 2-year intervals as the heart matures.[8] There is little evidence to support any of the prescribed interval recommendations between 1 year and 4 years for the PPE or for routine health care.[4]

The AAP recommends an annual comprehensive health supervision visit from age 6 years to age 21 years for healthy children, adolescents, and young adults.[9] The AAFP recommends a preventive health visit every 1 to 3 years as necessary for adolescents and young adults. An important reason for performing a complete PPE annually is that many individuals and their parents or guardians use the PPE as their only visit for health care.[10]

When a PCP performs annual health supervision visits in the medical home, the PPE authoring societies recommend incorporating required elements of the PPE into the health supervision encounter every 1 to 2 years to maintain continuity of care so that a separate visit for a PPE is not needed. Given the time constraints of a typical health supervision visit, the goal of integrating the PPE may be more easily achieved if the PPE portion of the evaluation is addressed every 2 years, rather than annually, to allow a different focus for evolving child and adolescent risk at each visit.

Incorporating the PPE into the routine health supervision screening after age 6 years may promote physical activity and sports safety of children and adolescents before they reach the age of interscholastic competition. In addition, doing so may potentially identify any risk for activity-related sudden cardiac death or other medical conditions affecting the physical activity of all children, not just those involved in organized sports.

College athletic departments generally determine the PPE frequency policies for their athletes using National Collegiate Athletic Association, National Association of Intercollegiate Athletics, and National Junior College Athletic Association recommendations and regulations. College student-athletes are often away from their medical home. Colleges also assume some financial risk for athletes during practice and competition; hence, more comprehensive health examinations at entry into a collegiate athletic program are often the norm. Once a comprehensive evaluation has been conducted, college student-athletes usually undergo abbreviated annual evaluations that focus on injuries or medical problems that have occurred since the comprehensive entry examination and have not resolved. The team physician at the collegiate level needs to be familiar with the health history of the student-athletes and will typically perform the examinations or review the information from examinations and yearly updates completed by providers who are not associated with the college program. It is the opinion of the PPE authoring societies that this frequency is appropriate for the college age group.

In 2025, the National Federation of State High School Associations conducted a survey of its 51 state associations. The federation received 42 responses. Of the respondents, 95% reported requiring a PPE prior to school-sponsored sports and/or activity participation. There is no universal agreement on the required interval between these evaluations. Seventy-five percent of respondents reported requiring the PPE be completed every 12 to 15 months, 2.5% require completion every 18 months, 17.5% reported a 2-year interval, and 5% reported requiring the PPE to be completed every 3 years (a follow-up question about the requirement of annual updates was not asked).

Seventy-five percent of respondents reported modifying the PPE forms to meet their specific needs, such as addressing questions on COVID-19 as the pandemic evolved, sex/gender questions, and subtle edits to address state-specific requirements. Seventy-five percent of respondents reported the PPE being used below the high school level.

The implementation of a nationwide format for PPEs and a data-based recommendation regarding frequency of examination has been hampered by a lack of research and other factors. Some issues that have influenced these decisions include (1) the requirements set by each state governing body and by specific schools; (2) the cost, especially out-of-pocket expenses for students; and (3) the availability of qualified personnel.

No outcomes-based research indicates that more frequent PPEs lessen the risk of injury or death in student-athletes, so an optimal frequency for the examination has not been established.[6,11–15]

The consensus of the PPE authoring societies is to have

- A comprehensive PPE at a minimum of every 2 years for grade school, middle school, and high school athletes.
- Annual updates including both a history questionnaire focused on heart, head, heat injury, and mental health issues and, if needed, a problem-focused examination based on any concerns detected in the history.

The basis for this recommendation is that individuals pass through stages of development that involve both physiological changes and psychological changes that merit monitoring. Careful cardiac auscultation at least every other year may help screen for previously undetected cardiac conditions. The annual history review also allows an opportunity to address new concerns that may have developed since the last comprehensive PPE. The individual and parents or guardians need to confirm with the school when the next PPE for medical eligibility is due.

INTERIM ANNUAL EVALUATIONS

An interim annual evaluation takes place between comprehensive examinations, either face-to-face or by questionnaire, usually before the first competitive season of the academic year. All individuals need to complete the history form and undergo an evaluation for any area indicated by the history. The purpose of the interim evaluation is to assess problems that have occurred since an individual's comprehensive PPE. When done in the provider's office, it also serves as an opportunity to discuss lifestyle issues and risk-taking behaviors and repeat critical questions regarding conditions such as syncope and concussion.

The provider reviews the history form and determines what parts of the physical examination to perform. While this may be a very brief visit, a more detailed examination would be performed when the provider identifies a potentially serious issue. For example, for an individual reporting syncope during exercise, a complete cardiovascular assessment would be required before medical eligibility is determined. In some states, the history form is reviewed by the school nurse or school athletic trainer, who sends individuals with positive responses to the appropriate provider of record for reevaluation and medical eligibility determination. This requires good communication between the schools and the providers.

CONFIDENTIALITY

Individuals, parents, providers' office staff, and school personnel need a clearly informed process for managing the PPE medical eligibility forms so that the information sent to the school is free of confidential information and properly stored at the school. The history and physical examination forms are intended to remain a part of an individual's confidential medical record at the PCP's office or, if completed in the school or in a group examination, in a secure area that can be accessed only by designated medical providers on a "need to know" basis in accordance with the Health Insurance Portability and Accountability Act and the Family Educational Rights and Privacy Act (see Chapter 3).

REFERENCES

1. Herring SA. Kibler WB, Putukian M. Team physician consensus statement: 2013 update. *Med Sci Sports Exerc.* 2013;45(8):1618–1622. Accessed May 12, 2025. https://journals.lww.com/acsm-msse/fulltext/2013/08000/team_physician_consensus_statement__2013_update.24.aspx
2. Pickham D, Chan G, Carey M. Pre-participation screening for athletes and the role of advanced practice providers. *J Electrocardiol.* 2015;48(3):339–344. PMID: 25791248 doi:10.1016/j.jelectrocard.2015.03.003
3. Herring SA, Kibler W, Putukian M. Sideline preparedness for the team physician: a consensus statement—2012 update. *Med Sci Sports Exerc.* 2012;44(12):2442–2445. PMID: 23160347 doi:10.1249/MSS.0b013e318275044f
4. Roberts WO, Löllgen H, Matheson GO, et al; American College of Sports Medicine (ACSM); Fédération Internationale du Médicine du Sport (FIMS). Advancing the preparticipation physical evaluation: an ACSM and FIMS joint consensus statement. *Clin J Sport Med.* 2014;24(6):442–447. PMID: 25347259 doi:10.1097/JSM.0000000000000168
5. LaBotz M, Bernhardt DT. Preparticipation physical examination: is it time to stop doing the sports physical? *Br J Sports Med.* 2017;51(3):151–152. PMID: 27935485 doi:10.1136/bjsports-2016-096892
6. Maron BJ, Friedman RA, Kligfield P, et al; American Heart Association Council on Clinical Cardiology; Advocacy Coordinating Committee; Council on Cardiovascular Disease in the Young; Council on Cardiovascular Surgery and Anesthesia; Council on Epidemiology and Prevention; Council on Functional Genomics and Translational Biology; Council on Quality of Care and Outcomes Research, and American

College of Cardiology. Assessment of the 12-lead electrocardiogram as a screening test for detection of cardiovascular disease in healthy general populations of young people (12-25 years of age): a scientific statement from the American Heart Association and the American College of Cardiology. *J Am Coll Cardiol.* 2014;64(14):1479–1514. PMID: 25234655 doi:10.1016/j.jacc.2014.05.006

7. Ljungqvist A, Jenoure PJ, Engebretsen L, et al. The International Olympic Committee (IOC) consensus statement on periodic health evaluation of elite athletes, March 2009. *Clin J Sport Med.* 2009;19(5):347–365. PMID: 19741306 doi:10.1097/JSM.0b013e3181b7332c
8. Maron BJ, Thompson PD, Ackerman MJ, et al. Recommendations and considerations related to preparticipation screening for cardiovascular abnormalities in competitive athletes: 2007 update: a scientific statement from the American Heart Association Council on Nutrition, Physical Activity, and Metabolism: *Endorsed by the American College of Cardiology Foundation.* 2007;115(12):1643–1655. doi:10.1161/circulationaha.107.181423
9. American Academy of Pediatrics Committee on Practice and Ambulatory Medicine; Bright Futures Periodicity Schedule Workgroup. 2017 recommendations for preventive pediatric health care. *Pediatrics.* 2017;139(4):e20170254. PMID: 28213605
10. Krowchuk DP, Krowchuk HV, Hunter DM, et al. Parents' knowledge of the purposes and content of preparticipation physical examinations. *Arch Pediatr Adolesc Med.* 1995;149(6):653–657. PMID: 7767421 doi:10.1001/archpedi.1995.02170190063011
11. Wingfield K, Matheson GO, Meeuwisse WH. Preparticipation evaluation: an evidence-based review. *Clin J Sport Med.* 2004;14(3):109–122. PMID: 15166898 doi:10.1097/00042752-200405000-00002
12. Brukner P, White S, Shawdon A, Holzer K. Screening of athletes: Australian experience. *Clin J Sport Med.* 2004;14(3):169–177. PMID: 15166906 doi:10.1097/00042752-200405000-00010
13. Metzl JD. Preparticipation examination of the adolescent athlete: part 1. *Pediatr Rev.* 2001;22(6):199–204. PMID: 11389307 doi:10.1542/pir.22-6-199
14. Stickler GB. Are yearly physical examinations in adolescents necessary? *J Am Board Fam Pract.* 2000;13(3):172–177. PMID: 10826864 doi:10.3122/15572625-13-3-172
15. O'Connor FG, Kugler JP, Oriscello RG. Sudden death in young athletes: screening for the needle in a haystack. *Am Fam Physician.* 1998;57(11):2763–2770. PMID: 9636339

CHAPTER 3

Legal, Ethical, and Privacy Issues of the PPE

The legal, ethical, and privacy issues of the preparticipation evaluation (PPE) are numerous and complex. Federal, state, and jurisdictional laws, regulations, and rules are inconsistent and add to the complexity. Individual institutions have widely discrepant policies and procedures. This chapter is intended as a general overview and *should not* be considered a legal opinion. The onus is on the medical community to navigate this landscape while adhering to the broad principles of privacy, inclusion, and equity and promoting health through activity and participation.

■ LEGAL ISSUES

Legal Requirements for PPE

Laws enacted that require participants to have a PPE before engaging in sports and other activities are reportedly intended to enhance safety, to increase the number of individuals accessing health care, and to create more touchpoints between participants and the health care system. It is unclear if PPEs do any of these.[1–4]

PPEs have not yet been demonstrated to reliably predict the risk of injury or health issues, and their effectiveness remains unclear.[2–4] Further, they may result in overmedicalization, overdiagnosis, and excessive testing of the intended participants. While participant safety is important, unwarranted testing or exclusion can needlessly reduce opportunities for physical activity and personal development, especially since it may disproportionately affect individuals in underresourced communities, those with poorer access to medical care, those with disabilities, and those already at risk for low physical activity. This occurs because testing that is necessary as a result of abnormal findings on PPE screening may be expensive or difficult to access. In one study, only 15% of the participants who were required to have a follow-up evaluation received the indicated follow-up.[1]

It is unclear why a requirement for PPEs exists for interscholastic sports and certain other activities but not for other forms of exercise, such as running, playing on a playground, or playing basketball or soccer with friends. PPE requirements may serve more to reduce liability for institutions, organizations, and schools, and to mitigate risk for their insurers, rather than to meaningfully protect participants. These concerns grow as evidence suggests that PPEs may not meaningfully reduce the risk of injury or death for individual participants.

Whether a required, routine PPE leads to high-quality health care or serves as a meaningful touchpoint for long-term health management is indeterminate.[1,2] Since many participants receive a PPE outside their usual medical home (eg, in urgent care centers, in free clinics, or at station-based examinations at school), this process can, paradoxically, disrupt integration into a medical home and continuity of care.[1,2] Many parents and guardians believe a PPE is an adequate substitution for a routine health supervision visit.[4] There is a large degree of heterogeneity among the individuals performing the PPE with regard to training, skill, and knowledge. This variability may result in inconsistent standards of assessment and differing determinations of medical eligibility.[5] A large majority of states allow nonphysicians to perform the evaluation.[1] This may complicate matters if the nonphysician provider does not have authority to write prescriptions and an individual with a chronic medical condition may require routine prescription medication or the administration of an emergency medication, such as epinephrine, glucagon, or albuterol; this, in turn, may affect how schools manage these participants.

Laws requiring participants to undergo routine PPEs may compel them to disclose personal or mental health information as a condition of participation, without guarantees of privacy. Individuals may have legitimate concerns about how this information is handled, stored, and accessed. These concerns may be heightened in station-based evaluations, when large numbers of individuals are present in settings that may lack the privacy protections of a medical home, where Health Insurance Portability and Accountability Act (HIPAA) regulations apply. The fear of stigma, bullying, or potential participation restrictions may lead individuals to withhold critical information. Additionally, questions that require individuals to disclose sensitive personal details, such as sex assigned at birth (rather than current gender identity), the date of the last menstrual cycle, or use of hormonal medications (eg, hormonal contraception or gender-affirming treatments) may be particularly distressing for individuals at risk of having their health information exposed. Cross-state travel for competition may subject participants to additional regulatory requirements, particularly affecting transgender individuals.[2]

The primary purpose of this book is to educate health care professionals about conditions that may impact an individual's ability to participate in certain sports or activities and how they can help address an individual's medical needs to allow for participation. It does not seek to answer the question as to whether such assessments should be a mandatory prerequisite for participation in sports or activities.

Shared Decision-Making in Medical Eligibility for Participation

Most often, participants undergoing a PPE are permitted full activity without restrictions. However, situations arise where a provider performing a PPE will make a recommendation for the individual to not participate in a chosen activity. These cases can be challenging because the individual's (and sometimes their family's) desire to participate is in direct conflict with the provider's goal to reduce risk for the person.[2]

When a participant (and their parents or guardians) still desires participation, even though a recommendation has been made to not participate in a given activity, a shared decision-making approach is critical so all involved can more fully understand the risks and benefits of participation. Second opinions or outside consultations may be helpful in these situations.[2]

Although a shared decision-making approach may be helpful for a participant and the provider performing a PPE, an involved organization or institution may still make an alternate determination.[2]

Legal Aspects of Limiting Medical Eligibility

There is a prevailing opinion, supported by case law, that an organization or institution and its team physician have the legal right to restrict an individual from participating in athletics or other activities. For this to be true, the decision would usually be expected to be individualized and contextually based on medical evidence (to the degree it may be available). Individual institutions and their respective team physicians may quantify and assess risk differently within a given set of circumstances. Some may allow participation for a situation that would not be permitted at a different institution. Also, an institution and its team physician may have a different opinion from that of an individual's treating physician. In cases where opinions differ, the courts have generally sided with the institution and its team physician.[6]

When assessing medical eligibility, the team physician for the institution or organization should make an individual determination based on applicable medical literature, national guidelines (eg, the American Heart Association and American College of Cardiology scientific statement "Eligibility and Disqualification Recommendations for Competitive Athletes With Cardiovascular Abnormalities"[6]), or outside specialist consultations. It is important to note that national guidelines and consensus documents are often conservative; however, when a physician chooses to not follow the guidelines, there should be clearly documented medical justification. Alignment between the treating physician(s), any outside consultants, the organization (if applicable), and the participant (and their parents or guardians, if applicable) is important to limit liability exposure.[6]

While exculpatory waivers (waivers of liability to the organization, institution, or team physician) are often used, if an athlete chooses to participate against medical advice, such waivers may not offer sufficient protection for those involved as they are often interpreted narrowly and may not be enforceable in a lawsuit, especially if the participant is a minor.

It is important to note the Americans With Disabilities Act (ADA) creates legal protections for individuals with disabilities wishing to participate in sports and other activities. Participants with disabilities should be provided reasonable accommodations, where applicable and appropriate. This also implies that participation and restriction determinations must be based on objective medical information and not assumptions or generalizations about an individual's disability status. At the same time, a team physician or treating physician and institution should not feel pressured to allow participation simply to avoid lawsuits. The focus should always remain on the individual and their ability to safely participate in the chosen activity, with an effort to enable participation whenever reasonable.[6]

Mandatory Reporting Requirements

If a PPE uncovers instances of interpersonal violence, including emotional, physical, or sexual abuse or misconduct as it relates to sports, the laws governing mandatory reporting of suspected or reported abuse apply. Mandatory reporting laws require that health care professionals report child abuse and neglect to a proper authority, such as a law enforcement agency or child protective services. Other federal, state, and local jurisdictional laws and institutional or organizational policies may apply to mandated reporting of other aspects of interpersonal violence. It is essential for physicians conducting PPEs to be familiar with these reporting obligations and to have a plan in place to ensure timely and appropriate reporting when necessary. This topic is discussed further in Chapter 9.

LIABILITY AND RISKS

Good Samaritan Statutes and Charitable Immunity

The medicolegal liability of health care providers performing PPEs varies depending on the setting. When PPEs are conducted in a medical clinic as part of the physician's normal daily responsibilities, standard malpractice laws apply. However, when physicians perform PPEs on a voluntary basis, liability protections may differ.[7]

"Good Samaritan" statutes generally protect health care professionals providing emergency care in unexpected situations. Since PPEs are evaluations that are scheduled in advance, Good Samaritan statutes typically would not apply, and physicians should not rely on them for protection from liability.[7]

"Good Samaritan" statutes generally protect health care professionals providing emergency care in unexpected situations. Since PPEs are evaluations that are scheduled in advance, Good Samaritan statutes typically would not apply, and physicians should not rely on them for protection from liability.

"Charitable immunity" statutes, on the other hand, may be more applicable and may do more to protect physicians who are volunteering their services, without any remuneration in return. These are also state-specific laws and help shield health care providers from lawsuits when they are acting within their professional scope and volunteering for nonprofit organizations by either capping damages or limiting noneconomic claims.[7]

Also, the **Volunteer Protection Act of 1997**, a federal law, offers personal liability protection to volunteers working for nonprofit organizations or government entities, provided they act within their assigned duties.[7]

While various laws exist that may partially shield health care professionals from some aspects of liability, clinicians should not rely solely on these protections. Because primary care physicians performing PPEs would be considered practicing within their specialty, and because compensation may be either direct or indirect (and not necessarily recognized by the provider as compensation), the applicability of these immunity statutes may be limited.[7]

Separately, institutional malpractice insurance provided by an employer may not cover care provided outside the scope of an individual's employment contract. Physicians performing PPEs outside their usual practice setting should confirm whether their malpractice insurance covers these activities and, if not, arrange for additional liability coverage.

Because liability protections vary widely by state and employment status, it is essential for physicians to familiarize themselves with applicable local laws to ensure liability protection.

Maintaining Professional Standards in the PPE

Both the participant and the examiner should feel comfortable and safe during a PPE. This is often accomplished when the health care provider follows a consistent examination procedure and is clear about the purpose and scope of the evaluation. A chaperone may help the participant feel more comfortable and may help with liability protection for the provider, and is recommended for sensitive examinations. Notably, screening genital and breast examinations are not recommended as a routine part of the PPE. Maintaining these professional standards helps reinforce trust and respect and improves comfort and safety.

Other Considerations

Providing free or highly discounted services may trigger anti-kickback statutes, especially in cases where referrals may be directed to providers performing these services. There may, separately, be third-party payer concerns if a provider of services has an active contract with the payer and is charging for the completion of a PPE in a different setting.

HIPAA, FERPA, and Privacy

Both HIPAA and the Family Educational Rights and Privacy Act (FERPA) affect how personal health information (PHI) can be shared between health care providers and institutions (or their personnel). HIPAA applies to **health care providers in the clinical setting**. This law creates standards regarding the use and disclosure of PHI. FERPA, on the other hand, protects students' privacy within educational settings. FERPA regulates **student education records in schools** (in those schools receiving federal funds) and sets standards for those who can access educational records without consent.[8,9]

Because HIPAA and FERPA govern different aspects of privacy in different contexts, their rules can be confusing for participants, physicians, and institutions, especially when they do not align. For example, a PPE conducted in a health care setting, such as a physician's office, is protected by HIPAA rules. This means the participant's personal physical and mental health information cannot be shared without their consent, although the participant may still choose to share their full PPE with a school or an organization if they wish.

A PPE conducted in a health care setting is protected by HIPAA rules. A PPE performed in a school setting is protected under FERPA.

On the other hand, when the same PPE is performed in a school setting—in a school receiving federal funds (eg, a school-sponsored mass PPE screening event or when performed by a school-employed health care provider)—the records are considered part of the educational record and fall under FERPA protections. Unlike HIPAA, FERPA allows school staff and other authorized individuals, inside and outside the school, to access those records without specific consent from the student. Further complicating matters, if a PPE is conducted in a school that does not receive federal funds, neither HIPAA nor FERPA applies, meaning there may be no formal privacy protections governing the disclosure of those records.

Any contractual relationship that exists between health care providers and their employing institution may also affect privacy protections. For instance, providers (eg, athletic trainers, school nurses, and school physicians) directly employed (or contracted) by the school are subject to FERPA. On the other hand, health care providers contracted from medical practices or hospitals (such as athletic trainers in an outreach program) are still subject to HIPAA regulations. Before receiving a PPE, participants should be informed by the health care provider performing the evaluation of any implications the PPE location or setting may have on the privacy of their PHI.

Privacy Implications in Practice

Working in the context of these privacy laws is essential for those conducting PPEs. To ensure confidentiality and to limit the amount of personal information shared to the minimum necessary for participation decisions, **medical eligibility forms should be kept separate from detailed health histories and physical examination forms.**[2]

At the same time, it may be important for certain health data to be shared with the treatment team at the institution or school (eg, sharing information with athletic trainers about chronic health conditions or known allergies). In certain circumstances, such as when no medical provider will be present for an event, coaches or other responsible parties may need to access this PHI. In cases like this, it is best to obtain written consent from the participant (or their parent/guardian) to share the necessary information and for the physician to inform the participant and their guardian of what information should be expected to be shared. In schools with team physicians, students may be required to sign a form allowing essential medical information to be shared among the physician, athletic trainer, coaches, and school administrators as a condition of participation. In some states, this form is incorporated in the paperwork required to participate in school-sponsored activities. Since the records for school-based PPEs typically remain with the institution rather than with the participant's primary health care provider, collaboration between school-based and community health care providers is vital to promote consistent and comprehensive care.

Schools and organizations should train staff on privacy laws so they can correctly handle PHI in compliance with applicable HIPAA and FERPA rules. Physicians and nonphysician providers who perform PPEs in either the private office setting or the institutional/school setting should be familiar with the applicable privacy laws and protections.

Schools should make sure that paper forms are kept in locked storage, accessible only to authorized individuals in order to keep PHI secure and confidential. However, they also need to be accessible when necessary, such as during travel or in emergencies. If the PPE is in a digital format, the electronic storage and communication systems require digital protection.

When a participant is deemed medically ineligible to take part in a sport or activity, determining who needs to know what information, and how to communicate the restriction, can be challenging. Coaches and team administrators need only be informed of the participant's eligibility status and in which sports, if any, they would be permitted to participate. In many cases, participants or their guardians will choose to share additional details with the coach. **However, a signed medical release of information form is generally considered necessary for a health care provider to discuss case specifics, including PHI, with coaches or administrators.**

Physicians and nonphysician providers should be aware of state laws related to consent, age of majority, and privacy, especially for sensitive issues like mental or sexual health or pregnancy.

CONCLUSION

There are several challenging legal, ethical, and privacy issues related to the PPE, which are made more complex because of inconsistent laws and variable institutional policies and procedures. Because PPEs have not been consistently shown to reduce the risk of injury or death for participants, physicians should err on the side of promoting safe participation, while working to eliminate inequities and barriers for individuals. Physicians and nonphysician providers should empower participants by using a shared decision-making approach to medical eligibility, while also understanding that the respective institution and their own team physician(s) will likely make any final determinations. Privacy of PHI remains important, and just because an individual wants to participate in sports or other activities does not imply all PHI can be freely shared with schools or institutions. Participants, physicians, and organizations should be aware of differing rules related to permitted and nonpermitted disclosures of health information. Physicians performing PPEs in a setting outside their typical practice setting or outside of a standard employment contract should ensure they have malpractice liability protections since charitable immunity statutes and volunteer status may provide incomplete protection.

REFERENCES

1. Kennedy M, Comer F, Young JA, Valasek AE. Increasing primary care follow-up after preparticipation physical evaluations. *Pediatr Qual Saf.* 2020;5(6):e358. PMID: 33134760
2. MacDonald J, Schaefer M, Stumph J. The preparticipation physical evaluation. *Am Fam Physician.* 2021;103(9):539–546. PMID: 33929170
3. Weise A, Könsgen N, Joisten C, et al. Pre-participation evaluation of recreational and competitive athletes—a systematic review of guidelines and consensus statements. *Sports Med Open.* 2025;11(1):33. PMID: 40188235 doi:10.1186/s40798-025-00837-6
4. Daniels EW, Onks CA, Gallo RA, Silvis ML. Is the preparticipation physical examination replacing the annual well child examination among student athletes? *Perm J.* 2021;25(3):20.298. PMID: 35348075 doi:10.7812/TPP/20.298
5. Wingfield K, Matheson GO, Meeuwisse WH. Preparticipation evaluation: an evidence-based review. *Clin J Sport Med.* 2004;14(3):109–122. PMID: 15166898 doi:10.1097/00042752-200405000-00002
6. Mitten MJ, Zipes DP, Maron BJ, Bryant WJ; American Heart Association Electrocardiography and Arrhythmias Committee of Council on Clinical Cardiology, Council on Cardiovascular Disease in Young, Council on Cardiovascular and Stroke Nursing, Council on Functional Genomics and Translational Biology, and American College of Cardiology. Eligibility and disqualification recommendations for competitive athletes with cardiovascular abnormalities: task force 15: legal aspects of medical eligibility and disqualification recommendations: a scientific statement from the American Heart Association and American College of Cardiology. *Circulation.* 2015;132(22):e346–e349. PMID: 26621654 doi:10.1161/CIR.0000000000000251
7. Benrud L, Darrah J, Johnson A. Liability considerations for physician volunteers in the u.s. *AMA J Ethics.* 2010;12(3):207–212 PMID: 23140870 doi:10.1001/virtualmentor.2010.12.3.hlaw1-1003
8. Office for Civil Rights. The HIPAA Privacy Rule. US Department of Health and Human Services. Reviewed September 27, 2024. Accessed March 15, 2025. https://www.hhs.gov/hipaa/for-professionals/privacy/index.html
9. US Department of Education. Family Educational Rights and Privacy Act (FERPA). Accessed March 15, 2025. https://studentprivacy.ed.gov/ferpa

CHAPTER 4

General Considerations for the History, Physical Examination, and Medical Eligibility

KEY POINTS AND SUMMARY OF EVIDENCE

- The preparticipation evaluation (PPE) authoring societies recommend that the PPE be integrated into the annual health supervision visit along with preventive care strategies by an appropriate health care provider (see Chapter 2) from the individual's medical home who has current and past medical records (strength of recommendation [SOR]: Level C).
- Key findings during the musculoskeletal history will direct the focus of the musculoskeletal physical examination, as currently there are limited screening examinations that have been validated to reduce injury risk (SOR: Level B).
- Medical eligibility and sports participation decisions should be clearly outlined and supported by evidence-based or expert opinion guidelines, and they should include specialty consultation when needed (SOR: Level B).
- If an individual is not medically qualified for a given sport, alternative activities should be discussed, and it is important to monitor individuals for physical and emotional repercussions of not being allowed to participate in desired activities (SOR: Level C).

INTRODUCTION

The purpose of the PPE is not to disqualify an individual from physical activity or sport participation, but for early detection of and intervention for potential conditions that could adversely affect the individual during physical activity, sport-specific training, and competition. This information is necessary for the sideline health care team (ie, athletic trainers and team physicians) to adequately prepare for the potential needs of individuals throughout the course of their athletic careers. A systematic approach to the history, physical examination, and medical eligibility decision-making process will enable an examiner to meet the goals and objectives of the PPE in an effective and efficient manner. The PPE authoring societies recommend that the PPE be integrated into the scope of preventive screening during the annual health supervision visit by an individual's primary care provider in their medical home or by their team physician (eg, in college sports settings). An unintended consequence of requiring the PPE for sports eligibility is that the PPE encounter often becomes a substitute for the individual's annual health supervision visit with their primary care physician.

The challenge for the primary care workforce to routinely evaluate the incredibly large number of children and adolescents in the United States who participate in some form of organized sport is daunting, especially if required annually. Having a uniform process that is user-friendly and efficient can promote optimum accuracy and inclusiveness. Obstacles to performing the PPE within the structure of the annual health supervision visit include time and scheduling limitations, inadequate training in the PPE process and its implications, uncertainty regarding the relative importance of each PPE component, length of the PPE form, time needed for covering non-PPE topics, and lack of a standard approach to the evaluation.[1–3]

Integrating the standardized PPE history questions and physical examination into the annual health supervision visit will reduce the likelihood of missing key elements and improve encounter efficiency.[4] Incorporating the standardized PPE form into the electronic medical record increases the potential to collect meaningful data that can direct future guidelines with evidence-based and outcome-driven content.[5]

This chapter discusses general considerations of the preparticipation history, physical examination, and medical eligibility determination, and it will serve as a prelude to questions and concerns covered in the remainder of the book that are more organ-system specific.

HISTORY

The medical history may be the most important component of the PPE. In PPEs for high school and collegiate athletes, the medical history alone detects 88% of general medical conditions and 67% to 75% of musculoskeletal conditions, yet it has not been proven to improve or change individual outcomes.[6] While the goal of the history questions is to detect all conditions that confer unacceptable risks to participation, the questions have not been subjected to scientific investigation[7]; thus, it is impossible to achieve a zero-risk competitive sport environment that is based on the question responses.

For individuals younger than 18 years, both the individual and the parent or guardian are asked to respond to medical history questions. Involving parents in the history portion of the evaluation is essential to improve the accuracy of the evaluation, as concordance between child or adolescent responses and parent or guardian responses to the medical history questions ranges from only 19% to 39%.[8] Full access to an individual's medical records during an evaluation completed within the medical home improves the accuracy of the medical information available to the provider who is determining medical eligibility.

Illiteracy and limited English proficiency are major barriers to completing an accurate medical history.[9] The use of medical interpreters or forms translated into the native language of an individual and their family will result in a more accurate history.[10] Making the history forms available in advance of the evaluation date, to be completed by the individual and their parent or guardian, can improve the accuracy of the history data on the form and reduce the errors associated with a rushed form completed immediately before the evaluation. Completing the form in advance of the PPE visit allows the parent or guardian to identify issues that the individual is not aware of or has forgotten, especially family and early childhood history.

It is important to review the medical history in a private setting with both the individual and the parent or guardian (if present) and again with the individual alone for more sensitive questions when age and developmentally appropriate. Any available medical records believed to be pertinent should be reviewed for past injuries or illnesses that may not have been reported in the current medical history or to clarify responses on the History Form. Positive responses to the medical history questions serve as a platform to pursue the secondary questions associated with the issue and to determine whether further medical evaluation is warranted. It is also prudent to orally clarify negative answers to key questions involving the heart, the head, and mental health issues to underscore the importance of truthful responses.

Questions regarding mental health concerns or high-risk behaviors are best addressed when the individual is alone to increase the chances of honest answers. While the written history forms may address some of these issues, many adolescents will not provide honest responses to questions that will be seen by parents or guardians.[11] Allowing the adolescent to complete validated supplemental questionnaires—such as the Patient Health Questionnaire versions 4, 9, or adolescent (PHQ-4, PHQ-9, or PHQ-A [ages 11–17 years]); the Generalized Anxiety Disorder 7-item (GAD-7) scale; or the PROMIS Depression instruments—on their own without a parent present can assist in screening for depression and anxiety during the examination and pave a path to appropriate evaluation and treatment resources.[12–14] The CRAFFT Screening Tool for Adolescent Substance Abuse 2.0 (https://crafft.org)[15] is designed for use with individuals younger than 21 years to address alcohol or other drug-use disorders and is endorsed by the American Academy of Pediatrics.[16]

The medical home provides the optimal setting for the most accurate medical history through continuity, records review, and a pathway for appropriate workup, along with the privacy of a medical office. A working relationship between the primary care physician and team physician provides the ideal situation for the individual participating in sport.

PHYSICAL EXAMINATION

The structured physical examination begins by measuring vital signs and visual acuity. Elevated blood pressure (discussed in Chapter 5A) and abnormal visual acuity are 2 of the most common abnormalities found during a PPE.[17]

Review of growth curve measurements can identify atypical weight loss or gain that may suggest disordered eating or insufficient energy availability, unhealthy weight-cutting behaviors in sports with weight classes, or performance-enhancing supplement use that may not be otherwise identified.[16] When height curves show reduced growth velocity, this suggests either insufficient caloric intake or delayed pubertal development that may place an athlete at higher risk for both overuse injury and contact or collision sport injury.[18] Decreased height velocity or delayed puberty may also indicate other medical problems such as endocrine or nutritional problems and deserves further evaluation. Body mass index curves should also be reviewed but may be falsely skewed toward overweight status by muscle development in some individuals who participate regularly in sport and exercise.

The physical examination builds on information elicited in the medical history. For example, key musculoskeletal history findings are then followed by a careful physical examination of involved joints and musculoskeletal regions. Unfortunately, no validated set of screening tests exists to predict injury risk in elite-level athletes,[19] although in adolescents who are transitioning through puberty, poor neuromuscular control of the lower extremity may be a risk factor for anterior cruciate ligament injury and patellofemoral joint pain. The components of each segment of the physical examination are discussed in the system sections of Chapter 5.

If conditions discovered during the evaluation cannot be fully addressed because of time constraints, the medical eligibility decision should be postponed until a full evaluation, including any necessary tests and referrals, can be completed.

DETERMINING MEDICAL ELIGIBILITY

Determination of medical eligibility is an important and sometimes difficult decision-making process, often pressured by time constraints associated with the start of team workouts or practice sessions. When additional evaluation is needed, the medical eligibility decision should be deferred until the necessary data are obtained. While up to 14% of athletes require further evaluation before medical eligibility status can be determined, more than 98% of athletes eventually qualify to participate in their desired sport.[20] For younger adolescents, temporary eligibility restrictions are mainly in response to growth-dependent musculoskeletal findings that require rehabilitation.[21]

Reports of prior restricted medical eligibility are significant findings that require additional investigation. To establish current medical eligibility, records of past evaluations or hospitalizations may be required to clarify past medical eligibility decisions and direct the current evaluation.

When a condition limits medical eligibility, the practitioner, youth, and parent or guardian should discuss risks and benefits of participation in desired activities, potential use of assistive devices or accommodations, risk to other participants, and selection of alternative activities that may be a better fit for the individual (ie, shared decision-making). Problems that limit medical eligibility usually require more time than is allotted to a standard PPE appointment, and additional visits are often needed to complete the investigation. Diligent review of previous records, completion of additional tests and treatment, appropriate referrals to specialists, and scheduling of follow-up visits to determine medical eligibility take precedence over sport schedule pressures or the individual's desire to participate in a certain sport.

The initial medical eligibility for sports status of an individual can be divided into the following 5 categories:

1. Medically eligible for all sports and activities without restriction
2. Medically eligible for all sports and activities without restriction, with recommendations for further evaluation or treatment of ______ (eg, "Check blood pressure in 1 month.")
3. Medically eligible *after* evaluation and clearance for ______

4. Medically eligible for certain sports and activities (list the specific sports or type of sports)
5. Not medically eligible for any sports or activities

A form for recording medical eligibility status is available in the Forms section of this book (p 301).

MEDICAL ELIGIBILITY CONSIDERATIONS

- The PPE may promote safe participation within the dynamic and static capabilities of an individual, rather than prevent all physical activity participation. Static capabilities refer to more anaerobic activities that cause firing of large skeletal muscle groups, resulting in sustained increased blood pressure that can further increase with any incorporation of Valsalva maneuvers (eg, weightlifting, rock climbing, water skiing). Dynamic capabilities refer to more aerobic activities that will increase blood flow and cardiac output in proportion to the metabolic demand of the activity (eg, cross-country skiing or running, cycling, boxing)[22] (see Figure 4-1).
- Activity restrictions can be supplemented with alternative activities that fit within the individual's medical eligibility.
- It is the opinion of the authoring societies that PPE sport qualification status is best determined using a single-examiner model in the medical home. If multiple providers conduct the PPE, one provider familiar with the demands of the activity and the current medical literature should render the sport qualification decision after reviewing the entire history and physical evaluation findings. It is often challenging to determine final medical eligibility in a station-based format if there are any questionable findings, if there is a lack of medical records, or if there are time constraints. In addition, arranging referrals in a timely manner may be difficult in the station-based setting.
- In cases where there is uncertainty regarding medical eligibility, consultation with appropriate subspecialist(s) should be obtained.
- When considering any abnormality or condition found during the PPE that may influence participation, the practitioner should consider the following questions:
  - —Does participation put the individual at risk for illness or injury above the inherent hazards of the activity?
  - —Does participation increase the risk of injury or illness for other participants?
  - —Will treatment of the underlying condition allow safe participation (eg, medication, rehabilitation, bracing, and padding)?
  - —Can limited participation be allowed while treatment or evaluation is completed?
  - —If medical eligibility is denied for certain sports because of medical or safety concerns, can the individual safely participate in their sport with modifications or in other activities or sports?
- Medical eligibility decisions should be based on pertinent clinical guidelines and reviews, an understanding of how specific medical conditions affect sports participation, and the classification of the sports being pursued (eg, static vs dynamic demands, degree and type of contact, specific positions [eg, goalie vs midfielder]).

- Shared decision-making among individuals and their parents or guardians, primary care physician, and team physician is needed when a condition limits medical eligibility. The practitioner and individual should discuss risks and benefits of participation in desired activities, potential use of assistive devices or accommodations, risk to other participants, and selection of alternative activities that may be a better fit for the individual.
- Sport activities can be risk stratified by the degree of contact or collision (Table 4-1). Contact and collision sports have a higher risk of serious trauma-related injury and can have high demands, both static and dynamic.
- **Using a Medical Eligibility Form that is separate from the history and physical examination forms will help protect confidential medical information.**
- When a school or an organization has a designated team physician or an athletic trainer, permission to share important medical information with these medical team members needs to be obtained from individuals and their parents or guardians (if a minor), even for personal data that might influence safe participation or restrict sports participation. With that in mind, the designated athletic trainer and team physician are the day-to-day and sideline medical management and health care team for these individuals participating in school sports and physical activities. They will be responsible for acute evaluation and management of any illnesses or injuries, as well as for referrals back to the medical home. They are held to the same confidentiality standards as the medical home. A working relationship between the medical home and these providers is beneficial for the individual participating in sport.
- An individual with restricted medical eligibility in a desired sport may experience the loss of physical and emotional benefits of regular physical activity, and those with serious or potentially lethal cardiac disease may be at risk for significant psychological distress. A restricted individual may experience a loss of perceived identity and self-esteem. It is important to address these factors as part of the sports qualification decision and monitor individuals who do not qualify for their sport for both psychological and physical status, as well as provide consistent emotional support.[23] Individuals with restricted medical eligibility may be assessed by a team of physicians or other providers. The medical home, parents, and medically related school personnel need to work together to monitor any individual with restricted medical eligibility. For individuals who are strongly connected with a team, an alternative nonplaying role (such as manager, student-coach, or a similar position) may allow them to continue their affiliation and identity as a team member.
- Medical eligibility may change with time depending on new injuries, new illnesses, new family medical issues, or newly disclosed personal or family history not previously reported. In such cases, the change in participation status needs to be communicated to team or institution officials, but the specifics of medical conditions resulting in the loss of safe participation status should not be shared unless the individual and family grant permission.
- Medical recommendations for participation surrounding a given condition may change with time.

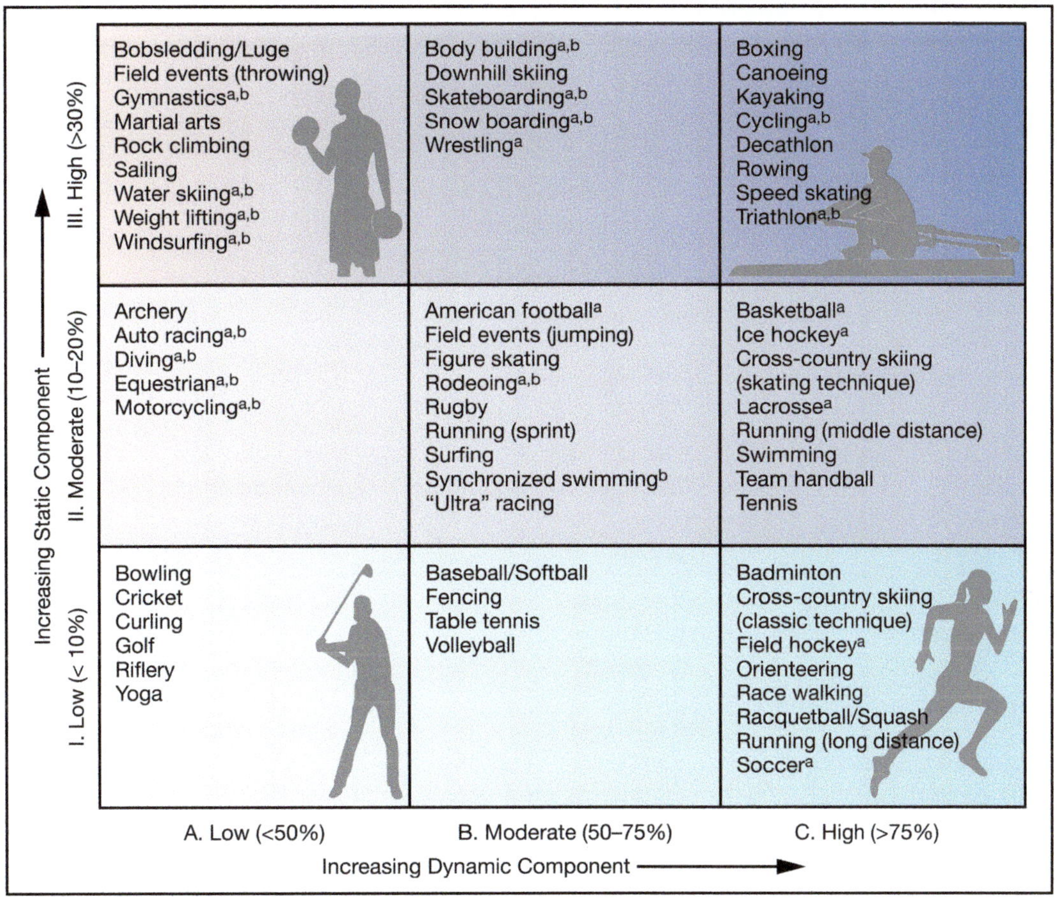

Figure 4-1. Classification of Sports

This classification is based on peak static and dynamic components achieved during competition; however, higher values may be reached during training. The increasing dynamic component is defined in terms of the estimated percentage of maximal oxygen uptake (VO_{2max}) achieved and results in an increasing cardiac output. The increasing static component is related to the estimated percentage of maximal voluntary contraction reached and results in an increasing blood pressure load. The lowest total cardiovascular demands (cardiac output and blood pressure) are shown in the palest color, with increasing dynamic load depicted by increasing blue intensity, and increasing static load depicted by increasing red intensity. Note the graded transition between categories, which should be individualized on the basis of player position and style of play.

[a] Danger of bodily collision.

[b] Increased risk if syncope occurs.

Adapted with permission from Mitchell JH, Haskell W, Snell P, et al. Task force 8: classification of sports. *J Am Coll Cardiol.* 2005;45(8):1364–1367.

Table 4-1. Classification of Sports Based on Impacts

LOW	MODERATE	HIGH
Badminton Bowling	Adventure racing (A combination of ≥2 disciplines, including orienteering and navigation, cross-country running, mountain biking, paddling, and climbing and rope skills)	Basketball Boxing[a]
Canoeing/kayaking (flat water) Rowing	Baseball Softball	Diving
Curling Dance Drill team	Canoeing/kayaking (white water) Cycling	Field hockey Ice hockey[b] American football
eSports: Archery Baseball Chess Cycling Dance Motorsport Sailing Shooting Taekwondo Tennis	Equestrian: Dressage Jumping Riding Martial arts: (Some forms are contact sports and others are limited-contact sport) Aikido Judo Jujitsu Karate Kung fu Taekwondo	Martial arts: (Some forms are contact sports and others are limited-contact sport) Aikido Judo Jujitsu Karate Kung fu Taekwondo
Field events: Discus Javelin Shot put	Field events: High jump Long jump/triple jump Pole vault	Lacrosse Rodeo Roller derby Rugby
Disc golf Golf Marching band Orienteering (A race in which competitors use a map and a compass to find their way through unfamiliar territory)	Floor hockey Football, flag or touch Handball	Skiing: Downhill racing Ski jumping Snowboarding
Pickleball Table tennis Tennis	Racquetball Squash Volleyball	Soccer Team handball Ultimate frisbee

Table 4-1. Classification of Sports Based on Impacts (*continued*)

LOW	MODERATE	HIGH
Powerlifting Body building	Weightlifting Tug of war Skateboarding	Water polo Wrestling
Race walking Riflery Rope jumping Rock climbing	Skiing: Alpine Cross-country Slalom racing Waterskiing	Gymnastics: Acrobatic Artistic Parkour Rhythmic Trampoline and tumbling
Running (regardless of distance) Track	Skating: In-line Roller Ice skating	Cheerleading
Sailing Scuba diving Swimming	Skydiving Surfing Windsurfing	

[a] The American Academy of Pediatrics opposes participation in boxing for children, adolescents, and young adults.

[b] The American Academy of Pediatrics recommends limiting the amount of body checking allowed for hockey players aged ≤ 15 years to reduce injuries.

REFERENCES

1. Madsen NL, Drezner JA, Salerno JC. The preparticipation physical evaluation: an analysis of clinical practice. *Clin J Sport Med.* 2014;24(2):142–149. PMID: 24231928 doi:10.1097/JSM.0000000000000008
2. Wingfield K, Matheson GO, Meeuwisse WH. Preparticipation evaluation: an evidence-based review. *Clin J Sport Med.* 2004;14(3):109–122. PMID: 15166898 doi:10.1097/00042752-200405000-00002
3. Johnson KE, McRee AL. Calling the shots: primary care providers discuss addressing health-risk behaviors during sports physicals. *J Pediatr Health Care.* 2020;34(2):109–116. PMID: 31548141 doi:10.1016/j.pedhc.2019.07.008
4. LaBotz M, Bernhardt DT. Preparticipation physical examination: is it time to stop doing the sports physical? *Br J Sports Med.* 2017;51(3):151–152. PMID: 27935485 doi:10.1136/bjsports-2016-096892
5. Kriz PK, Clyne A, Ford SR. Preparticipation physical exams: the Rhode Island perspective, a call for standardization. *R I Med J.*·2016;99(10):19–22. PMID: 27706273
6. Koester MC, Amundson CL. Preparticipation screening of high school athletes: are recommendations enough? *Phys Sportsmed.* 2003;31(8):35–38. PMID: 20086484 doi:10.3810/psm.2003.08.460
7. Best TM. The preparticipation evaluation: an opportunity for change and consensus. *Clin J Sport Med.* 2004;14(3):107–108. PMID: 15166897 doi:10.1097/00042752-200405000-00001
8. Carek PJ, Futrell M, Hueston WJ. The preparticipation physical examination history: who has the correct answers? *Clin J Sport Med.* 1999;9(3):124–128. PMID: 10512339 doi:10.1097/00042752-199907000-00002
9. Berkman ND, Sheridan SL, Donahue KE, Halpern DJ, Crotty K. Low health literacy and health outcomes: an updated systematic review. *Ann Intern Med.* 2011;155(2):97–107. PMID: 21768583 doi:10.7326/0003-4819-155-2-201107190-00005
10. Powers BJ, Trinh JV, Bosworth HB. Can this patient read and understand written health information? *JAMA.* 2010;304(1):76–84. PMID: 20606152 doi:10.1001/jama.2010.896

11. Chang C, Putukian M, Aerni G, et al. Mental health issues and psychological factors in athletes: detection, management, effect on performance and prevention: American Medical Society for Sports Medicine Position Statement—Executive Summary. *Br J Sports Med.* 2020;54(4):216–220. PMID: 31810972
12. Lewandowski RE, O'Connor B, Bertagnolli A, et al. Screening for and diagnosis of depression among adolescents in a large health maintenance organization. *Psychiatr Serv.* 2016;67(6):636–641. PMID: 26876655
13. Maurer DM. Screening for depression. *Am Fam Physician.* 2012;85(2):139–144. PMID: 22335214
14. Depression: a brief guide to PROMIS Depression instruments. Assessment Center website. September 9, 2015. Accessed October 5, 2024. http://www.healthmeasures.net/images/PROMIS/manuals/PROMIS_Depression_Scoring_Manual_02222017.pdf
15. CRAFFT. Accessed October 5, 2024. http://crafft.org
16. Hagan JF Jr, Shaw JS, Duncan PM, eds. *Bright Futures: Guidelines for Health Supervision of Infants, Children, and Adolescents.* 4th ed. American Academy of Pediatrics; 2017
17. Dixit S, DiFiori J. Prevalence of hypertension and prehypertension in collegiate student athletes. *Clin J Sport Med.* 2006;16(5):440
18. Kriz PK, Stein C, Kent J, et al. Physical maturity and concussion symptom duration among adolescent ice hockey players. *J Pediatr.* 2016;171:234–239.e2. PMID: 26781190
19. Bahr R. Why screening tests to predict injury do not work-and probably never will ...: a critical review. *Br J Sports Med.* 2016;50(13):776–780. PMID: 27095747 doi:10.1136/bjsports-2016-096256
20. Smith J, Laskowski ER. The preparticipation physical examination: Mayo Clinic experience with 2,739 examinations. *Mayo Clin Proc.* 1998;73(5):419–429. PMID: 9581581 doi:10.1016/S0025-6196(11)63723-3
21. Mayer F, Bonaventura K, Cassel M, et al. Medical results of preparticipation examination in adolescent athletes. *Br J Sports Med.* 2012;46(7):524–530. PMID: 22576783 doi:10.1136/bjsports-2011-090966
22. Levine B, Baggish A, Kovacs R, et al. Eligibility and disqualification recommendations for competitive athletes with cardiovascular abnormalities: task force 1: classification of sports: dynamic, static, and impact: a scientific statement from the American Heart Association and American College of Cardiology. *Circulation.* 2015;132(22):e262–e266. doi:10.1161/CIR.0000000000000237
23. Maron BJ, Zipes DP, Kovacs RJ; American Heart Association Electrocardiography and Arrhythmias Committee of the Council on Clinical Cardiology, Council on Cardiovascular Disease in the Young, Council on Cardiovascular and Stroke Nursing, Council on Functional Genomics and Translational Biology, American College of Cardiology. Eligibility and disqualification recommendations for competitive athletes with cardiovascular abnormalities: preamble, principles, and general considerations: a scientific statement from the American Heart Association and American College of Cardiology. *Circulation.* 2015;132(22):e256–e261. PMID: 26621642 doi:10.1161/CIR.0000000000000236

CHAPTER 5

Systems-Based Examination

A: Cardiovascular Problems

HISTORY FORM QUESTIONS

Heart Health Questions About You

1. *Have you ever had pain, discomfort, or shortness of breath in your chest during exercise?*
2. *Have you ever passed out or nearly passed out during or after exercise, or in response to sudden loud noises?*
3. *Has a doctor ever told you that you have any heart problem, heart murmur, or high blood pressure?*
4. *Has a doctor ever ordered a test for your heart (for example, electrocardiography [ECG/EKG] or echocardiography)?*
5. *Have you ever had a seizure?*

Heart Health Questions About Your Family

6. *Has any family member or relative died or had a disability from heart problems before age 50 years, or had any unexpected or sudden unexplained death (SUD) before age 50 years (including drowning, unexplained car accident, or sudden infant death syndrome)?*
7. *Does anyone in your family have hypertrophic cardiomyopathy (HCM), dilated cardiomyopathy, Marfan syndrome, arrhythmogenic cardiomyopathy (ACM), long QT syndrome (LQTS), short QT syndrome, Brugada syndrome, or catecholaminergic polymorphic ventricular tachycardia (CPVT) or have a pacemaker or an implanted defibrillator?*

Secondary Questions

- Have you ever had excessive or unexplained fatigue with exercise?
- Do you ever have heart beats that feel abnormal or irregular at rest or during exercise?
- Has anyone in your family been diagnosed with a congenital heart condition or heart condition at birth?

KEY POINTS

- Sudden cardiac arrest (SCA) and sudden cardiac death (SCD) are rare events in athletes.
- SCA/SCD in young athletes and children is caused by a diverse group of congenital or acquired structural, valvular, and electrical diseases of the heart.
- SCA/SCD may be the first manifestation of underlying cardiac disease; warning symptoms that require cardiac workup include syncope and/or chest pain during exercise, unexplained breathlessness during exercise, and unexplained seizures.
- A detailed personal and family history may help identify individuals at risk for SCD.
- A family history of sudden unexpected or unexplained death, sudden death before the age of 50 years due to cardiac problems, sudden infant death, unexplained drowning, unexplained near drowning, car crashes caused by unexplained driver's loss of consciousness, or unexplained seizures may indicate the presence of a genetic cardiovascular disorder placing the athlete at increased risk for SCD.
- Physical examination should focus on detecting hypertension, pathological heart murmurs, and any physical findings suggestive of Marfan syndrome or other connective tissue disorders.
- **Performing a preparticipation evaluation (PPE) every 1 to 2 years may lead to the identification of new cardiovascular concerns because of the variability in expression and onset of cardiac conditions associated with SCA/SCD during growth and maturation.**
- Athletes with suspected or identified risk for SCD should be evaluated by a cardiologist, preferably a cardiologist who has experience taking care of athletes.

SCD remains the leading medical cause of death in young athletes during exertion.[1–3] Identifying young athletes at risk is difficult because SCD may be the first manifestation of an inherited cardiac condition in asymptomatic individuals.[1] The estimated incidence of SCA or SCD (SCA/SCD) among young competitive athletes varies widely between studies[2] but overall is rare.

Preparticipation cardiovascular evaluation attempts to identify individuals with abnormalities that may provoke SCD on the basis of personal and family history.[4] The American Heart Association (AHA), the American College of Cardiology (ACC), and The American Medical Society for Sports Medicine (AMSSM) indicate that the principal objective of PPE from a cardiovascular perspective is to reduce the risk of sudden death related to a heart-related condition associated with physical activity and enhance the safety of athletes during exercise by using red flag symptoms and family history to detect the potential for SCD.[4,5] This is reflected in the 2015 AHA and ACC consensus statement on preparticipation cardiovascular screening in athletes, with specific recommendations for a detailed personal and family history and physical examination broken down into 15 task forces (9 disease related and 6 on relevant topics and issues).[4,6–20] In 2024, the Heart Rhythm Society published its expert consensus statement on arrhythmias in the athlete, with the recommendation that a history and physical examination be included for cardiovascular screening.[21] Because SCA/SCD can occur outside of activity in individuals with these cardiac conditions, the American Academy of Pediatrics (AAP) developed a policy statement that was updated in 2021 with 4 modified SCA/SCD screening questions to be used for all children regardless of their activity status.[22] **The *PPE: Preparticipation Evaluation*, 6th Edition, includes updated heart health questions to align with the AHA 14 points for assessing cardiovascular risk in athletes and the 4 modified screening questions recommended by the AAP.**

This section:

- Reviews the incidence of SCD in young athletes
- Defines a comprehensive cardiovascular assessment using personal and family history
- Identifies cardiac conditions associated with positive responses to the heart health questions
- Describes signs and symptoms of underlying cardiac pathology
- Discusses the diagnostic investigation for concerning history or examination findings
- Examines the concept of differential risk for SCD in certain athletic populations
- Explores the role of electrocardiography (ECG) and other noninvasive cardiovascular screening of athletes
- Provides guidelines, references, and resources for management of, and medical eligibility decisions for, athletes with cardiovascular disorders

INCIDENCE OF SUDDEN CARDIAC DEATH IN YOUNG ATHLETES

The exact incidence of SCD among athletes and nonathletes in the United States is unknown. Both the number of cardiac arrests and the number of athletes at risk are elusive and often not uniformly defined in studies. Additionally, there are no specific guidelines for the approach to the cardiac examination during autopsy in SCD cases in the United States.[23,24] Some studies include only deaths that meet the definition of exercise-associated sudden death (collapse during or within 1 hour of activity), while others include all athletes who die, independent of activity. A study from the province of Ontario, Canada,[25] showed an incidence of 1.167 SCA/SCDs per 100,000 athlete-years in 12- to 17-year-olds during or within 1 hour of participation in physical activity. A comparable rate for the general population in the same area of Canada was lower at 0.69 SCA/SCDs per 100,000 person-years in 12- to 17-year-olds.[26] Studies in the United States report an annual incidence of 1.5 cases of SCA/SCD per 100,000 high school athletes compared to 1.4 SCAs per 100,000 persons in the general population aged 14 to 24 years.[27,28]

The rate may be as high as 6.8 per 100,000 athletes per year in individuals participating at the elite level, as suggested by a study of English soccer players screened at ages 15 to 17 years with both ECG and echocardiography.[29] In this targeted screening of soccer players, 6 of the 8 deaths occurred in players who had tested negative for cardiac risk, suggesting that screening is *not sensitive* enough to detect all potential cases, in contrast to concerns about *specificity* that dominate the discussion in the United States. For collegiate athletes, a 20-year review of a National Collegiate Athletic Association (NCAA) database in the United States demonstrated an overall SCA/SCD incidence of 1.6 per 100,000 athletes per year.[2] Studies that included all athletes who died indicated that roughly half of cardiac-related deaths occurred during exertion, and the remainder occurred at rest or during sleep.[30–32]

Athletes may have different SCA/SCD risk based on age, genetics, sport, or level of play.[1,24] Sudden cardiac death in athletes is more common in those assigned male at birth, with male to female ratios ranging from 5:1 to 10:1.[1,33] Although SCA/SCD can occur in any sport, basketball and football players have the highest incidence of SCA/SCD at the college level (5.22 and 3.15 per 100,000 athletes per year, respectively).[2] About half of SCA/SCDs in collegiate athletes occur during exertion, which is similar to the study findings in younger athletes.[2] Over the past 20 years, SCA/SCD rates have decreased in NCAA athletes, likely the result of many factors including improved primary and secondary prevention through better screening and widespread implementation of emergency action plans. Despite improved survival rates following SCA events, more intensive screening strategies may be warranted in high-risk populations, but prospective outcomes-based studies are lacking. A large, multicentered randomized trial to evaluate the usefulness of ECG in PPE screening would define the utility of the intervention and provide an evidence-based solution to the controversy; however, the numbers needed to reach a reasonable conclusion are daunting.

CAUSES OF SUDDEN CARDIAC DEATH IN YOUNG ATHLETES

Sudden cardiac arrest or death may have a variety of congenital or acquired causes primarily involving structural and electrical problems[24,34–36] (Box 5A-1). Exercise is a known trigger for SCA/SCD at all ages, especially in sedentary populations. The most commonly reported causes of SCA/SCD in young athletes include hypertrophic cardiomyopathy (HCM), coronary artery anomalies, arrhythmogenic cardiomyopathy (ACM), dilated cardiomyopathy, myocarditis, long QT syndrome (LQTS), ventricular preexcitation or Wolff-Parkinson-White (WPW) syndrome, aortic dissection, and atherosclerotic coronary artery disease (CAD).[1,24,35–37] In studies with autopsy data, up to 63% of adolescent athletes and 19% of collegiate athletes with sudden death during exercise had no structural or anatomical abnormalities.[2,38] These cases, known as autopsy-negative sudden unexplained death (ANSUD), are likely caused by arrhythmias. Some may be caused by genetic abnormalities, but the exact mechanism remains unclear for many because of the lack of a genetic autopsy. Additionally, autopsies are not always done in the setting of SCD. In a recent European review, autopsies were not performed in up to 40% of individuals younger than 50 years who had SCD.[39] Similar trends have been seen in young athletes. A recent report from the FIFA Sudden Death Registry showed a total of 617 cases of sudden death in players from 67 countries, but autopsies were performed in only 124 cases.[40] A study using data from the National Center for Catastrophic Sports Injury Research in the United States reported 173 fatalities in young athletes from 2014 to 2018, with autopsy reports available for only 96 cases.[27]

The combined incidence of all cardiovascular conditions known to cause SCA/SCD in the young athletic population is estimated to be 1 in 80,000 to 1 in 200,000 athletes per year.[7] However, identifying conditions associated with SCA/SCD has not been shown to change the outcomes. Many athletes with preexisting cardiovascular conditions must be competing without a problem given the roughly 100- to 150-fold difference in prevalence between cardiovascular conditions and athlete deaths.

PERSONAL AND FAMILY HISTORY

A comprehensive personal and family history is critical to identifying athletes with red flag conditions that may result in SCA/SCD. The PPE cardiovascular questions were

Box 5A-1. Causes of Sudden Cardiac Death in Young Athletes

Structural or Functional
- Hypertrophic cardiomyopathy: 2%–36%
- Idiopathic left ventricular hypertrophy: 1%–16%
- Coronary artery anomalies: 5%–17%
- Myocarditis: 2%–9%
- Arrhythmogenic cardiomyopathy: 4%–22%
- Dilated cardiomyopathy: 1%–3%
- Aortic rupture (Marfan syndrome/connective tissue disorders): 3%–5%
- Bicuspid aortic valve/aortic stenosis: 1%
- Atherosclerotic coronary artery disease: 3%

Electrical
- Long QT syndrome[a]: 5%–10%
- Catecholaminergic polymorphic ventricular tachycardia[a]: 1%
- Wolff-Parkinson-White syndrome: 2%–3%
- Brugada syndrome[a]: 1%

Other
- Drugs and stimulants: 30% in users
- Commotio cordis: 1%
- Autopsy-negative sudden unexplained death: 42%

[a] Familial or genetic.

developed to elicit responses that may indicate the presence of a serious cardiac condition and prompt further investigation. Parent or guardian verification of personal and family history is recommended for high school and middle school athletes. Use of a standardized and detailed questionnaire (such as the History Form on pp 293–294) is strongly recommended to assist health care professionals in performing a comprehensive cardiovascular risk assessment. For a detailed review of the approach to positive history or physical examination findings, the Special Communication series in *Current Sports Medicine Reports* (May/June 2015 and July/August 2015) is a recommended resource.[41,42]

Personal History

The medical history focuses on exertional-related symptoms that suggest underlying cardiovascular disease. The *PPE: Preparticipation Evaluation*, 6th Edition, follows the AHA recommendations to include heart health questions about exertional chest pain or discomfort, unexplained syncope or near syncope, excessive exertional or unexplained dyspnea/fatigue associated with exercise, prior recognition of a heart murmur, and a history of elevated systemic blood pressure (BP).[7] A history of palpitations or an irregular heartbeat related to exercise or history of a seizure, which are not included in the AHA recommendations, are also considered relevant to SCA/SCD risk.[43]

Secondary questions with the potential to affect cardiovascular risks may include those pertaining to current or past illicit drug use (ie, cocaine, amphetamines, or ecstasy), ergogenic substances (ie, anabolic steroids, human growth hormone, or stimulants), or a recent acute viral syndrome (risk of myocarditis). Questions to ask in follow-up to an abnormal history response can be found in Table 5A-1.

Table 5A-1. Abnormal History Follow-Up Questions

Follow-Up Question	Additional Follow-Up Questions
Have you ever experienced chest pain or discomfort with exercise?	• How would you describe your pain? What does it feel like? Where is it located? • Are there things other than exercise or how hard you exercise that cause your chest discomfort? • When does your chest discomfort occur during exercise? Beginning, middle, end, or after? • How long does your chest discomfort last after you stop exercising? • Have you ever passed out or felt like you were about to pass out while you had your chest discomfort? • Is there anything else associated with your exertional chest discomfort? • Does the discomfort in your chest make you slow down or stop your exercise? • Has anyone in your family (parents, sisters, brothers, grandparents, uncles, aunts, or cousins) died of heart attack or heart problems? • Has anyone in your family had an unexplained death? • Was anyone in your family born with a heart condition? • Has anyone in your family been told they cannot play sports? • Does anyone in your family have an implantable cardiac defibrillator? • Do you take any medications or supplements? • Do you use any street or recreational drugs? • Do you use any nutritional supplements or drugs to improve your performance? • What do you use to improve your performance?
Have you ever nearly lost or actually lost consciousness?	• Did the collapse occur during or immediately after exercise? • If the collapse occurred immediately after exercise, were you already stopped or still moving? • Did you feel anything that warned you or made you feel like something was wrong, such as chest pain, palpitations (irregular heartbeat), visual changes, wheezing/shortness of breath, nausea, or itching? • What happened after the collapse? Did you wake up quickly, or were you out for a long time? How long? Did you have a seizure? Did you wet your pants, pass stool, or bite your tongue? Did anyone check your breathing, heart rate, or temperature at the time of your collapse? • What medications and supplements were you using before the event? • Were you ill in the few days before your collapse? • Have you ever collapsed like this before? • Is there a family history of collapse during exercise or of sudden cardiac arrest or death?
Have you ever had excessive shortness of breath or fatigue with exercise beyond what is expected for your level of fitness?	• Is the shortness of breath recent or new for you or has it been there for a long time (weeks or months)? • Does this occur every time you exercise or only when you exercise hard? • Do you experience chest discomfort along with the shortness of breath? • Do you get light-headed or dizzy? • Have you passed out during exercise? • Does anyone in your family have a serious heart condition or has anyone died suddenly? • Do you have a history of exercise asthma or allergies? • Have you recently moved to a different home or recently moved to the area? • Are you not playing as well as you should or could because of excessive fatigue? Are you getting tired during regular or usual daily activities?

Table 5A-1. Abnormal History Follow-Up Questions *(continued)*

Follow-Up Question	Additional Follow-Up Questions
Have you ever been told that you have a heart murmur?	• What can you tell me about your heart murmur? • Were you born with the murmur? Is it still present? • Have you been told it is an innocent murmur and not to worry about it? Have you been told it should be fixed or watched closely? • Do you experience chest pain, shortness of breath at rest or with exercise, or racing, pounding, or skipped heartbeats that you can feel in your chest? • Does anyone else in your family have a heart murmur?
Do you experience the skipped, irregular, or racing heartbeats (palpitations) with exercise?	• Are the palpitations associated with passing out (syncope) or near passing out (presyncope)? • Do the palpitations have an abrupt onset and end (termination)? • Is there anything that stops or starts the palpitations consistently?
Has anyone in your family < 35 years of age died suddenly or unexpectedly of heart disease?	• What is your relationship with the family member who died? • At what age did the death occur, especially if < 35 years old? • Do you know what caused the death? Was it a heart attack? • Do you know anything about the death (signs, symptoms, and circumstances)?
Has anyone in your family < 35 years of age been disabled from heart disease or had cardiac treatments including surgery?	• Can you name the heart disease that caused your family member's disability? • What treatments or surgical procedures has your family member had? • Can you describe the disability?
Are there any cardiac conditions in your extended family members such as hypertrophic or dilated cardiomyopathy, long QT syndrome or other ion channelopathies, Marfan syndrome, or arrhythmias?	• What is the diagnosis, who has it, and at what age did the diagnosis occur? • How was the diagnosis made? • Has anyone in your family had genetic testing for these heart conditions? • Have any of your family members had pacemakers or defibrillators implanted? • Has anyone in your family died unexpectedly or had surgery for these conditions?

Chest Pain

Exertional chest discomfort, pain, pressure, or tightness may indicate the presence of myocardial ischemia with exercise, especially if associated with syncope, near syncope, or palpitations. Chest pain during exercise, especially when associated with other symptoms, is very concerning and warrants careful cardiac investigation. In young athletes, chest discomfort is most often caused by exercise-induced asthma, gastroesophageal reflux, or costochondritis, but exertional angina can occur.

Exertional chest pain may be the result of ischemic chest pain in individuals with certain congenital or acquired cardiovascular diseases. Intramural tunneling (myocardial bridging), where a segment of coronary artery is completely surrounded by myocardium, is seen in about one-third of individuals with **HCM.**[44] Impaired coronary perfusion may occur during exercise because of compression of the segment in the setting of hypertrophied myocardium. **Coronary artery anomalies**, which account for 2% to 17% of SCA/SCD in athletes, may also present with exertional chest pain. In one study, 12 of 27 athletes (44%) who died of an anomalous coronary artery had prodromal symptoms such as exertional syncope, chest pain, or palpitations in the 24 months before their death.[45] Exertional chest discomfort and angina is also present in about 5% of individuals with **aortic stenosis,** which is responsible for 3% of SCA/SCDs in US athletes.[46] The compensatory increase in left ventricular (LV) mass affects coronary microvascular function. Reduced diastolic perfusion time and increased hemodynamic load on the LV in moderate to severe aortic stenosis can lead to coronary microvascular dysfunction and ischemia, especially during exercise when there is an increase in myocardial oxygen demand.[47]

Chest pain can also be present in individuals with myocarditis. **Myocarditis** accounts for 2% to 9% of SCA/SCDs in adolescent athletes.[1,48] The risk of SCA/SCD is higher in those with LV dysfunction, but SCA/SCD may occur as the result of a tachyarrhythmia in the setting of normal cardiac function.[48,49] The most common causes of acute myocarditis are viral infections, with parvovirus B19 and human herpesvirus 6 having the highest prevalence, followed by adenovirus and enteroviruses (Coxsackieviruses A and B).[49,50] During the COVID-19 pandemic, some children developed shock with ventricular dysfunction termed *multisystem inflammatory syndrome in children*, with autopsy evidence of myocardial inflammation.[49] Additional infectious etiologies include bacterial, fungal, and parasitic infections, and noninfectious etiologies include autoimmune, hypersensitivity, medications, and toxins.[49] The acute phase of myocarditis appears with an influenza-like illness that may lead to dilated cardiomyopathy with signs and symptoms of congestive heart failure such as shortness of breath or fatigue.

CAD may also present with exertional chest pain, light-headedness, palpitations, or dyspnea. Newer research suggests that the presence of atherosclerotic CAD begins to increase around age 20 years and accounts for 6% to 10% of SCA/SCDs in college-aged athletes; CAD is the most frequent cause of SCA/SCD in athletes older than 35 years.[30] Atherosclerotic plaque development is progressive and related to coronary risk factors such as hypertension, diabetes, dyslipidemia, tobacco use, illicit drug or anabolic steroid use, and a family history of premature atherosclerotic disease. Exercise may cause myocardial ischemia with risk of plaque disruption, arrhythmia, and SCA/SCD.

Fatigue, Syncope, and Palpitations

In addition to myocarditis, excessive unexplained dyspnea or fatigue associated with exercise may indicate other cardiovascular conditions such as hypertrophic or dilated cardiomyopathy. Palpitations or irregular heartbeats may signify arrhythmias or conduction abnormalities, such as supraventricular tachyarrhythmias, ion channel disorders, or WPW syndrome. These symptoms warrant further investigation before determining medical eligibility for sports participation.

Exertional syncope or near syncope can occur during or immediately following exercise and involves a transient loss of both consciousness and postural tone. Careful questioning of the athlete is important to distinguish between syncope occurring during exercise (ie, the athlete collapses while running toward the finish line or during play) and syncope occurring after exercise (ie, the athlete collapses shortly after crossing the finish line). Exertional syncope that occurs during exercise is a red flag symptom and an ominous sign of potential underlying cardiovascular disease, warranting a thorough investigation before allowing an athlete to return to sport.[51] Exercise-associated collapse (EAC) refers to syncope occurring after the finish line. EAC is not always due to a benign cause. The absence of prodromal symptoms before a syncopal event also warrants a higher level of suspicion for a pathological cause, because a sudden, abrupt loss of consciousness is more likely associated with the sudden onset of a ventricular arrhythmia as seen in patients with underlying ion channel disorders or other structural cardiac diseases that can lead to arrhythmias.

Exertional syncope that occurs during exercise is a red flag symptom and an ominous sign of potential underlying cardiovascular disease, warranting a thorough investigation before allowing an athlete to return to sport.

Ion channel disorders are primary electrical diseases of the heart that predispose to potentially lethal ventricular arrhythmias; they are characterized by mutations in ion channels that lead to dysfunctional sodium, potassium, calcium, and other ion transport across cell membranes. Channelopathy-related SCA/SCDs in athletes are underestimated as most are generally associated with a structurally normal heart, and less than half are confirmed with postmortem genetic testing.[21] **LQTS** is the most common ion channelopathy, with an estimated 1 in 2,000 affected individuals, and accounts for 5% to 10% of SCD cases and up to 15% of resuscitated SCA cases.[15,52] It is characterized by prolongation of the QT interval corrected for heart rate on ECG. Most arrhythmias from LQTS are triggered by emotional stress, physical exertion, or sudden arousal and appear with syncope or near syncope, seizures, or sudden death (Table 5A-2).[53] Syncope is usually caused by torsades de pointes, a specific form of polymorphic ventricular tachycardia.

Catecholaminergic polymorphic ventricular tachycardia (**CPVT**) is a rare ion channelopathy that affects approximately 1 in 10,000 individuals. Although rarer than LQTS, it is likely responsible for up to 15% of unexplained SCA/SCDs in individuals younger than 35 years.[54] CPVT can present with syncope, drowning or near drowning, seizure, or sudden death triggered by vigorous physical exertion or acute emotion. Syncope is the most

Table 5A-2. Signs and Symptoms of Cardiac Ion Channel Disorders

Disorder	Trigger	Event
LQTS-1	Emotional stress, physical exercise, swimming, or diving into water	Syncope, sudden death, seizure, drowning or near drowning, or motor vehicle crash
LQTS-2	Emotional stress, physical exercise, or auditory stimuli (loud noises)	Syncope, sudden death, seizure, or motor vehicle crash
LQTS-3	Rest or sleep	Sudden death or sudden infant death
CPVT	Emotional stress or vigorous physical exercise	Syncope, sudden death, seizure, or drowning or near drowning

Abbreviations: CPVT, catecholaminergic polymorphic ventricular tachycardia; LQTS-, long QT syndrome type.

common initial symptom, with more than 60% of affected individuals experiencing their first event by the age of 20 years (mean age at first event, 7–12 years).[54,55] Diagnosis of ion channel disorders may be delayed because of the misdiagnosis of epilepsy or vasovagal events.

Syncope, palpitations, or chest pain may be the first symptoms in individuals with **ACM**, formerly called arrhythmogenic right ventricular cardiomyopathy (ARVC). ACM was originally thought to be a congenital defect in the development of the right ventricle; however, with improvement in genetic and diagnostic testing it is now understood that both ventricles can be affected, leading to the use of the broader term ACM.[56] Myocardial electrical instability caused by fibrofatty replacement of the ventricular wall leads to ventricular arrhythmias that can precipitate cardiac arrest.[1] ACM affects 1 in 100,000 to 1 in 5,000 in the general population and typically presents in adults, with one large study reporting a mean age of 36 ± 14 years at presentation.[57] However, in a study of 108 individuals with confirmed ACM, there was an association between competitive sports participation and earlier onset of symptoms, with 40% of individuals in competitive sports experiencing symptoms 10 years after initiation of sports participation. This same study also showed that individuals who participated in competitive sports were significantly younger at sports participation initiation than those who only participated in recreational sports, with a mean age of 15 versus 21 years, respectively.[58] Studies in young athletes have reported ACM as the leading cause of SCA/SCD in 8% to 22% of cases.[38,57]

Malignant arrhythmias may also be the result of ventricular preexcitation in individuals with **WPW syndrome.** The estimated prevalence of WPW in the general population is 1 to 3 per 1,000 individuals and up to 5.5 per 1,000 in those with a first-degree relative diagnosed with WPW.[59] In a recent meta-analysis of 1,869 individuals with asymptomatic WPW, the incidence of SCA/SCD was 1.93 in individuals younger than 18 years and 0.86 in those older than 18 years.[60] In 3 of the largest series of resuscitated individuals with WPW, most events occurred between 20 and 30 years of age; 73% of individuals had prior symptoms (palpitations, chest pain, syncope, documented arrythmia), and 27% were asymptomatic.[60] Ventricular preexcitation is caused by abnormal electrical conduction through an accessory pathway bypassing the atrioventricular node and leading to the characteristic ECG pattern of a short PR interval, prolonged QRS complex, and a slurred delta wave. The presence of an accessory pathway allows for the development of a tachyarrhythmia with the potential to degenerate into ventricular fibrillation and cardiac arrest.

Syncope or near syncope (dizziness or light-headedness) occurring after exercise is much more common than syncope occurring during exercise, and is unlikely to represent underlying cardiovascular disease, especially if preceded by light-headedness, diaphoresis, nausea, or tunnel vision, all of which suggest a neurally mediated event (ie, vasovagal syncope). EAC is commonly observed at endurance events and involves athletes who are unable to stand or walk unaided as a result of light-headedness, faintness, dizziness, or syncope.[61] During exercise, increases in heart rate and stroke volume result in a substantial rise in cardiac output and offset diminished systemic vascular resistance from vasodilatation in exercising muscles. After exercising, without muscle contraction in the legs (muscle pump) to maintain venous return, cardiac filling may be dramatically reduced. Forceful ventricular contractions against a diminished ventricular volume are postulated to excessively stimulate ventricular mechanoreceptors, causing not only reflex vasodilatation and bradycardia but subsequent hypotension and syncope (exercise-associated postural hypotension).[62] Neurally mediated syncope, also known as neurocardiogenic syncope, is generally regarded as the most common mechanism of syncope or near syncope in young adults, and it can be triggered by situational stressors as well as exercise stressors. Nonetheless, EAC, or any suspected neurocardiogenic syncope associated with a complete loss of consciousness or near syncope, warrants a diagnostic workup to exclude an underlying cardiac disorder. In addition, it is recommended that recurrent cases of apparently benign vasovagal syncope be investigated with ECG at a minimum.

A clear history of either an abrupt increase in heart rate disproportional to activity or palpitations associated with syncope or near syncope may require further investigation with ECG, echocardiography, exercise stress testing to exhaustion, cardiac event monitoring, and potentially consultation with an electrophysiologist.

A history of previously performed cardiac testing such as ECG, echocardiography, or exercise treadmill testing may indicate a previously suspected cardiac disorder, and a careful review of past medical records may establish the outcomes of the evaluation. This may preclude repeating the studies.

Family History

A family history of nontraumatic sudden death before age 50 years is likely cardiac related and may be caused by inheritable cardiac conditions. This is why the 6th edition of *PPE: Preparticipation Evaluation* has continued to include the family history questions that align with the recommended AHA family history questions on (1) premature death (sudden and unexpected, or otherwise) before age 50 years caused by heart disease in one or more relatives, (2) disability from heart disease in a close relative younger than 50 years, and (3) specific knowledge of family members with cardiac conditions known to cause SCA/SCD in athletes.[6] In addition, a family history of unexplained syncope, unexplained near drowning or drowning, unexplained motor vehicle crash, unexplained seizure activity, or sudden infant death syndrome may indicate the presence of an inherited ion channel disorder that could put an individual at risk of a fatal ventricular arrythmia in the setting of exertional activity.

A detailed family history may help identify athletes with a predisposition to underlying cardiac disease. A careful family history of sudden unexplained death (SUD) to identify athletes at risk of inherited cardiac conditions known to cause SCA/SCD during exertion is an important part of the PPE. Family history is particularly important in primary electrical disease of the heart. Inherited arrhythmia syndromes include LQTS, CPVT, and Brugada syndrome.[15] The 3 most common LQTS subtypes are inherited in an autosomal dominant manner. Family history of an early unexplained death, especially in the setting of exercise (especially swimming), auditory stimuli, emotional stress, or during sleep are concerning for LQTS and need further investigation.

CPVT is a familial disorder characterized by stress-induced ventricular arrhythmias that result in SCA/SCD in children and young adults. CPVT is typically inherited in an autosomal dominant fashion; however, autosomal recessive transmission has been observed.[54] A family history of stress-related events (syncope, seizure, or SCD) is present in approximately 30% to 60% of those diagnosed with CPVT.[54,63]

Unlike LQTS and CPVT, most SCA/SCD events in **Brugada syndrome** occur during sleep; however, there may be an increased risk of arrythmia during exercise given the association of arrythmias with fevers. Brugada syndrome is an autosomal dominant disorder affecting 1 in 2,000 individuals, with those assigned male at birth being more commonly affected.[1,64] Most individuals with Brugada syndrome experience their first event between the ages of 30 and 50 years.[64]

Electrical abnormalities being identified as the cause of SCA/SCD in athletes are rarely diagnosed given that most have a structurally normal heart.[21] In the United Kingdom, SCA/SCD cases examined between 1994 and 2021 as part of a national autopsy database demonstrated positive genetic testing findings for a pathogenic or likely pathogenic variant in 64% of cases of ANSUD.[65] Only 36% of individuals in this study had symptoms prior to death, with a majority experiencing syncope and/or seizures and 19% having a family history of SCA/SCD at younger than 50 years of age. The frequency of a positive family history of either SCA/SCD or syncope has been as high as 53% in smaller studies.[55] The high frequency of familial SCA/SCD or syncope in people who have ANSUD emphasizes the need for careful evaluation of athletes with a family history of SUD.

Structural heart diseases known to increase the risk of SCA/SCD can be caused by inheritable genetic disorders. A family history of nontraumatic sudden death before age 50 years or a family member with a diagnosis of heart disease indicates the need for further questioning to determine the risk of an inherited cardiac condition, such as HCM, ACM, and connective tissue disorders, that can lead to SCA/SCD during exertion.

Variable expression is seen in individuals with HCM, which is an autosomal dominant disorder. Although HCM may appear in childhood, the morphological expression typically develops in early adolescence to young adulthood and is characteristically present by the end of physical maturity in most individuals who are genetically predisposed to the disorder.[66] The phenotypic expression of HCM and other cardiomyopathies in adolescence is the primary rationale supporting the recommendation that preparticipation cardiovascular evaluation be performed every 1 to 2 years while in high school and at matriculation to college, although there are no data to support this interval. A positive family history of an enlarged, thick, or even athletic heart, especially in the setting of early SCA/SCD, indicates the need for further investigation for possible HCM. Similarly, confirmed ACM in a first-degree relative is a major diagnostic criterion. In up to 66% of people with clinically diagnosed ACM, there is a pathogenic variant in genes encoding cardiac desmosomal proteins.[1,57,67]

The phenotypic expression of HCM and other cardiomyopathies in adolescence is the primary rationale supporting the recommendation that preparticipation cardiovascular evaluation be performed every 1 to 2 years while in high school and at matriculation to college, although there are no data to support this interval.

A rarer cause of SCA/SCD is **aortic dissection**, which is most commonly preceded by aortic dilation. Aortic dilation is caused by degenerative changes in the elastic properties of the aortic wall. The progressive loss of elasticity and compliance of the aorta occurs normally with aging; however, it can be seen in younger people with inherited connective tissue diseases (Marfan syndrome, Ehlers-Danlos syndrome, Loeys-Dietz syndrome, familial/thoracic aortic aneurysm and dissection), aortic valvulopathies like bicuspid aortic valve (BAV), or certain inflammatory diseases (infectious and autoimmune).[68,69]

There are several inheritable connective tissue diseases that cause cystic medial necrosis leading to progressive aortic dilation.[51] Marfan syndrome is the most common connective tissue disorder inherited through autosomal dominant transmission in 75% of cases, and 25% are de novo mutations with a prevalence of 20 to 30 per 100,000 individuals.[70] Cardiovascular complications are the major cause of morbidity and mortality in patients with Marfan syndrome. The risk of aortic rupture or dissection increases during adolescence, and 50% of patients with undiagnosed Marfan syndrome will die by 40 years of age.[70]

Valvulo-aortopathies are responsible for 3% to 5% of SCA/SCDs. Bicuspid aortic valve (BAV) is the most common congenital heart disease and the most common valvulo-aortopathy, occurring in 0.7% to 1.4% of the general population.[71] Aortic stenosis can be as high as 50% in individuals with BAV, and the prevalence of dilation can be as high as 80%.[72] The incidence of aortic dissection is low in BAV, but it is higher than that in the general population. Risk factors for dissection include hypertension, family history of aortic dissection, family history of unexplained early SCA/SCD, and an increase in aortic diameter at a rate of > 3 mm/year.[71]

PHYSICAL EXAMINATION

The AHA recommends that the PPE include (1) auscultation for heart murmurs, (2) a brachial artery BP taken in the sitting position, (3) palpation of femoral pulses to exclude coarctation of the aorta (if there is a need to remove clothing to palpate femoral pulses, a chaperone is recommended), and (4) examination for the physical stigmata of Marfan syndrome.[6] However, normal physical examination findings do not exclude conditions that predispose individuals to SCA/SCD.

Auscultation of the heart should be performed in the supine and standing positions (or with Valsalva maneuver), specifically to identify pathological murmurs. Particular attention is paid to the presence and character of any murmurs, the timing of murmurs in relation to S_1 and S_2, extra heart sounds (S_3 and S_4), and clicks (Table 5A-3). The inability of physicians to distinguish pathological murmurs from physiological murmurs by auscultation, regardless of experience or level of training, is well known.[62] Simplifying the physical examination allows better differentiation between benign murmurs and pathological murmurs. Characteristics of pathological murmurs that require further evaluation or referral include loud (>grade 2/6) or harsh murmurs; radiation of the murmur laterally, rather than upward; presence in middle to late systole, accompanied by a click; or any murmur that becomes louder (or changes quality) with dynamic maneuvers (standing or squatting) or Valsalva maneuver. In addition, any holosystolic or diastolic murmur requires further evaluation. In the absence of concerning symptoms or family history, innocent murmurs require no further investigation. If doubt persists, either cardiac imaging with echocardiography or consultation with a cardiovascular specialist is recommended.

Table 5A-3. Significance of Abnormal Heart Murmurs

Auscultatory Finding	Significance
• Harsh, loud (usually ≥ grade 3), systolic ejection murmur • Loudest right upper sternal border • Increases with maneuvers that decrease venous return (ie, Valsalva, or moving from squatting to standing)	HCM-associated LV outflow tract obstruction
• Systolic ejection murmur heard best at right upper sternal border • Radiation to neck • Diminishes with maneuvers that decrease venous return (ie, Valsalva) and increases with maneuvers that increase venous return (ie, squatting)	Aortic stenosis
• Holosystolic murmur heard best at the apex • Radiation to axilla	Mitral valve regurgitation and possible dilated cardiomyopathy or HCM
• Diastolic murmur heard at right upper sternal border • Murmur accentuated with hand grip (increased systemic vascular resistance)	Aortic valve insufficiency and possible Marfan syndrome or bicuspid aortic valve
• High-frequency diastolic murmur heard best at left upper sternal border	Pulmonary valve insufficiency from primary pulmonary hypertension (Graham Steele murmur)
• Soft early systolic murmur heard best at the upper sternal border while supine (increased venous return) • Murmur often absent or diminished when standing or sitting and with Valsalva maneuver	Physiological (hyperdynamic) flow murmur in a well-trained athlete

Abbreviations: HCM, hypertrophic cardiomyopathy; LV, left ventricular.

Brachial artery BP is best measured in the sitting position with the cuff on the bare arm at heart level after the patient has been at rest for several minutes in a quiet area. Measuring BP with an appropriately sized cuff is required for accurate BP measurements (see Figure 5A-1). Proper cuff size requires the bladder length to be 80% to 100% of the arm circumference and the bladder width to be at least 40% of the arm circumference. An inappropriately sized cuff can falsely elevate or lower the BP measurement.[64] If the BP is initially elevated, it is recommended that the measurement be repeated after the individual rests in a quiet, calm environment for 5 to 10 minutes. The diagnosis of hypertension in athletes younger than 18 years requires BP readings at 3 different visits, with values from 90% to 95% of age-, sex-, and height-based reference ranges defined as prehypertension; values from 95% to 99% plus 5 mm Hg defined as stage 1 hypertension; and values greater than 99% plus 5 mm Hg defined as stage 2 hypertension. An average of 2 auscultatory measurements are recommended to define the BP category if elevated BP is found using *oscillometric* readings. Tables based on sex, age, and height, with systolic and diastolic BP values listed for prehypertension, stage 1 hypertension, and stage 2 hypertension, can be found in *A Pocket Guide to Blood Pressure Measurement in Children*, published by the National Heart, Lung, and Blood Institute (http://www.nhlbi.nih.gov/health/public/heart/hbp/bp_child_pocket/bp_child_pocket.pdf).

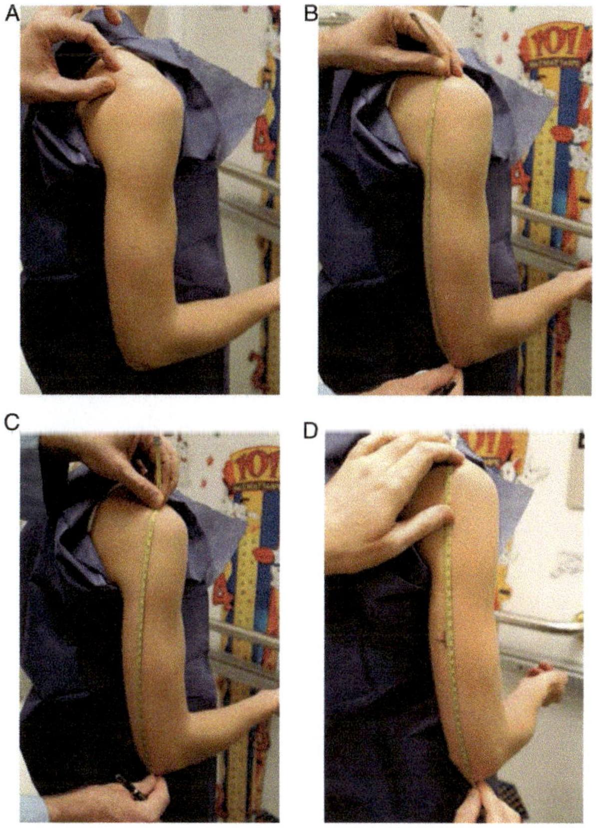

Figure 5A-1. Determination of Proper BP Cuff Size

A, Marking spine extending from acromion process. B, Correct tape placement for upper arm length. C, Incorrect tape placement for upper arm length. D, Marking upper arm length midpoint.

Reproduced from Centers for Disease Control and Prevention, National Center for Health Statistics. *2021 Anthropometry Procedures Manual*. Updated May 2021. Accessed February 10, 2026. https://wwwn.cdc.gov/nchs/data/nhanes/public/2021/manuals/2021-Anthropometry-Procedures-Manual-508.pdf

If elevated readings persist, evaluation by an experienced hypertension provider is recommended to confirm the diagnosis with ambulatory BP monitoring, screen for secondary causes, and assess for target organ damage using echocardiography. Individuals with stage 1 hypertension without target organ damage (LVH, proteinuria, retinopathy) can participate in all sports with periodic monitoring, whereas those with stage 2 hypertension or target organ damage should be restricted from high-static (isometric) sports (see Table 4-1 in Chapter 4, General Considerations for the History, Physical Examination, and Medical Eligibility) until BP is adequately controlled.

Simultaneous palpation of radial and femoral artery pulses is an important component of the physical examination. In the presence of systemic arterial hypertension, delayed femoral artery pulses when compared with radial artery pulses may indicate the presence of coarctation of the aorta, which requires additional evaluation.

Physical examination findings in connective tissue disorders can be highly variable. The physical examination focuses on hypermobility of the wrist or thumb (or both), chest wall deformities, murmur associated with mitral valve prolapse, hindfoot deformities, and other features associated with a marfanoid appearance and connective tissue disorders (Table 5A-4). While physical examination features alone are not sufficient for diagnosis, they may raise suspicion and warrant a more detailed family history and cardiovascular evaluation according to the rules presented in Table 5A-5.

Table 5A-4. Systemic Score Suggestive of Marfan Syndrome

Feature	Score[a]
Wrist *and* thumb sign	+3
Wrist *or* thumb sign	+1
Pectus carinatum deformity	+2
Pectus excavatum or chest asymmetry	+1
Hindfoot deformity	+2
Plain flatfoot	+1
Spontaneous pneumothorax	+2
Dural ectasia	+2
Protucia acetabulae	+2
Scoliosis or thoracolumbar kyphosis	+1
Reduced elbow extension	+1
3 of 5 facial features	+1
Skin striae	+1
Severe myopia	+1
Mitral valve prolapse	+1
Reduced upper segment/lower segment & increased arm span to height ratio	+1

[a] A score of ≥7 is considered a positive systemic score.

Used with permission from The Marfan Foundation. Calculation of systemic score. The Marfan Foundation website. Accessed July 1, 2026. https://www.marfan.org/dx/score

Table 5A-5. Diagnostic Criteria for Marfan Syndrome

The diagnosis of Marfan syndrome relies on a set of defined clinical criteria (the 2010 Ghent nosology) developed to facilitate accurate recognition of the syndrome and improve patient treatment and counseling. The diagnostic criteria put more weight onto the cardiovascular manifestations of the disorder. Aortic root aneurysm and ectopia lentis (dislocated lenses) are now cardinal features.

- In the absence of any family history, the presence of these 2 features is sufficient for the unequivocal diagnosis of Marfan syndrome.
- In the absence of 1 of these 2 cardinal features, the presence of either an *FBN1* mutation or a positive systemic score is required.
- In some cases, genetic testing can be helpful.

Experts expect that while use of new diagnostic criteria lengthens the time to a definitive diagnosis of Marfan syndrome, it decreases the risk of a premature or missed diagnosis.

In the Absence of Family History	In the Presence of Family History
1. Aortic root dilatation *z* score ≥ 2 *and* ectopia lentis = Marfan syndrome 2. Aortic root dilatation *z* score ≥ 2 *and* an *FBN1* mutation = Marfan syndrome 3. Aortic root dilatation *z* score ≥ 2 *and* a systemic score ≥ 7 points = Marfan syndrome 4. Ectopia lentis *and* an *FBN1* mutation associated with aortic root dilatation = Marfan syndrome	1. Ectopia lentis *and* family history of Marfan syndrome (as defined to the left) = Marfan syndrome 2. A systemic score ≥ 7 points *and* family history of Marfan syndrome (as defined to the left) = Marfan syndrome 3. Aortic root dilatation *z* score ≥ 2 if patient age ≥ 20 y, or ≥ 3 if patient age < 20 y, *and* family history of Marfan syndrome (as defined to the left) = Marfan syndrome

Adapted with permission from The Marfan Foundation. Summary of diagnostic criteria. The Marfan Foundation website. Accessed December 1, 2025. https://www.marfan.org/dx/rules

INVESTIGATION OF ATHLETES WITH CARDIOVASCULAR SYMPTOMS

Athletes identified with cardiovascular symptoms or signs such as exertional syncope or near syncope, chest pain, palpitations, or excessive exertional dyspnea require a thorough cardiovascular evaluation to exclude underlying heart disease before they are allowed to participate in vigorous physical activity. The diagnostic workup of athletes with red flag symptoms or physical findings may include ECG, echocardiography, stress ECG, ambulatory rhythm monitoring, or other advanced cardiac imaging (such as magnetic resonance imaging or computed tomography) to evaluate for the presence of structural abnormalities such as ACM or congenital coronary artery anomalies, and consultation with a cardiologist may be required to determine appropriate testing. The investigation of rapid or irregular heartbeats concerning for tachyarrhythmias or ion channel disorders may include similar studies and consultation with an electrophysiologist.

LIMITATIONS OF THE PREPARTICIPATION CARDIOVASCULAR EVALUATION

No outcomes-based studies demonstrate that the PPE is effective in preventing or detecting the rare instance of an athlete's being at risk for SCA/SCD; however, many abnormalities have been found during the evaluations. Disease-specific presentations are important warning symptoms, and concerning family history requires investigation. Some athletes who experience SCA/SCD have red flag conditions that are not recognized, and some have no red flag conditions at the time of their PPE screening.[1,64,73,74] To be effective medical evaluation tools, the PPE questionnaires require that athletes and parents complete the forms honestly. Previous studies have demonstrated a lack of concordance between answers supplied by parents and those of the student-athletes, so parental involvement is crucial for best outcomes.[75] The ability of providers to distinguish physiological cardiac murmurs from pathological cardiac murmurs with cardiac auscultation is limited[62]; however, access to echocardiography allows those in doubt to easily determine the cause of a heart murmur.

NONINVASIVE CARDIOVASCULAR SCREENING OF ATHLETES

The value of adding ECG or echocardiography screening to determine the medical eligibility of athletes is highly debated, and the issue is magnified by the fact that the prevalence and incidence of both SCA and SCD in athletes are very low and may not differ from those in the general population.[76,77] The AHA and ACC continue to recommend against the routine use of ECG and echocardiography for screening of young athletes in the United States. The American Medical Society for Sports Medicine has published a position statement on PPE cardiac screening to help sports medicine physicians decide whether to use ECG as a screening tool, rather than as a "case finding" study.[26] The statement suggests a new paradigm for determining medical eligibility using ECG as a screening tool on the basis of the perceived risk of the athlete population, the individual physician's ability to accurately interpret findings from the screening and subsequent evaluation studies, and the available cardiology infrastructure to complete the evaluations generated by positive test results in a timely manner.

Outcomes From Cardiovascular Screening

The outcomes for individuals who have had cardiovascular screening beyond history and physical examination, and the natural course of those diseases screened for, are not well-known for athletes or nonathletes. The PPEs that included resting ECG in 12-year-old boys (n = 415) and girls (n = 318) before entering competitive sports programs resulted in restricted medical eligibility for 5.5% of athletes.[78] A longitudinal observational cohort study of more than 11,000 elite-level, adolescent English Football (soccer) Association athletes screened with a required ECG and echocardiography at age 16.4 (±1.2) years, from 1996 through 2006, showed that the prevalence of cardiovascular diseases that may be associated with sudden death was 0.38% (42 per 11,168 athletes or 376 per 100,000 athletes).[29] Eight deaths were attributed to cardiac disease among the screened athletes. The mean time between screening and SCA/SCD was 6.8 years. Cardiomyopathy accounted for

7 of 8 SCA/SCDs. Six of the 8 athletes with SCA/SCD had normal preparticipation ECG and echocardiographic (false-negative) screening results. These results call into question the efficacy of the single-time screening model used in this study and suggest that perhaps the frequency of screening needs to increase, or the athlete's age at initial screening needs to increase. Without appropriately trained individuals to interpret additional cardiac screening test results, it is likely that more frequent ECG and echocardiographic screening will lead to increased cost of the evaluation program. More research is needed on the natural course of diseases associated with sudden death in elite-level athletes compared with that in both non–elite-level athletes and nonathletes, as well as models and modalities used for cardiovascular screening.

The decision to add screening tests to the PPE requires careful consideration of the actual differential risk of SCA/SCD in the targeted population compared with the expected false-positive and false-negative aspects of the proposed screening test. A study evaluating cardiovascular screening in collegiate athletes from Pacific-12 Conference institutions from 2009 to 2017 found that the addition of an ECG to the history and physical examination improved the identification of SCA/SCD-associated conditions by 6-fold when adequate resources and clinical expertise were available.[79] Individual providers performing the PPE or the institutions requiring the PPE may choose to add a screening test to the medical eligibility evaluation when the benefit to the population at risk is greater than the potential harm (Figure 5A-2). Continual quality control and improvement is needed if a screening test, such as ECG, is added to the PPE. In an era of "choosing wisely," adhering to the principles of population screening and considering the additional cost to the health care system add to the complexity of this decision.

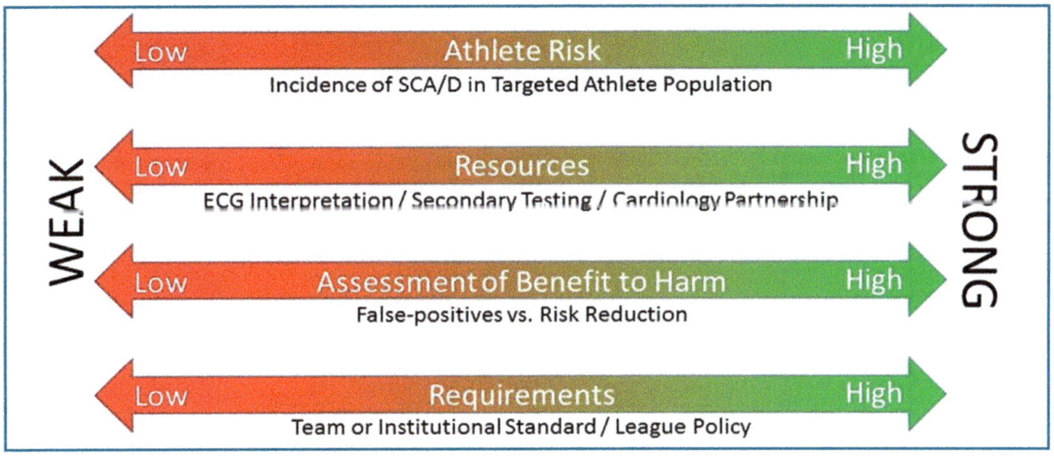

Figure 5A-2. Strength of Rationale for ECG Screening

Abbreviations: ECG, electrocardiographic; SCA/SCD, sudden cardiac arrest or death.

When assessing the benefit of adding an ECG to athlete screening, the perceived location on each of the above scales may help determine the answer for a specific population. The rationale to add an ECG is not supported by answers that tend toward the weak end of each scale.

Reprinted with permission from Drezner JA, O'Connor FG, Harmon KG, et al. AMSSM position statement on cardiovascular preparticipation screening in athletes: current evidence, knowledge gaps, recommendations and future directions. *Br J Sports Med.* 2017;51(3):153–167.

If ECG is added to the PPE as a screening test, using the most current athlete-specific criteria for ECG interpretation is recommended to decrease the number of false-positive test results and minimize additional testing, cost to the health care system, and undue stress for the individual athlete and family. For individual practitioners interested in including the ECG in the preparticipation evaluation or in offering ECG screening within the model of informed decision-making with athletes and families, a summary of the ECG criteria and next steps from the "International Consensus Standards for ECG Interpretation in Athletes"[80] is provided in Figure 5A-3.

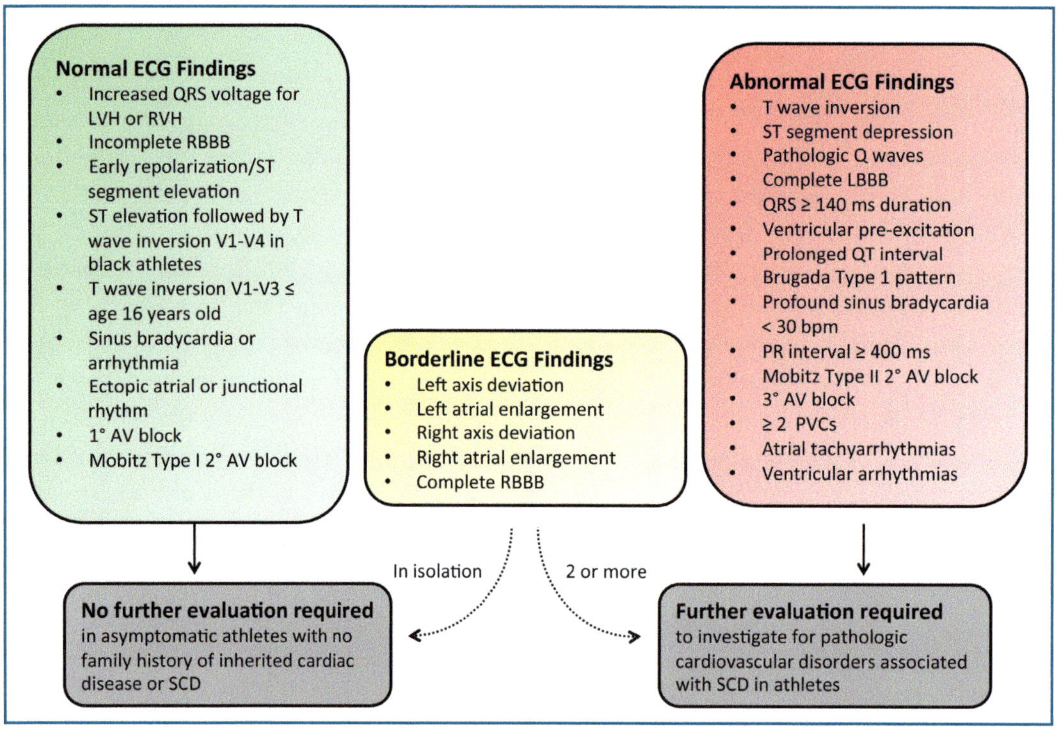

Figure 5A-3. International Consensus Standards for ECG Interpretation in Athletes

Abbreviations: AV, atrioventricular; ECG, electrocardiographic; LBBB, left bundle branch block; LVH, left ventricular hypertrophy; PVC, premature ventricular contraction; RBBB, right bundle branch block; RVH, right ventricular hypertrophy; SCD, sudden cardiac death.

Reprinted with permission from Drezner JA, Sharma S, Baggish A, et al. International criteria for electrocardiographic interpretation in athletes: consensus statement. *Br J Sports Med*. 2017;51(9):704–731.

MEDICAL ELIGIBILITY RECOMMENDATIONS FOR ATHLETES WITH IDENTIFIED CARDIOVASCULAR DISEASE

Activity recommendations involving temporary or permanent sports disqualification or restrictions for athletes with identified cardiovascular disease should be made in consultation with a cardiologist, preferably one with expertise in working with athletes. The AHA and ACC scientific statement "Eligibility and Disqualification Recommendations for Competitive Athletes With Cardiovascular Abnormalities"[7] provides participation recommendations for competitive athletes with cardiovascular abnormalities, and the most recent version of this document should be used for decision-making. These expert consensus recommendations provide a framework for determining medical eligibility for patients who have various cardiovascular abnormalities by using the dynamic and static components of sport activities. The AHA and ACC scientific statement recommendations take into account the severity of disease, the potential for sudden death or disease progression, and the type and intensity of exercise involved in a particular sport.[7]

Cardiopulmonary risk can be estimated by using the dynamic and static components of an activity (Figure 5A-4). The cardiopulmonary demands of physical activity are defined by the effects on the left ventricle (LV) of the heart. Static exercises produce a pressure load on the LV, while dynamic exercises produce a volume load on the LV. The combination of static loads and dynamic loads varies by sport.

Medical eligibility recommendations have become increasingly complex with the addition of newer technologies for the evaluation and treatment of cardiovascular conditions in children and young adults. From a best practice perspective, determining medical eligibility may seem straightforward on the basis of the AHA and ACC scientific statement. However, disqualification from sport is life altering, from both a physical health perspective and a mental health perspective. A less active lifestyle, limited to low-intensity activities, may lead to weight gain, depression, and a paradoxical increase in other cardiovascular conditions. New medical advances combined with shared decision-making involving the athlete, family members, physicians, and other members of the interdisciplinary health care team may allow changes in medical eligibility.[24,41,81–84] In the shared decision-making model, all parties contribute information to the problem at hand, and the health care team provides the risk and benefit analysis of the different approaches. Ultimately, in a shared decision-making model, both parties (athlete and physician) share responsibility for the resolution of the health-related issue with an acceptable level of potential risk and potential long-term benefit for the athlete (see Chapter 3).

New medical advances combined with shared decision-making involving the athlete, family members, physicians, and other members of the interdisciplinary health care team may allow changes in medical eligibility.

REFERENCES

1. Finocchiaro G, Westaby J, Sheppard MN, Papadakis M, Sharma S. Sudden cardiac death in young athletes: JACC state-of-the-art review. *J Am Coll Cardiol.* 2024;83(2):350–370. PMID: 38199713 doi:10.1016/j.jacc.2023.10.032
2. Petek BJ, Churchill TW, Moulson N, et al. Sudden cardiac death in National Collegiate Athletic Association athletes: a 20-year study. *Circulation.* 2024;149(2):80–90. PMID: 37955565 doi:10.1161/circulationaha.123.065908
3. Martinez KA, Bos JM, Baggish AL, et al. Return-to-play for elite athletes with genetic heart diseases predisposing to sudden cardiac death. *J Am Coll Cardiol.* 2023;82(8):661–670. PMID: 37587576 doi:10.1016/j.jacc.2023.05.059
4. Maron BJ, Zipes DP, Kovacs RJ; American Heart Association Electrocardiography and Arrhythmias Committee of Council on Clinical Cardiology, Council on Cardiovascular Disease in Young, Council on Cardiovascular and Stroke Nursing, Council on Functional Genomics and Translational Biology, and American College of Cardiology. Eligibility and disqualification recommendations for competitive athletes with cardiovascular abnormalities: preamble, principles, and general considerations: a scientific statement from the American Heart Association and American College of Cardiology. *Circulation.* 2015;132(22):e256–e261. PMID: 26621642 doi:10.1161/cir.0000000000000236
5. Drezner JA, O'Connor FG, Harmon KG, et al. AMSSM Position Statement on Cardiovascular Preparticipation Screening in Athletes: current evidence, knowledge gaps, recommendations and future directions. *Br J Sports Med.* 2017;51(3):153–167. PMID: 27660369 doi:10.1136/bjsports-2016-096781
6. Levine BD, Baggish AL, Kovacs RJ, Link MS, Maron MS, Mitchell JH; American Heart Association Electrocardiography and Arrhythmias Committee of Council on Clinical Cardiology, Council on Cardiovascular Disease in Young, Council on Cardiovascular and Stroke Nursing, Council on Functional Genomics and Translational Biology, and American College of Cardiology. Eligibility and disqualification recommendations for competitive athletes with cardiovascular abnormalities: task force 1: classification of sports: dynamic, static, and impact: a scientific statement from the American Heart Association and American College of Cardiology. *Circulation.* 2015;132(22):e262–e266. PMID: 26621643 doi:10.1161/cir.0000000000000237
7. Maron BJ, Levine BD, Washington RL, Baggish AL, Kovacs RJ, Maron MS; American Heart Association Electrocardiography and Arrhythmias Committee of Council on Clinical Cardiology, Council on Cardiovascular Disease in Young, Council on Cardiovascular and Stroke Nursing, Council on Functional Genomics and Translational Biology, and American College of Cardiology. Eligibility and disqualification recommendations for competitive athletes with cardiovascular abnormalities: task force 2: preparticipation screening for cardiovascular disease in competitive athletes: a scientific statement from the American Heart Association and American College of Cardiology. *Circulation.* 2015;132(22):e267–e272. PMID: 26527714 doi:10.1161/cir.0000000000000238
8. Maron BJ, Udelson JE, Bonow RO, et al; American Heart Association Electrocardiography and Arrhythmias Committee of Council on Clinical Cardiology, Council on Cardiovascular Disease in Young, Council on Cardiovascular and Stroke Nursing, Council on Functional Genomics and Translational Biology, and American College of Cardiology. Eligibility and disqualification recommendations for competitive athletes with cardiovascular abnormalities: task force 3: hypertrophic cardiomyopathy, arrhythmogenic right ventricular cardiomyopathy and other cardiomyopathies, and myocarditis: a scientific statement from the American Heart Association and American College of Cardiology. *Circulation.* 2015;132(22):e273–e280. PMID: 26621644 doi:10.1161/cir.0000000000000239
9. Van Hare GF, Ackerman MJ, Evangelista JA, et al; American Heart Association Electrocardiography and Arrhythmias Committee of Council on Clinical Cardiology, Council on Cardiovascular Disease in Young, Council on Cardiovascular and Stroke Nursing, Council on Functional Genomics and Translational Biology, and American College of Cardiology. Eligibility and disqualification recommendations for competitive athletes with cardiovascular abnormalities: task force 4: congenital heart disease: a scientific statement from the American Heart Association and American College of Cardiology. *Circulation.* 2015;132(22):e281–e291. PMID: 26621645 doi:10.1161/cir.0000000000000240
10. Bonow RO, Nishimura RA, Thompson PD, Udelson JE. Eligibility and disqualification recommendations for competitive athletes with cardiovascular abnormalities: task force 5: valvular heart disease: a scientific statement from the American Heart Association and American College of Cardiology. *J Am Coll Cardiol.* 2015;66(21):2385–2392. PMID: 26542667 doi:10.1016/j.jacc.2015.09.037

11. Black HR, Sica D, Ferdinand K, White WB. Eligibility and disqualification recommendations for competitive athletes with cardiovascular abnormalities: task force 6: hypertension: a scientific statement from the American Heart Association and the American College of Cardiology. *J Am Coll Cardiol.* 2015;66(21):2393–2397. PMID: 26542658 doi:10.1016/j.jacc.2015.09.038
12. Braverman AC, Harris KM, Kovacs RJ, Maron BJ; American Heart Association Electrocardiography and Arrhythmias Committee of Council on Clinical Cardiology, Council on Cardiovascular Disease in Young, Council on Cardiovascular and Stroke Nursing, Council on Functional Genomics and Translational Biology, and American College of Cardiology. Eligibility and disqualification recommendations for competitive athletes with cardiovascular abnormalities: task force 7: aortic diseases, including Marfan syndrome: a scientific statement from the American Heart Association and American College of Cardiology. *Circulation.* 2015;132(22):e303–e309. PMID: 26621648 doi:10.1161/cir.0000000000000243
13. Thompson PD, Myerburg RJ, Levine BD, Udelson JE, Kovacs RJ; American Heart Association Electrocardiography and Arrhythmias Committee of Council on Clinical Cardiology, Council on Cardiovascular Disease in Young, Council on Cardiovascular and Stroke Nursing, Council on Functional Genomics and Translational Biology, and American College of Cardiology. Eligibility and disqualification recommendations for competitive athletes with cardiovascular abnormalities: task force 8: coronary artery disease: a scientific statement from the American Heart Association and American College of Cardiology. *Circulation.* 2015;132(22):e310–e314. PMID: 26621649 doi:10.1161/cir.0000000000000244
14. Zipes DP, Link MS, Ackerman MJ, Kovacs RJ, Myerburg RJ, Estes NA III; American Heart Association Electrocardiography and Arrhythmias Committee of Council on Clinical Cardiology, Council on Cardiovascular Disease in Young, Council on Cardiovascular and Stroke Nursing, Council on Functional Genomics and Translational Biology, and American College of Cardiology. Eligibility and disqualification recommendations for competitive athletes with cardiovascular abnormalities: task force 9: arrhythmias and conduction defects: a scientific statement from the American Heart Association and American College of Cardiology. *Circulation.* 2015;132(22):e315–e325. PMID: 26621650 doi:10.1161/cir.0000000000000245
15. Ackerman MJ, Zipes DP, Kovacs RJ, Maron BJ; American Heart Association Electrocardiography and Arrhythmias Committee of Council on Clinical Cardiology, Council on Cardiovascular Disease in Young, Council on Cardiovascular and Stroke Nursing, Council on Functional Genomics and Translational Biology, and American College of Cardiology. Eligibility and disqualification recommendations for competitive athletes with cardiovascular abnormalities: task force 10: the cardiac channelopathies: a scientific statement from the American Heart Association and American College of Cardiology. *Circulation.* 2015;132(22):e326–e329. PMID: 26527716 doi:10.1161/cir.0000000000000246
16. Estes NA III, Kovacs RJ, Baggish AL, Myerburg RJ; American Heart Association Electrocardiography and Arrhythmias Committee of Council on Clinical Cardiology, Council on Cardiovascular Disease in Young, Council on Cardiovascular and Stroke Nursing, Council on Functional Genomics and Translational Biology, and American College of Cardiology. Eligibility and disqualification recommendations for competitive athletes with cardiovascular abnormalities: task force 11: drugs and performance-enhancing substances: a scientific statement from the American Heart Association and American College of Cardiology. *Circulation.* 2015;132(22):e330–e333. PMID: 26621651 doi:10.1161/cir.0000000000000247
17. Link MS, Myerburg RJ, Estes NA III; American Heart Association Electrocardiography and Arrhythmias Committee of Council on Clinical Cardiology, Council on Cardiovascular Disease in Young, Council on Cardiovascular and Stroke Nursing, Council on Functional Genomics and Translational Biology, and American College of Cardiology. Eligibility and disqualification recommendations for competitive athletes with cardiovascular abnormalities: task force 12: emergency action plans, resuscitation, cardiopulmonary resuscitation, and automated external defibrillators: a scientific statement from the American Heart Association and American College of Cardiology. *Circulation.* 2015;132(22):e334–e338. PMID: 26621652 doi:10.1161/cir.0000000000000248
18. Link MS, Estes NA III, Maron BJ; American Heart Association Electrocardiography and Arrhythmias Committee of Council on Clinical Cardiology, Council on Cardiovascular Disease in Young, Council on Cardiovascular and Stroke Nursing, Council on Functional Genomics and Translational Biology, and American College of Cardiology. Eligibility and disqualification recommendations for competitive athletes with cardiovascular abnormalities: task force 13: commotio cordis: a scientific statement from the American Heart Association and American College of Cardiology. *Circulation.* 2015;132(22):e339–e342. PMID: 26621653 doi:10.1161/cir.0000000000000249
19. Maron BJ, Harris KM, Thompson PD, Eichner ER, Steinberg MH; American Heart Association Electrocardiography and Arrhythmias Committee of Council on Clinical Cardiology, Council on

Cardiovascular Disease in Young, Council on Cardiovascular and Stroke Nursing, Council on Functional Genomics and Translational Biology, and American College of Cardiology. Eligibility and disqualification recommendations for competitive athletes with cardiovascular abnormalities: task force 14: sickle cell trait: a scientific statement from the American Heart Association and American College of Cardiology. *Circulation*. 2015;132(22):e343–e345. PMID: 26527715 https://www.ahajournals.org/doi/pdf/10.1161/cir.0000000000000250

20. Mitten MJ, Zipes DP, Maron BJ, Bryant WJ. Eligibility and disqualification recommendations for competitive athletes with cardiovascular abnormalities: task force 15: legal aspects of medical eligibility and disqualification recommendations: a scientific statement from the American Heart Association and American College of Cardiology. *J Am Coll Cardiol*. 2015;66(21):2447–2450. PMID: 26542663 doi:10.1016/j.jacc.2015.09.047
21. Lampert R, Chung EH, Ackerman MJ, et al. 2024 HRS expert consensus statement on arrhythmias in the athlete: evaluation, treatment, and return to play. *Heart Rhythm*. 2024;21(10):e151–e252. PMID: 38763377 doi:10.1016/j.hrthm.2024.05.018
22. Erickson CC, Salerno JC, Berger S, et al; American Academy of Pediatrics Section on Cardiology and Cardiac Surgery, Pediatric and Congenital Electrophysiology Society (PACES) Task Force on Prevention of Sudden Death in the Young. Sudden death in the young: information for the primary care provider. *Pediatrics*. 2021;148(1):e2021052044. PMID: 34155130 doi:10.1542/peds.2021-052044
23. Kelly KL, Lin PT, Basso C, et al. Sudden cardiac death in the young: a consensus statement on recommended practices for cardiac examination by pathologists from the Society for Cardiovascular Pathology. *Cardiovasc Pathol*. 2023;63:107497. PMID: 36375720 doi:10.1016/j.carpath.2022.107497
24. Lampert R, Harmon KG. Sudden cardiac arrest in athletes. *N Engl J Med*. 2026;394(3):268–280. PMID: 41534044 doi:10.1056/NEJMra2312555
25. Landry CH, Allan KS, Connelly KA, Cunningham K, Morrison LJ, Dorian P; Rescu Investigators. Sudden cardiac arrest during participation in competitive sports. *N Engl J Med*. 2017;377(20):1943–1953. PMID: 29141175
26. Allan KS, Morrison LJ, Pinter A, Tu JV, Dorian P; Rescu Epistry Investigators. "Presumed cardiac" arrest in children and young adults: a misnomer? *Resuscitation*. 2017;117:73–79. PMID: 28602695
27. Peterson DF, Kucera K, Thomas LC, et al. Aetiology and incidence of sudden cardiac arrest and death in young competitive athletes in the USA: a 4-year prospective study. *Br J Sports Med*. 2021;55(21):1196–1203. PMID: 33184114 doi:10.1136/bjsports-2020-102666
28. Meyer L, Stubbs B, Fahrenbruch C, et al. Incidence, causes, and survival trends from cardiovascular-related sudden cardiac arrest in children and young adults 0 to 35 years of age: a 30-year review. *Circulation*. 2012;126(11):1363–1372. PMID: 22887927 doi:10.1161/CIRCULATIONAHA.111.076810
29. Malhotra A, Dhutia H, Finocchiaro G, et al. Outcomes of cardiac screening in adolescent soccer players. *N Engl J Med*. 2018;379(6):524–534. PMID: 30089062 doi:10.1056/NEJMoa1714719
30. Harmon KG, Asif IM, Maleszewski JJ, et al. Incidence, cause, and comparative frequency of sudden cardiac death in National Collegiate Athletic Association athletes: a decade in review. *Circulation*. 2015;132(1):10–19. PMID: 25977310
31. Maron BJ, Doerer JJ, Haas TS, Tierney DM, Mueller FO. Sudden deaths in young competitive athletes: analysis of 1866 deaths in the United States, 1980-2006. *Circulation*. 2009;119(8):1085–1092. PMID: 19221222
32. Maron BJ, Friedman RA, Kligfield P, et al; American Heart Association Council on Clinical Cardiology; Advocacy Coordinating Committee; Council on Cardiovascular Disease in the Young; Council on Cardiovascular Surgery and Anesthesia; Council on Epidemiology and Prevention; Council on Functional Genomics and Translational Biology; Council on Quality of Care and Outcomes Research, and American College of Cardiology. Assessment of the 12-lead electrocardiogram as a screening test for detection of cardiovascular disease in healthy general populations of young people (12-25 years of age): a scientific statement from the American Heart Association and the American College of Cardiology. *J Am Coll Cardiol*. 2014;64(14):1479–1514. PMID: 25234655
33. Drezner JA, Chun JS, Harmon KG, Derminer L. Survival trends in the United States following exercise-related sudden cardiac arrest in the youth: 2000-2006. *Heart Rhythm*. 2008;5(6):794–799. PMID: 18486566
34. Drezner JA, Courson RW, Roberts WO, Mosesso VN Jr, Link MS, Maron BJ; Inter-Association Task Force. Inter-association task force recommendations on emergency preparedness and management of sudden cardiac arrest in high school and college athletic programs: a consensus statement. *Heart Rhythm*. 2007;4(4):549–565. PMID: 17399652
35. Corrado D, Basso C, Rizzoli G, Schiavon M, Thiene G. Does sports activity enhance the risk of sudden death in adolescents and young adults? *J Am Coll Cardiol*. 2003;42(11):1959–1963. PMID: 14662259

36. Ha FJ, Han HC, Sanders P, et al. Sudden cardiac death related to physical exercise in the young: a nationwide cohort study of Australia. *Intern Med J*. 2023;53(4):497–502. PMID: 34719841 doi:10.1111/imj.15606
37. Bagnall RD, Singer ES, Tfelt-Hansen J. Sudden cardiac death in the young. *Heart Lung Circ*. 2020;29(4):498–504. PMID: 32029328 doi:10.1016/j.hlc.2019.11.007
38. Finocchiaro G, Radaelli D, D'Errico S, et al. Sudden cardiac death among adolescents in the United Kingdom. *J Am Coll Cardiol*. 2023;81(11):1007–1017. PMID: 36922085 doi:10.1016/j.jacc.2023.01.041
39. Banner J, Basso C, Tolkien Z, Kholova I, Michaud K, Gallagher PJ. Autopsy examination in sudden cardiac death: a current perspective on behalf of the Association for European Cardiovascular Pathology. *Virchows Arch*. 2021;478(4):687–693. PMID: 33111163 doi:10.1007/s00428-020-02949-8
40. Egger F, Scharhag J, Kästner A, Dvořák J, Bohm P, Meyer T. FIFA Sudden Death Registry (FIFA-SDR): a prospective, observational study of sudden death in worldwide football from 2014 to 2018. *Br J Sports Med*. 2022;56(2):80–87. PMID: 33361135 doi:10.1136/bjsports-2020-102368
41. Asif IM, Roberts WO, Fredericson M, Froelicher V, eds. The cardiovascular preparticipation evaluation (PPE) for the primary care and sports medicine physician, part I. *Curr Sports Med Rep*. 2015;14(3):246–267. PMID: 25968861
42. Asif IM, Roberts WO, Fredericson M, Froelicher V, eds. The cardiovascular preparticipation evaluation (PPE) for the primary care and sports medicine physician, part II. *Curr Sports Med Rep*. 2015;14(4):333.
43. Asif IM, Yim ES, Hoffman JM, Froelicher V. Update: causes and symptoms of sudden cardiac death in young athletes. *Phys Sportsmed*. 2015;43(1):44–53. PMID: 25656358 doi:10.1080/00913847.2015.1001306
44. Bruce C, Ubhi N, McKeegan P, Sanders K. Systematic review and meta-analysis of cardiovascular consequences of myocardial bridging in hypertrophic cardiomyopathy. *Am J Cardiol*. 2023;188:110–119. PMID: 36512852 doi:10.1016/j.amjcard.2022.10.059
45. Basso C, Maron BJ, Corrado D, Thiene G. Clinical profile of congenital coronary artery anomalies with origin from the wrong aortic sinus leading to sudden death in young competitive athletes. *J Am Coll Cardiol*. 2000;35(6):1493–1501. PMID: 10807452
46. Stefani L, Galanti G, Toncelli L, et al. Bicuspid aortic valve in competitive athletes. *Br J Sports Med*. 2008;42(1):31–35. PMID: 17548371
47. Wiegerinck EM, van de Hoef TP, Rolandi MC, et al. Impact of aortic valve stenosis on coronary hemodynamics and the instantaneous effect of transcatheter aortic valve implantation. *Circ Cardiovasc Interv*. 2015;8(8):e002443. PMID: 26245891 doi:10.1161/circinterventions.114.002443
48. Pelliccia A, Solberg EE, Papadakis M, et al. Recommendations for participation in competitive and leisure time sport in athletes with cardiomyopathies, myocarditis, and pericarditis: position statement of the Sport Cardiology Section of the European Association of Preventive Cardiology (EAPC). *Eur Heart J*. 2019;40(1):19–33. PMID: 30561613 doi:10.1093/eurheartj/ehy730
49. Law YM, Lal AK, Chen S, et al; American Heart Association Pediatric Heart Failure and Transplantation Committee of the Council on Lifelong Congenital Heart Disease and Heart Health in the Young and Stroke Council. Diagnosis and management of myocarditis in children: a scientific statement from the American Heart Association. *Circulation*. 2021;144(6):e123–e135. PMID: 34229446 doi:10.1161/cir.0000000000000100133
50. Halle M, Binzenhöfer L, Mahrholdt H, Johannes Schindler M, Esefeld K, Tschöpe C. Myocarditis in athletes: a clinical perspective. *Eur J Prev Cardiol*. 2021;28(10):1050–1057. PMID: 33611403 doi:10.1177/2047487320909670
51. O'Connor FG, Oriscello RG, Levine BD. Exercise-related syncope in the young athlete: reassurance, restriction or referral? *Am Fam Physician*. 1999;60(7):2001–2008. PMID: 10569503
52. Krahn AD, Laksman Z, Sy RW, et al. Congenital Long QT syndrome. *JACC Clin Electrophysiol*. 2022;8(5):687–706. PMID: 35589186 doi:10.1016/j.jacep.2022.02.017
53. Harvey A, Curnier D, Dodin P, Abadir S, Jacquemet V, Caru M. The influence of exercise and postural changes on ventricular repolarization in the long QT syndrome: a systematic scoping review. *Eur J Prev Cardiol*. 2022;29(12):1633–1677. PMID: 35537006 doi:10.1093/eurjpc/zwac081
54. Aggarwal A, Stolear A, Alam MM, et al. Catecholaminergic polymorphic ventricular tachycardia: clinical characteristics, diagnostic evaluation and therapeutic strategies. *J Clin Med*. 2024;13(6):1781. PMID: 38542006 doi:10.3390/jcm13061781
55. Tester DJ, Spoon DB, Valdivia HH, Makielski JC, Ackerman MJ. Targeted mutational analysis of the RyR2-encoded cardiac ryanodine receptor in sudden unexplained death: a molecular autopsy of

49 medical examiner/coroner's cases. *Mayo Clin Proc.* 2004;79(11):1380–1384. PMID: 15544015 doi:10.4065/79.11.1380

56. Corrado D, Zorzi A, Cipriani A, et al. Evolving diagnostic criteria for arrhythmogenic cardiomyopathy. *J Am Heart Assoc.* 2021;10(18):e021987. PMID: 34533054 doi:10.1161/jaha.121.021987
57. McNally E, MacLeod H, Dellefave-Castillo L. Arrhythmogenic right ventricular cardiomyopathy overview. In: Adam MP, Feldman J, Mirzaa GM, et al, eds. *GeneReviews(®)* [Internet]. University of Washington, Seattle. Updated May 11, 2023. https://www.ncbi.nlm.nih.gov/books/NBK1131/
58. Ruwald AC, Marcus F, Estes NA III, et al. Association of competitive and recreational sport participation with cardiac events in patients with arrhythmogenic right ventricular cardiomyopathy: results from the North American multidisciplinary study of arrhythmogenic right ventricular cardiomyopathy. *Eur Heart J.* 2015;36(27):1735–1743. PMID: 25896080 doi:10.1093/eurheartj/ehv110
59. Cohen MI, Triedman JK, Cannon BC, et al; Pediatric and Congenital Electrophysiology Society (PACES); Heart Rhythm Society (HRS); American College of Cardiology Foundation (ACCF); American Heart Association (AHA); American Academy of Pediatrics (AAP); Canadian Heart Rhythm Society (CHRS). PACES/HRS expert consensus statement on the management of the asymptomatic young patient with a Wolff-Parkinson-White (WPW, ventricular preexcitation) electrocardiographic pattern: developed in partnership between the Pediatric and Congenital Electrophysiology Society (PACES) and the Heart Rhythm Society (HRS). Endorsed by the governing bodies of PACES, HRS, the American College of Cardiology Foundation (ACCF), the American Heart Association (AHA), the American Academy of Pediatrics (AAP), and the Canadian Heart Rhythm Society (CHRS). *Heart Rhythm.* 2012;9(6):1006–1024. PMID: 22579340 doi:10.1016/j.hrthm.2012.03.050
60. Delise P, Sciarra L. Sudden cardiac death in patients with ventricular preexcitation. *Card Electrophysiol Clin.* 2020;12(4):519–525. PMID: 33162000 doi:10.1016/j.ccep.2020.08.002
61. Roberts WO. Exercise-associated collapse in endurance events: a classification system. *Phys Sportsmed.* 1989;17(5):49–59. PMID: 27447266
62. O'Connor FG, Johnson JD, Chapin M, Oriscello RG, Taylor DC. A pilot study of clinical agreement in cardiovascular preparticipation examinations: how good is the standard of care? *Clin J Sport Med.* 2005;15(3):177–179. PMID: 15867562
63. Leenhardt A, Lucet V, Denjoy I, Grau F, Ngoc DD, Coumel P. Catecholaminergic polymorphic ventricular tachycardia in children: a 7-year follow-up of 21 patients. *Circulation.* 1995;91(5):1512–1519. PMID: 7867192
64. Drezner JA, Fudge J, Harmon KG, Berger S, Campbell RM, Vetter VL. Warning symptoms and family history in children and young adults with sudden cardiac arrest. *J Am Board Fam Med.* 2012;25(4):408–415. PMID: 22773708 doi:10.3122/jabfm.2012.04.110225
65. Sheppard MN, Westaby J, Zullo E, Fernandez BVE, Cox S, Cox A. Sudden arrhythmic death and cardiomyopathy are important causes of sudden cardiac death in the UK: results from a national coronial autopsy database. *Histopathology.* 2023;82(7):1056–1066. PMID: 36799099 doi:10.1111/his.14889
66. Maron BJ, Haas TS, Ahluwalia A, Murphy CJ, Garberich RF. Demographics and epidemiology of sudden deaths in young competitive athletes: from the United States National Registry. *Am J Med.* 2016;129(11):1170–1177. PMID: 27039955
67. Alblaihed L, Kositz C, Brady WJ, Al-Salamah T, Mattu A. Diagnosis and management of arrhythmogenic right ventricular cardiomyopathy. *Am J Emerg Med.* 2023;65:146–153. PMID: 36638611 doi:10.1016/j.ajem.2022.12.010
68. Monda E, Verrillo F, Rubino M, et al. Thoracic aortic dilation: implications for physical activity and sport participation. *Diagnostics (Basel).* 2022;12(6):1392. PMID: 35741202 doi:10.3390/diagnostics12061392
69. Cozijnsen L, Braam RL, Waalewijn RA, et al. What is new in dilatation of the ascending aorta? Review of current literature and practical advice for the cardiologist. *Circulation.* 2011;123(8):924–928. PMID: 21357847 doi:10.1161/circulationaha.110.949131
70. Loeys BL, Dietz HC, Braverman AC, et al. The revised Ghent nosology for the Marfan syndrome. *J Med Genet.* 2010;47(7):476–485. PMID: 20591885
71. Rodríguez-Palomares JF, Dux-Santoy L, Guala A, Galian-Gay L, Evangelista A. Mechanisms of aortic dilation in patients with bicuspid aortic valve: JACC state-of-the-art review. *J Am Coll Cardiol.* 2023;82(5):448–464. PMID: 37495282 doi:10.1016/j.jacc.2022.10.042
72. Evangelista A, Isselbacher EM, Bossone E, et al; IRAD Investigators. Insights from the International Registry of Acute Aortic Dissection: a 20-year experience of collaborative clinical research. *Circulation.* 2018;137(17):1846–1860. PMID: 29685932 doi:10.1161/circulationaha.117.031264

73. Alapati S, Strobel N, Hashmi S, Bricker JT, Gupta-Malhotra M. Sudden unexplained cardiac arrest in apparently healthy children: a single-center experience. *Pediatr Cardiol.* 2013;34(3):639–645. PMID: 23052663
74. Sealy DP, Pekarek L, Russ D, Sealy C, Goforth G. Vital signs and demographics in the preparticipation sports exam: do they help us find the elusive athlete at risk for sudden cardiac death? *Curr Sports Med Rep.* 2010;9(6):338–341. PMID: 21068565
75. Carek PJ, Futrell M, Hueston WJ. The preparticipation physical examination history: who has the correct answers? *Clin J Sport Med.* 1999;9(3):124–128. PMID: 10512339
76. Asplund CA, O'Connor FG. The evidence against cardiac screening using electrocardiogram in athletes. *Curr Sports Med Rep.* 2016;15(2):81–85. PMID: 26963014
77. Asif IM, Drezner JA. Cardiovascular screening in young athletes: evidence for the electrocardiogram. *Curr Sports Med Rep.* 2016;15(2):76–80. PMID: 26963013
78. Mayer F, Bonaventura K, Cassel M, et al. Medical results of preparticipation examination in adolescent athletes. *Br J Sports Med.* 2012;46(7):524–530. PMID: 22576783 doi:10.1136/bjsports-2011-090966
79. Harmon KG, Suchsland MZ, Prutkin JM, et al. Comparison of cardiovascular screening in college athletes by history and physical examination with and without an electrocardiogram: efficacy and cost. *Heart Rhythm.* 2020;17(10):1649–1655. PMID: 32380289 doi:10.1016/j.hrthm.2020.04.032
80. Drezner JA, Sharma S, Baggish A, et al. International criteria for electrocardiographic interpretation in athletes: consensus statement. *Br J Sports Med.* 2017;51(9):704–731. PMID: 28258178 doi:10.1136/bjsports-2016-097331
81. James PA, Oparil S, Carter BL, et al. 2014 evidence-based guideline for the management of high blood pressure in adults: report from the panel members appointed to the Eighth Joint National Committee (JNC 8). *JAMA.* 2014;311(5):507–520. PMID: 24352797
82. Flynn JT, Kaelber DC, Baker-Smith CM, et al; American Academy of Pediatrics Subcommittee on Screening and Management of High Blood Pressure in Children. Clinical practice guideline for screening and management of high blood pressure in children and adolescents. *Pediatrics.* 2017;140(3):e20171904. PMID: 28827377
83. Kim JH, Baggish AL, Levine BD, et al; American Heart Association Leadership Committee of the Council on Clinical Cardiology; Council on Basic Cardiovascular Sciences; Council on Cardiovascular and Stroke Nursing; Council on Cardiovascular Surgery and Anesthesia; Council on Peripheral Vascular Disease; and American College of Cardiology. Clinical considerations for competitive sports participation for athletes with cardiovascular abnormalities: a scientific statement from the American Heart Association and American College of Cardiology. *Circulation.* 2025;151(11):e716–e761. PMID: 39973614 doi:10.1161/CIR.0000000000001297
84. Baggish AL, Ackerman MJ, Putukian M, Lampert R. Shared decision making for athletes with cardiovascular disease: practical considerations. *Curr Sports Med Rep.* 2019;18(3):76–81. PMID: 30855305 doi:10.1249/JSR.0000000000000575

B: Nervous System

HISTORY FORM QUESTIONS

1. *Have you ever had a hit or blow that caused confusion, prolonged headache, or memory problems, or been diagnosed with a concussion?*
2. *Have you ever had numbness, tingling, weakness in your arms or legs, or been unable to move your arms or legs after being hit or falling?*

SECONDARY QUESTIONS

- What can you tell me about your head injury or concussion?
- Have you ever had an unexplained seizure?
- Has anyone in your family had unexplained fainting, seizures, or near drowning?
- Do you have headaches with exercise?
- What can you tell me about the symptoms in your arms or legs?
- Have you had any test or imaging for the problem?

KEY POINTS

- Concussions are common across all sports (not just collision sports) and are both underrecognized and underreported.
- After sustaining a concussion, an individual should not return to contact/collision sport or high-risk activity for head injury until they have complete symptom resolution, have normal physical examination findings, and have successfully completed a return to learn process and a graduated return to sport strategy.
- Postconcussion return to play decisions require an individualized approach.
- Individuals younger than 18 years may take longer to recover after concussion than older individuals.
- Females with a sport-related concussion may be more symptomatic and may take longer to recover.
- Sequelae of concussion may include persisting symptoms that can last from weeks to months.
- Cervical spinal cord neurapraxia (CCN) is a spinal cord injury that presents with motor and/or sensory changes in more than one extremity (bilateral arms or legs or 1 arm and 1 leg) and is a spinal cord injury.
- An individual with CCN should be evaluated for cervical spinal stenosis, and neurosurgical consultation should be considered.
- Return to play with cervical spinal stenosis is controversial.
- Stingers or burners are unilateral and transient.
- Individuals with brachial plexus injuries may return to play when asymptomatic.
- Seizures should not preclude individuals from physical activity.
- Headaches can be triggered or worsened by exercise and may prohibit physical activity.
- Primary exertion headache can occur with aerobic exercise.

INTRODUCTION

A goal of the preparticipation evaluation (PPE) is to detect neurological conditions that may limit or preclude medical eligibility, require modified athletic participation, place individuals at higher risk for injury, or affect athletic performance.

Neurological conditions that affect sports participation and physical activity include sport-related concussion (SRC) and its sequelae, CCN (transient paraparesis, quadriparesis, or tetraparesis), brachial plexus injuries ("stingers/burners"), seizure disorders, and headache disorders. A history of head trauma, cervical spine injury, or neurological symptoms during competition indicates the need for a more detailed neurological examination including assessment of cranial nerves, motor and sensory examination, deep tendon reflexes, cognitive function, and cerebellar function.[1] This section will review the PPE questions that address current or previous neurological issues and discuss appropriate workup, management, and medical eligibility concerns for each condition.

SPORT-RELATED CONCUSSION

Sport-related concussion is an injury to the brain. The term *mild traumatic brain injury* (mTBI) is often used interchangeably with concussion, which may not be accurate. mTBI is a broader term that includes concussions and other mild traumatic brain injuries. In 2022, the 6th International Conference on Concussion in Sport Group modified its definition of SRC as follows:

> Sport-related concussion is a traumatic brain injury caused by a direct blow to the head, neck, or body resulting in an impulsive force being transmitted to the brain that occurs in sports and exercise-related activities. This initiates a neurotransmitter and metabolic cascade, with possible axonal injury, blood flow change, and inflammation affecting the brain. Symptoms and signs may present immediately, or evolve over minutes or hours, and commonly resolve within days, but may be prolonged. No abnormality is seen on standard structural neuroimaging studies (computed tomography or magnetic resonance imaging T1- and T2-weighted images), but in the research setting, abnormalities may be present on functional, blood flow or metabolic imaging studies. Sport-related concussion results in a range of clinical symptoms and signs that may or may not involve loss of consciousness. The clinical symptoms and signs of concussion cannot be explained solely by (but may occur concomitantly with) drug, alcohol, or medication use, other injuries (such as cervical injuries, peripheral vestibular dysfunction) or other comorbidities (such as psychological factors or coexisting medical conditions).[2]

SRC neurological signs and symptoms caused by mechanical acceleration or deceleration are not related to macroscopic neural damage, but are believed to be caused by a disturbance in the neurochemical pathways or microstructural injury.[3–5] The pathophysiology of concussion, as described in animal models and some recent human studies, involves a neurometabolic cascade of events.[5–7]

Since this injury occurs at the cellular level, the vast majority of individuals with SRC show no changes with computed tomography or magnetic resonance imaging (MRI) and do not require neuroimaging. Standard neuroimaging may be necessary to evaluate for a structural brain injury such as a subdural hematoma.[8,9]

There are 2 primary considerations for medical eligibility when an individual has a history of SRC noted during the PPE. First, the most recent concussion must be completely resolved, and, second, a prior concussion places an individual at a higher risk for future SRC. For individuals with a history of SRC, it is important to ask secondary concussion-related questions including those pertaining to the number, frequency, severity, treatment, and length of recovery from past SRC, and the presence of mood, learning, attention, sleep, or headache disorders. Before an individual is allowed to participate in contact sports or other activities that might increase their risk of additional brain injury, a synthesis of the clinical data to determine medical eligibility and a thorough discussion of the potential risk to the brain with the individual (and parents or guardian, if a minor) are essential. Concussion evaluation and treatment in special populations is reviewed in Chapter 7.

There are potential health risks of returning an individual with ongoing concussion symptoms to play, including increased susceptibility to an additional, possibly more severe concussion, prolonged duration of symptoms, and second impact syndrome (SIS). In animal laboratory models, when a second injury occurs before the brain has fully recovered from the first injury, this results in worsening cellular metabolic changes and significantly decreased cognitive function, which accounts for worsening symptoms.[8,10–15] SIS is a controversial and rare condition described as occurring when an individual sustains a second head injury before the symptoms of the initial SRC injury have fully cleared.[2,16–18] SIS has a mortality rate approaching 50% and a morbidity rate nearing 100%, which emphasizes the importance of allowing the brain to completely heal before returning to contact/collision sports and other activities that pose a risk for head injury.[19] SIS is an exceedingly rare phenomenon, but the majority of cases have involved high school–aged and younger individuals.[20] Even in the absence of SIS, repeated head injuries during the time that the brain is still recovering from a concussion can lead to worse and more prolonged symptoms, and thus activities that pose a risk for head trauma should be avoided. The potential risk for SIS supports the recommendation to immediately remove an individual from play following a suspected SRC and to withhold medical eligibility while symptomatic.

The diagnosis of concussion continues to be based on clinical assessment as there is no single confirmatory sign, symptom, or objective test. Recovery patterns and time frames vary from individual to individual. There is no single objective test that determines when an individual has recovered from a concussion. Recovery is also based on clinical assessment. An individual is clinically recovered from SRC when asymptomatic at rest, with normal physical examination results, normal cognitive function, and the ability to participate in usual activities without symptoms, including school, work, activities of daily living, recreation, and sport.[3]

An individual is clinically recovered from SRC when asymptomatic at rest, with normal physical examination results, normal cognitive function, and the ability to participate in usual activities without symptoms, including school, work, activities of daily living, recreation, and sport.[3]

Return to sport recommendations for children have been extrapolated from adult consensus guidelines, and further research is required to refine a child-specific program. Studies demonstrate a longer recovery period for younger individuals compared to college-age and older individuals; thus, a more conservative approach to the return of younger individuals to full participation is reasonable for contact and collision sports.[21–28]

The baseline comparison method, in which the individual's postconcussion performance is compared to a healthy baseline evaluation from preseason, is still being investigated. It has been described as the "gold standard" in concussion management by some,[29,30] while other expert groups have not advocated for this position.[3] Several tools have been suggested as adjuncts to the PPE including, but not limited to, baseline computerized neurocognitive testing (CNT), the Sport Concussion Assessment Tool (SCAT), graded symptom checklists, Balance Error Scoring System (BESS), tandem gait, and Vestibular/Ocular Motor Screening (VOMS) testing.[31–35] Some advocate for obtaining baseline symptom scores on a "regular basis," as an individualized baseline is a more meaningful benchmark for managing a future concussion. No universal agreement exists on whether baseline CNT should be used routinely.[36] Obtaining baseline SCAT and/or BESS measures for large numbers of individuals is time intensive and likely cost prohibitive.[30,32,37] The utility of the SCAT decreases 3 to 5 days after injury (after which the Sport Concussion Office Assessment Tool is suggested)[38] and when used serially to evaluate SRC should be done under the same or similar conditions as the baseline assessment.[32,39–41] Impaired tandem gait performance has been noted in pediatric participants with prolonged concussion recovery; however, normative data are not available.[34,42] Tools such as the VOMS have demonstrated some usefulness in the evaluation of SRC.[33,43–45] At this time, there are not enough studies of adequate quality to recommend its inclusion in the SCAT or the PPE.[21,36,46]

The National Collegiate Athletic Association (NCAA) recommends a one-time, preparticipation baseline concussion assessment for all college varsity student-athletes that includes but is not necessarily limited to:

- Brain injury/concussion history
- Symptom evaluation
- Cognitive assessment
- Balance evaluation[47]

There is no consensus agreement on the definition of postconcussion syndrome. The 6th International Conference on Concussion in Sport Group suggests the term *persisting symptoms*, rather than *postconcussion syndrome*, for failure of normal clinical recovery beyond the expected time frame of more than 1 month in all ages.[2] In individuals with persisting symptoms, it is important to evaluate for cervical strains, vestibular injuries, oculomotor disorders, sleep cycle disturbances, and mental health issues that may confound the diagnosis and benefit from other interventions. These coexisting conditions can mimic and/or amplify symptoms of a concussion and may prolong recovery and return to participation. Young patients with persisting symptoms are more likely to have high preinjury somatization.[48,49] Individuals with persisting symptoms may benefit from additional evaluation by a concussion specialist[21] and should not return to sport participation until all symptoms have resolved.

The absolute number of concussions an individual can sustain and continue to participate in contact sports has not been defined.[8] High school students with a history of concussions who have no physical, medical, or cognitive difficulties are generally allowed to participate in all sports. Sustained attention and cognitive function deficits following a concussion may persist long after the injury, limiting medical eligibility.[50] The evidence available regarding concussion recovery in children is sparse.[51] Most young patients experience resolution of their symptoms within 4 weeks.[21,52] Providers managing young individuals with a history of multiple concussions may adopt a more conservative strategy regarding medical eligibility or return to play. When repeat concussions occur with lesser force, are more severe, take longer to fully recover, or show changes in baseline brain function, withholding medical eligibility for contact/collision sports or "sports with high risk" should be considered.

Females with SRC may be more symptomatic and may take longer to recover. In addition, concussed women are at increased risk for postconcussion symptoms compared to men, but this has not been shown in girls younger than 18 years.[53]

Clinicians should be aware of the potential for long-term consequences from multiple subconcussive impacts.[51] There is increasing concern that head impact exposure and recurrent concussions contribute to long-term neurological sequelae including chronic traumatic encephalopathy and chronic neurocognitive impairment.[8] Two studies found no increased risk of dementia, Parkinson disease, amyotrophic lateral sclerosis, or cognitive or depressive problems in former high school football players compared to classmates who did not play football.[54,55]

Several biomarkers are being investigated for concussion evaluation.[56,57] These biomarkers are not yet suited for routine clinical practice and have not been advanced for clinical use.[2,58] Nutritional supplements are also being investigated for potential preventive or therapeutic roles in concussion.[59,60] There is no evidence that supplements can prevent or treat concussions.[60]

There are no evidence-based guidelines for disqualifying or retiring an athlete from their sport after concussion,[8,21,61] although there are expert opinion publications that provide some considerations for limiting medical eligibility.[62,63] When considering retirement from sport, the opportunity for shared decision-making cannot be overemphasized. It may be prudent to refer an athlete to a specialist with expertise in SRC when contemplating retiring an individual from a particular sport.

CERVICAL SPINAL CORD NEURAPRAXIA

CCN, also called *transient quadriplegia/tetraplegia* or *transient paraplegia*, is characterized by an acute, transient impairment of sensory and/or motor function in more than one extremity. The pathology is named for the number of extremities affected. Symptoms include burning pain, numbness, tingling, or loss of sensation with or without motor weakness or paralysis. Symptoms usually resolve within 10 to 15 minutes but may last up to 48 hours.[64] The most common cause of CCN is cervical spinal stenosis due to narrowing of the spinal canal, which can be congenital or acquired (degenerative changes, cervical instability, or intervertebral disc protrusion).[65]

The physical examination, unless conducted at the time of injury, results in normal findings. An MRI of the cervical spine is recommended to evaluate for an underlying spinal abnormality such as cervical spinal stenosis.[66] Cervical spinal stenosis can be defined by a cervical canal measurement of less than 14 mm at C4.[67] However, the concept of functional spinal stenosis or a canal so small as to obliterate the protective cerebral spinal fluid cushion is more frequently used.[67]

There is debate as to whether individuals who have had an episode of CCN should be allowed to return to play in athletic events.[68] A review of 110 MRI images of adolescent and adult athletes with CCN who were followed for 3 years showed a 56% risk of a recurrent episode. Recurrence was strongly associated with the degree of stenosis; the authors concluded that cervical spinal stenosis was a risk factor for CCN.[69] A single, uncomplicated episode of CCN did not increase the risk of incurring permanent neurological sequelae.[69,70] Other experts strongly disagree and contend that functional spinal stenosis is an absolute contraindication to participation in contact or collision sports after an episode of CCN.[66,67]

Before adolescence, CCN is not due to congenital cervical spinal stenosis. Rather, CCN in these individuals is attributed to the increased mobility of the pediatric spine rather than the presence of cervical stenosis.[68,71,72] Long-term follow-up of a small pediatric cohort with CCN showed full return to previous activities, including sports, and none of the children experienced a subsequent permanent neurological injury.[71]

Given the medicolegal risk and controversy, following an episode of CCN with documented cervical spinal stenosis, it is advised to seek neurosurgical consultation and use shared decision-making prior to allowing return to play, particularly in collision sports.

BRACHIAL PLEXUS INJURIES

Transient brachial plexus injuries, commonly referred to as stingers, burners, or *transient brachial plexopathy*, involve unilateral upper extremity pain and paresthesia following a blow to the neck or shoulder, and the symptoms resolve rapidly. Individuals typically complain of burning dysesthesias beginning in the shoulder region and radiating down the arm and hand.

These injuries are most common in contact and collision sports, such as football, rugby, and wrestling. Injury rates in football players are reported as high as 26% in a single season[73] and 50% across a career.[74] Approximately 50% to 60% of college and 30% of high school football players reported a brachial plexus injury over the course of their playing career.[75,76]

There are 2 typical injury mechanisms for stingers: tensile stretch and compressive force. Tensile injuries occur when the neck is forcibly stretched away from the ipsilateral shoulder as the shoulder is simultaneously depressed, stretching a portion of the nerve. Tensile injuries are more common in high school–aged or younger individuals. Stingers from compression forces occur when the neck is forcibly flexed in a posterolateral direction or by direct compression on the affected side, "pinching" the nerve tissues.[72,77] Compression stingers are more common in individuals 20 years and older who have more degenerative disc changes and foraminal narrowing.

Stingers are likely an injury to the proximal cervical nerve root of the spinal nerve complex. The cervical nerve roots do not have a protective epineurium or perineurium to help absorb either compressive or tensile forces. Recurrent stingers are more common when degenerative disc disease is present,[77] and degenerative changes in the spine that occur with aging place the nerve root at greater risk.[78]

When there is a history of stingers, secondary questions are asked to clarify the frequency of previous episodes, the location of symptoms (unilateral vs bilateral), and the current reduction strategies (eg, neck collars, strengthening). An individual may, at separate times, have stingers in different arms; however, concurrent bilateral symptoms are by definition due to CCN pathology and require further evaluations as outlined in the previous section.

Physical examination to assess the involved and contralateral upper extremity includes muscle strength (myotomes C4–C8), sensation in C3–T1 dermatomes, reflexes (biceps, triceps, brachioradialis), muscle mass symmetry (ruling out muscle atrophy), neck range of motion, and provocation tests to reproduce symptoms (brachial plexus traction test, shoulder abduction test, shoulder distraction, cervical compression test, Spurling test, upper limb tension tests, and Valsalva). Spurling test is the most common radiculopathy examination technique and is performed by extending the head in a lateral direction and then rotating it while applying axial pressure (Figure 5B-1). Any reproduction of radiating pain, tingling, or numbness down the arm during neck rotation, extension, and compression is a positive test result suggesting cervical root impingement. Positive results for 2 or more provocation tests are considered to increase the accuracy of the diagnosis of cervical radiculopathy (Table 5B-1).[79]

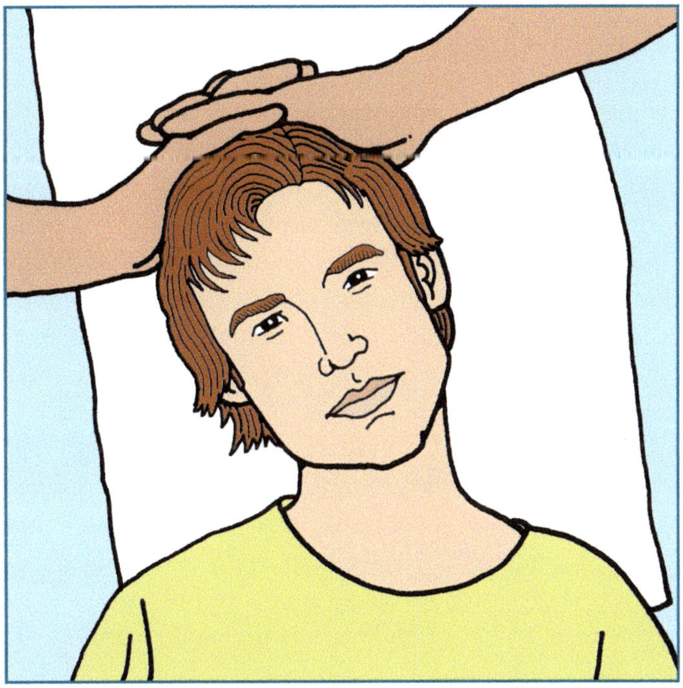

Figure 5B-1. Spurling Test

Table 5B-1. Sensitivity and Specificity of Conventional Provocative Tests in Cervical Radiculopathy

Variable	Sensitivity (%)	Specificity (%)
Spurling	30–50	74–93
Shoulder abduction	17–78	75–92
Valsalva	22	94
Distraction	44	90–97
Upper limb tension test	72–97	11–33

Reproduced from Kang KC, Lee HS, Lee JH. Cervical radiculopathy focus on characteristics and differential diagnosis. *Asian Spine J.* 2020;14(6):921–930. doi:10.31616/asj.2020.0647

Upper limb nerve tension tests that are used for ruling out radiculopathy—the median, ulnar, and radial bias maneuvers—are analogous to the straight leg raise in the lower extremity. The tests put a stretch on the brachial plexus and nerve, and when this reproduces the symptoms, the test is considered positive. The tests are shown in Figure 5B-2.

Abnormal findings on neurological examination or a history of recurrent stingers indicates the need for cervical radiography, with or without adjuvant cervical MRI, to evaluate for possible cervical spinal stenosis.[1] When numbness, weakness, or both persist for longer than 4 weeks, electromyography can be done to define the nature and location of the injury. Electromyography performed prior to 4 weeks has a high incidence of false-negative results.[80,81]

Players with a history of stingers or burners may return to activity when free of any neck or radicular pain and when they have full range of motion and strength.[82] An individual who recovers from serial stingers quickly can be allowed to participate without restrictions. Long-term, significant nerve injury is a rare outcome, but it does occur. More than 3 episodes of stingers may be a relative contraindication for return to play.[83]

Neck strengthening may benefit individuals with a history of stingers. In addition, protective equipment that limits lateral neck flexion and hyperextension may be helpful.[84] Tackling technique in football can be reviewed by the coaching staff to prevent dangerous practices, in particular, spear tackling or "leading with the head."[85]

Congenital cervical fusion, also known as Klippel-Feil syndrome (KFS), is a rare condition that can place individuals at increased risk for spinal cord injury after minor trauma. The classic triad of low posterior hairline, short neck, and limited cervical range of motion is seen in less than 50% of patients.[86] There is no clear consensus in the literature regarding the criteria for or against participation in contact sports by individuals with KFS, but there does appear to be agreement that instability of the upper (occiput-1/NC2) cervical spine as well as craniocervical abnormalities are absolute contraindications for contact sports. For stable fusions, especially caudal to C3, patients can compete without restrictions.[86]

Because of the high-energy nature of contact sports, it is important to perform flexion-extension imaging studies as well as careful neurological and musculoskeletal examinations to assess for hypermobility, instability, and neurological deficits before clearing patients with KFS for participation. In addition, athletic participation criteria as they pertain to

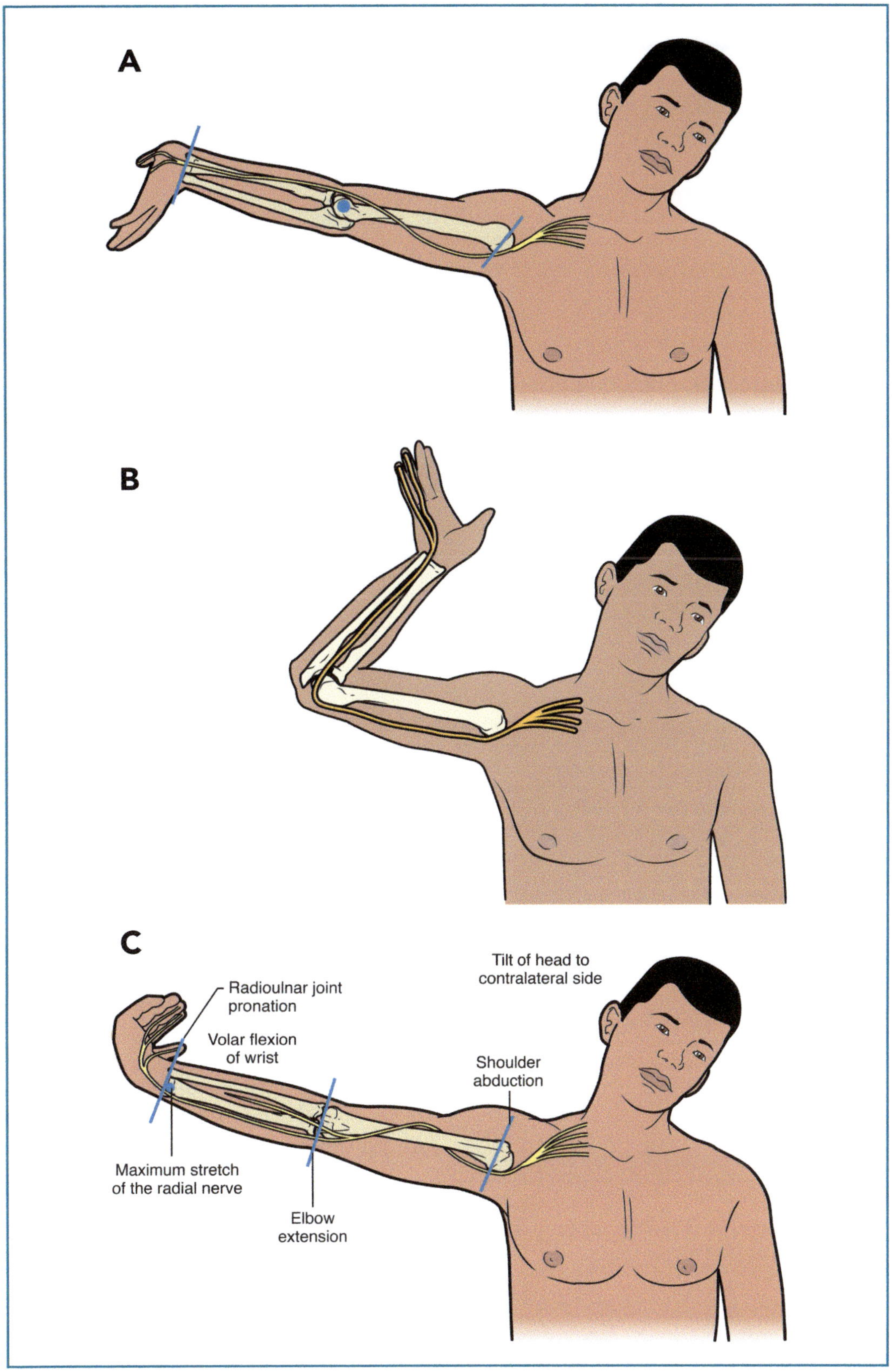

Figure 5B-2. Upper Limb Nerve Tension Tests for the Median (a), Ulnar (b), and Radial Nerves (c)

abnormalities associated with KFS, such as renal agenesis, hearing loss, and cardiovascular defects, need to be considered.[86,87]

While detailed discussions of specific disabilities/syndromes are also included in Chapter 7, sports participation with other spine conditions is outlined in Table 5B-2.[88]

Table 5B-2. Return-to-Play Recommendations

Absolute Contraindications	Level of Evidence[a]
Clinical	
Second stinger in the same game	IV
Persistent neurological deficits on clinical exam	IV
Symptoms in bilateral or multiple extremities	IV
Suspicion of neck injury	IV
Continued neck pain or discomfort	IV
Lack of full cervical range of motion	IV
Radiologic	
Cervical spine fracture	V
Ligamentous laxity or injury	V
Cervical spinal cord edema or abnormality	V
Neural compression	V
Evidence of spear-tackler's spine	V
Multilevel fusion from Klippel-Feil syndrome	V
Ankylosing spondylitis or diffuse idiopathic skeletal hyperostosis	IV
Evidence of rheumatoid arthritis	IV
Relative Contraindications	**Level of Evidence[a]**
Persistence of symptoms beyond 1 h	IV
Second stinger in the same season	V
Three or more prior episodes of stingers with full return to baseline cervical range of motion and neurological status and without an increase in baseline neck discomfort	V

Table 5B-2. Return-to-Play Recommendations (*continued*)

No Contraindications	Level of Evidence[a]
First-time stinger that is transient (less than 1 h) with full resolution of symptoms	V
Second-time stinger not in the same game or season that is transient (less than 1 h) with full resolution of symptoms	V
Less than 3 previous episodes of stingers lasting less than 24 h, with full cervical range of motion and no evidence of neurological deficit	V
Single-level Klippel-Feil anomaly, without involvement of the C0–C1 articulation	IV
Spina bifida occulta	IV
Torg ratio < 0.8 and asymptomatic	IV

[a] Based on the *Journal of Bone & Joint Surgery* levels of evidence,[88] level I indicates good evidence for or against recommending intervention (ie, randomized clinical trials); level II indicates fair evidence for or against recommending intervention (ie, prospective cohort studies); level III indicates conflicting or poor-quality evidence for or against recommending intervention (ie, retrospective cohort and case-control studies); level IV indicates insufficient or conflicting evidence for or against intervention (ie, case series/reports); and level V is mechanism-based reasoning, often from expert opinion (ie, surveys).

Reproduced from Bowles DR, Canseco JA, Alexander TD, Schroeder GD, Hecht AC, Vaccaro AR. The prevalence and management of stingers in college and professional collision athletes. *Curr Rev Musculoskelet Med.* 2020;13(6):651–662. doi:10.1007/s12178-020-09665-5

SEIZURES

Seizures are not common among athletes, in part because patients with seizure disorder may be incorrectly discouraged from participating in strenuous exercise and team sports for fear of exacerbating the disorder.[89,90] Athletes with well-controlled seizure disorders can participate in collision and contact sports without affecting seizure frequency.[89] However, concussion may exacerbate seizure disorders in athletes.[91]

New-onset seizures or seizures occurring after head injury require a thorough medical evaluation and seizure control prior to resuming sport participation. Syncope with myoclonic activity can easily be confused with seizure, and it is important to evaluate for potential cardiac causes of syncope prior to assuming a diagnosis of seizure disorder (see Chapter 5A). Some antiepileptic medications have side effects that may affect performance, including rash, weight gain, nausea, behavioral changes, and/or cognitive impairment.[92] The World Anti-Doping Agency (WADA) and the NCAA do not ban most antiepileptic drugs, but athletes and providers need to keep current with the banned medication lists, as updates to these lists can occur.[89,93]

Water sports, archery, riflery, strength training, weightlifting, power lifting, and sports involving heights can present unique challenges for athletes with seizures, and limitations may be indicated for some individuals.[94,95] Water sports carry the risk of drowning, and aerial sports carry the risk of falls; these risks must be discussed with the individual and parents or guardians. The individual must never swim, dive, or train in the water alone.[89] Coaches should be informed so they are aware of the risks. Patients should inform their physician about any seizure activity, so control can be improved.

HEADACHES

In a survey of male and female athletes, 35% reported headaches during activity.[2,21,96] Frequent headaches can be caused or worsened by intense or prolonged physical activity and interfere with sports participation. Providers should consider the primary and secondary reasons for headache, including sport-specific causes, when evaluating an individual, as outlined in Box 5B-1.[97] Physical examination is performed to evaluate for secondary causes of headache by assessing blood pressure, examining the retina for papilledema, and evaluating cranial nerve and cerebellar function.

Box 5B-1. International Headache Society Classification of Headaches[97]

Primary Headaches
Migraine[a]
Tension-type headache
Trigeminal autonomic cephalalgias
Other primary headache disorders
    a. Primary cough headache (benign exertion headache)
    b. Primary exertion headache (effort headache)

Secondary Headaches
Headaches attributed to head/neck trauma (postconcussive headache)
Headaches attributed to cranial or cervical vascular disorder
Headache attributed to nonvascular intracranial disorder
Headache attributed to substance or its withdrawal
Headache attributed to infection
Headache attributed to disorders of homeostasis
Headache or facial pain attributed to disorders of cranium, neck, eyes, ears, sinuses, teeth, mouth, or other facial or cranial structure
Headache attributed to psychiatric disorder

[a] May be triggered by exercise.

Migraine headaches occur more often in females and frequently develop during adolescence,[38] with a community prevalence of 12% to 18%.[98] Migraines do not limit medical eligibility but may hamper performance and day-to-day participation. Migraines may be triggered by the stress of competition, by head trauma or head impact (heading a soccer ball), or physical exertion alone. Individuals with a history of migraines may take longer to recover following concussion, and concussion may exacerbate migraine frequency.[99–101] It is important to ask about migraine headache triggers so preventive strategies can be implemented.

Neither WADA nor the NCAA ban ergot derivatives or triptans, but β-blockers are banned for some athletes.[93] Some medications used in migraine treatment may impair performance or slow reaction time, increasing the risk of injury in some sports. Most athletes can compete effectively and safely after taking a triptan. Some athletes require precompetition prophylaxis. If treatment is needed during competition, an injectable, rapid-onset triptan may facilitate more rapid return to play.

Primary exertion headache is categorized under "Other Primary Headache Disorders."[97] The pathophysiological mechanisms underlying primary exertion headache are unknown. Most investigators believe it is vascular in origin. It is hypothesized that venous or arterial distension, secondary to physical exertion, is the pain-inducing mechanism. On first occurrence, it is mandatory to exclude subarachnoid hemorrhage, arterial dissection, and reversible cerebral vasoconstriction syndrome.

Prophylactic treatment strategies for recurrent exertion headaches include indomethacin and graduated exercise programs that stay slightly below the headache-onset threshold.[98] When evaluating an individual with effort-related headaches, it is important to ask about prior/current concussion and head injury. Following a concussion, an individual may continue to have headaches with exertion related to the head injury. In these cases, if exertion-related headaches were not present prior to the concussion, it may indicate that the brain is not completely healed and the individual should be restricted from contact sports and high-risk activities until the symptoms have resolved.[3]

Primary cough headache is brought on suddenly by coughing, straining, or the Valsalva maneuver in the absence of other intracranial pathology such as cerebral aneurysm or Arnold-Chiari malformation.[97] Imaging, particularly of the posterior fossa, is required to rule out secondary forms of cough headache. Treatment strategies include using nonsteroidal anti-inflammatory medications such as indomethacin and altering breathing patterns during weightlifting.[98]

REFERENCES

1. Miller DJ, Blum AB, Levine WN, Ahmad CS, Popkin CA. Preparticipation evaluation of the young athlete: what an orthopaedic surgeon needs to know. *Am J Sports Med.* 2015;44(6):1605–1615. PMID: 26330569
2. Patricios JS, Schneider KJ, Dvorak J, et al. Consensus statement on concussion in sport: the 6th International Conference on Concussion in Sport–Amsterdam, October 2022. *Br J Sport Med.* 2023;57(11):695–711. doi:10.1136/bjsports-2023-106898
3. McCrory P, Meeuwisse W, Dvořák J, et al. Consensus statement on concussion in sport—the 5th international conference on concussion in sport held in Berlin, October 2016. *Br J Sports Med.* 2017;51(11):838–847. PMID: 28446457
4. Aubry M, Cantu R, Dvorak J, et al; Concussion in Sport (CIS) Group. Summary and agreement statement of the 1st International Symposium on Concussion in Sport, Vienna 2001. *Clin J Sport Med.* 2002;12(1):6–11. PMID: 11854582
5. Giza CC, Hovda DA. The new neurometabolic cascade of concussion. *Neurosurgery.* 2014;75:S24–S33. PMID: 25232881
6. Barkhoudarian G, Hovda DA, Giza CC. The molecular pathophysiology of concussive brain injury. *Clin Sports Med.* 2011;30(1):33–48. PMID: 21074080
7. Choe MC, Babikian T, DiFiori J, Hovda DA, Giza CC. A pediatric perspective on concussion pathophysiology. *Curr Opin Pediatr.* 2012;24(6):689–695. PMID: 23080130
8. Harmon KG, Drezner J, Gammons M, et al; American Medical Society for Sports Medicine. American Medical Society for Sports Medicine position statement: concussion in sport. *Clin J Sport Med.* 2013;23(1):1–18. PMID: 23269325

9. Herring SA, Cantu RC, Guskiewicz KM, et al; American College of Sports Medicine. Concussion (mild traumatic brain injury) and the team physician: a consensus statement—2011 update. *Med Sci Sports Exerc.* 2011;43(12):2412–2422. PMID: 22089299
10. Shrey DW, Griesbach GS, Giza CC. The pathophysiology of concussions in youth. *Phys Med Rehabil Clin N Am.* 2011;22(4):577–602. PMID: 22050937
11. Vagnozzi R, Tavazzi B, Signoretti S, et al. Temporal window of metabolic brain vulnerability to concussions: mitochondrial-related impairment—part I. *Neurosurgery.* 2007;61(2):379–389. PMID: 17762751
12. Vagnozzi R, Signoretti S, Cristofori L, et al. Assessment of metabolic brain damage and recovery following mild traumatic brain injury: a multicentre, proton magnetic resonance spectroscopic study in concussed patients. *Brain.* 2010;133(11):3232–3242. PMID: 20736189
13. Tavazzi B, Vagnozzi R, Signoretti S, et al. Temporal window of metabolic brain vulnerability to concussions: oxidative and nitrosative stresses—part II. *Neurosurgery.* 2007;61(2):390–395. PMID: 17806141
14. Longhi L, Saatman KE, Fujimoto S, et al. Temporal window of vulnerability to repetitive experimental concussive brain injury. *Neurosurgery.* 2005;56(2):364–374. PMID: 15670384
15. Kissick J, Johnston KM. Return to play after concussion: principles and practice. *Clin J Sport Med.* 2005;15(6):426–431. PMID: 16278546
16. Cantu RC. Second-impact syndrome. *Clin Sports Med.* 1998;17(1):37–44. PMID: 9475969
17. McLendon LA, Kralik SF, Grayson PA, Golomb MR. The controversial second impact syndrome: a review of the literature. *Pediatr Neurol.* 2016;62:9–17. PMID: 27421756 doi:10.1016/j.pediatmeurol.2016.03.009
18. Engelhardt J, Brauge D, Loiseau H. Second impact syndrome. Myth or reality? *Neurochirurgie.* 2021;67(3):265–275. PMID: 32169407 doi:10.1016/j.neuchi.2019.12.007
19. Casa DJ, Guskiewicz KM, Anderson SA, et al. National Athletic Trainers' Association position statement: preventing sudden death in sports. *J Athl Train.* 2012;47(1):96–118. PMID: 22488236
20. Mueller FO. Catastrophic head injuries in high school and collegiate sports. *J Athl Train.* 2001;36(3):312–315. PMID: 12937502
21. Halstead ME, Walter KD, Moffatt K; American Academy of Pediatrics Council on Sports Medicine and Fitness; et al. Sport-related concussion in children and adolescents. *Pediatrics.* 2018;142(6):e20183074
22. Nelson LD, Guskiewicz KM, Barr WB, et al. Age differences in recovery after sport-related concussion: a comparison of high school and collegiate athletes. *J Athl Train.* 2016;51(2):142–152. PMID: 26974186
23. Williams RM, Puetz TW, Giza CC, Broglio SP. Concussion recovery time among high school and collegiate athletes: a systematic review and meta-analysis. *Sports Med.* 2015;45(6):893–903. PMID: 25820456
24. Erlanger D, Kaushik T, Cantu R, et al. Symptom-based assessment of the severity of a concussion. *J Neurosurg.* 2003;98(3):477–484. PMID: 12650417
25. Lee YM, Odom MJ, Zuckerman SL, Solomon GS, Sills AK. Does age affect symptom recovery after sports-related concussion? A study of high school and college athletes. *J Neurosurg Pediatr.* 2013;12(6):537–544. PMID: 24063601
26. Purcell L, Harvey J, Seabrook JA. Patterns of recovery following sport-related concussion in children and adolescents. *Clin Pediatr (Phila).* 2016;55(5):452–458. PMID: 26063756
27. McClincy MP, Lovell MR, Pardini J, Collins MW, Spore MK. Recovery from sports concussion in high school and collegiate athletes. *Brain Inj.* 2006;20(1):33–39. PMID: 16403698
28. Schneider KJ, Patricios JS. Amsterdam 2022 International Consensus on Concussion in Sport: calling clinicians to action! *Br J Sports Med.* 2023;57(11):615–616. https://bjsm.bmj.com/content/bjsports/57/11/615.full.pdf
29. Lovell MR, Pardini JE. New developments in sports concussion management. In: Slobounov S, Sebastianelli W, eds. *Foundations of Sport-Related Brain Injuries.* Springer; 2006:111–136
30. Zimmer A, Marcinak J, Hibyan, Webbe F. Normative values of major SCAT2 and SCAT3 components for a college athlete population. *Appl Neuropsychol: Adult.* 2015;22(2):132–140. doi:10.1080/23279095.2013.867265
31. Kerr ZY, Snook EM, Lynall RC, et al. Concussion-related protocols and preparticipation assessments used for incoming student-athletes in National Collegiate Athletic Association member institutions. *J Athl Train.* 2015;50(11):1174–1181. PMID: 26540099
32. Schmidt JD, Register-Mihalik JK, Mihalik JP, Kerr ZY, Guskiewicz KM. Identifying impairments after concussion: normative data versus individualized baselines. *Med Sci Sports Exerc.* 2012;44(9):1621–1628. PMID: 22525765
33. Mucha A, Collins MW, Elbin RJ, et al. A brief Vestibular/Ocular Motor Screening (VOMS) assessment to evaluate concussions: preliminary findings. *Am J Sports Med.* 2014;42(10):2479–2486. PMID: 25106780

34. Oldham JR, DiFabio MS, Kaminski TW, DeWolf RM, Buckley TA. Normative tandem gait in collegiate student-athletes: implications for clinical concussion assessment. *Sports Health*. 2017;9(4):305–311. PMID: 27899680
35. Brooks MA, Snedden TR, Mixis B, Hetzel S, McGuine TA. Establishing baseline normative values for the Child Sport Concussion Assessment Tool. *JAMA Pediatr.* 2017;171(7):670–677. PMID: 28492862
36. Davis GA, Purcell L, Schneider KJ, et al. The Child Sport Concussion Assessment Tool 5th Edition (Child SCAT5): background and rationale. *Br J Sports Med.* 2017;51(11):859–861. doi:10.1136/bjsports-2017-097492
37. Randolph C. Implementation of neuropsychological testing models for the high school, collegiate, and professional sport settings. *J Athl Train.* 2001;36(3):288–296. PMID: 12937498
38. Lipton RB, Bigal ME, Steiner TJ, Silberstein SD, Olesen J. Classification of primary headaches. *Neurology.* 2004;63(3):427–435. PMID: 15304572
39. Yengo-Kahn AM, Hale AT, Zalneraitis BH, Zuckerman SL, Sills AK, Solomon GS. The Sport Concussion Assessment Tool: a systematic review. *Neurosurg Focus.* 2016;40(4):E6. PMID: 27032923
40. Alsalaheen B, McClafferty A, Haines J, Smith L, Yorke A. Reference values for the balance error scoring system in adolescents. *Brain Inj.* 2016;30(7):914–918. PMID: 27057617
41. Hansen C, Cushman D, Anderson N, et al. A normative dataset of the balance error scoring system in children aged between 5 and 14. *Clin J Sport Med.* 2016;26(6):497–501. PMID: 27783573
42. Corwin DJ, Wiebe DJ, Zonfrillo MR, et al. Vestibular deficits following youth concussion. *J Pediatr.* 2015;166(5):1221–1225. PMID: 25748568
43. Tjarks BJ, Dorman JC, Valentine VD, et al. Comparison and utility of King-Devick and ImPACT® composite scores in adolescent concussion patients. *J Neurol Sci.* 2013;334(1-2):148–153. PMID: 24007870
44. Pearce KL, Sufrinko A, Lau BC, Henry L, Collins MW, Kontos AP. Near point of convergence after a sport-related concussion: measurement reliability and relationship to neurocognitive impairment and symptoms. *Am J Sports Med.* 2015;43(12):3055–3061. PMID: 26453625
45. Vernau BT, Grady MF, Goodman A, et al. Oculomotor and neurocognitive assessment of youth ice hockey players: baseline associations and observations after concussion. *Dev Neuropsychol.* 2015;40(1):7–11. PMID: 25649773
46. Echemendia RJ, Meeuwisse W, McCrory P, et al. The Sport Concussion Assessment Tool 5th Edition (SCAT5): background and rationale. *Br J Sports Med.* 2017;51:848–850. doi:10.1136/bjsports-2017-097506
47. National Collegiate Athletic Association. Concussion Safety Protocol Checklist. Updated September 2023. https://ncaaorg.s3.amazonaws.com/ssi/concussion/SSI_ConcussionSafetyProtocolChecklist.pdf
48. Grubenhoff JA, Currie D, Comstock RD, Juarez-Colunga E, Bajaj L, Kirkwood MW. Psychological factors associated with delayed symptom resolution in children with concussion. *J Pediatr.* 2016;174:27–32.e1. PMID: 27079963
49. Root JM, Zuckerbraun NS, Wang L, et al. History of somatization is associated with prolonged recovery from concussion. *J Pediatr.* 2016;174:39–44.e1. PMID: 27059916
50. Moser RS, Schatz P, Jordan BD. Prolonged effects of concussion in high school athletes. *Neurosurgery.* 2005;57(2):300–306. PMID: 16094159
51. Broglio SP, Cantu RC, Gioia GA, et al; National Athletic Trainers' Association. National Athletic Trainers' Association position statement: management of sport concussion. *J Athl Train.* 2014;49(2):245–265. PMID: 24601910
52. Harmon KG, Clugston JR, Dec K, et al. American Medical Society for Sports Medicine position statement on concussion in sport. *Br J Sports Med.* 2019;53(4):213–225. PMID: 30705232 doi:10.1136/bjsports-2018-100338
53. Preiss-Farzanegan SJ, Chapman B, Wong TM, Wu J, Bazarian JJ. The relationship between gender and postconcussion symptoms after sport-related mild traumatic brain injury. *PM R.* 2009;1(3):245–253. PMID: 19627902
54. Savica R, Parisi JE, Wold LE, Josephs KA, Ahlskog JE. High school football and risk of neurodegeneration: a community-based study. *Mayo Clin Proc.* 2012;87(4):335–340. PMID: 22469346
55. Deshpande SK, Hasegawa RB, Rabinowitz AR, et al. Association of playing high school football with cognition and mental health later in life. *JAMA Neurol.* 2017;74(8):909–918. PMID: 28672325 doi:10.1001/jamaneurol.2017.1317
56. Smith AM, Stuart MJ, Roberts WO, et al. Concussion in ice hockey: current gaps and future directions in an objective diagnosis. *Clin J Sport Med.* 2017;27(5):503–509. doi:10.1097/JSM.0000000000000412

57. Papa L, Ramia MM, Edwards D, Johnson BD, Slobounov SM. Systematic review of clinical studies examining biomarkers of brain injury in athletes after sports-related concussion. *J Neurotrauma.* 2015;32(10):661–673. PMID: 25254425 doi:10.1089/neu.2014.3655
58. Kawata K, Liu CY, Merkel SF, Ramirez SH, Tierney RT, Langford D. Blood biomarkers for brain injury: what are we measuring? *Neurosci Biobehav Rev.* 2016;68:460–473. PMID: 27181909 doi:10.1016/j.neubiorev.2016.05.009
59. Petraglia AL, Winkler EA, Bailes JE. Stuck at the bench: potential natural neuroprotective compounds for concussion. *Surg Neurol Int.* 2011;2:146. PMID: 22059141
60. Ashbaugh A, McGrew C. The role of nutritional supplements in sports concussion treatment. *Curr Sports Med Rep.* 2016;15(1):16–19. PMID: 26745164
61. Ellis MJ, McDonald PJ, Cordingley D, Mansouri B, Essig M, Ritchie L. Retirement-from-sport considerations following pediatric sports-related concussion: case illustrations and institutional approach. *Neurosurg Focus.* 2016;40(4):E8. PMID: 27032925
62. Cantu RC, Register-Mihalik JK. Considerations for return-to-play and retirement decisions after concussion. *PM R.* 2011;3(10 suppl 2):S440–S444. PMID: 22035687
63. Concannon LG, Kaufman MS, Herring SA. The million dollar question: when should an athlete retire after concussion? *Curr Sports Med Rep.* 2014;13(6):365–369. PMID: 25391091
64. Torg JS, Pavlov H, Genuario SE, et al. Neurapraxia of the cervical spinal cord with transient quadriplegia. *J Bone Joint Surg Am.* 1986;68(9):1354–1370. PMID: 3782207
65. Pavlov H, Torg JS, Robie B, Jahre C. Cervical spinal stenosis: determination with vertebral body ratio method. *Radiology.* 1987;164(3):771–775. PMID: 3615879
66. Cantu RV, Cantu RC. Current thinking: return to play and transient quadriplegia. *Curr Sports Med Rep.* 2005;4(1):27–32. PMID: 15659276
67. Cantu RC. The cervical spinal stenosis controversy. *Clin Sports Med.* 1998;17(1):121–126. PMID: 9475976
68. Kurian PA, Light DI, Kerr HA. Burners, stingers, and cervical cord neurapraxia/transient quadriparesis. In: O'Brien M, Meehan WP, eds. *Head and Neck Injuries in Young Athletes. Contemporary Pediatric and Adolescent Sports Medicine.* Springer; 2016:121–149. https://doi.org/10.1007/978-3-319-23549-3_10
69. Torg JS, Corcoran TA, Thibault LE, et al. Cervical cord neurapraxia: classification, pathomechanics, morbidity, and management guidelines. *J Neurosurg.* 1997;87(6):843–850. PMID: 9384393
70. Hsu WK. Transient quadriparesis and cervical neuropraxia in elite athletes. *Clin Sports Med.* 2021;40(3):463–470. PMID: 34051940
71. Boockvar JA, Durham SR, Sun PP. Cervical spinal stenosis and sports-related cervical cord neurapraxia in children. *Spine (Phila Pa 1976).* 2001;26(24):2709–2712. PMID: 11740359 doi:10.1097/00007632-200112150-00015
72. Bowles DR, Canseco JA, Alexander TD, Schroeder GD, Hecht AC, Vaccaro AR. The Prevalence and management of stingers in college and professional collision athletes. *Curr Rev Musculoskelet Med.* 2020;13(6):651–662. PMID: 32691363 doi:10.1007/s12178-020-09665-5
73. Charbonneau RM, McVeigh SA, Thompson K. Brachial neuropraxia in Canadian Atlantic University sport football players: what is the incidence of "stingers"? *Clin J Sport Med.* 2012;22(6):472–477. PMID: 23006981
74. Starr HM Jr, Anderson B, Courson R, Seiler JG. Brachial plexus injury: a descriptive study of American football. *J Surg Orthop Adv.* 2014;23(2):90–97. PMID: 24875339
75. Clancy WG Jr, Brand RL, Bergfield JA. Upper trunk brachial plexus injuries in contact sports. *Am J Sports Med.* 1977;5(5):209–216. PMID: 907035
76. Sallis RE, Jones K, Knopp W. Burners. *Phys Sportsmed.* 1992;20(11):47–55. PMID: 29283810
77. Levitz CL, Reilly PJ, Torg JS. The pathomechanics of chronic, recurrent cervical nerve root neurapraxia: the chronic burner syndrome. *Am J Sports Med.* 1997;25(1):73–76. PMID: 9006696
78. Weinberg J, Rokito S, Silber JS. Etiology, treatment, and prevention of athletic "stingers." *Clin Sports Med.* 2003;22(3):493–500. PMID: 12852682
79. Kang K-C, Lee HS, Lee J-H. Cervical radiculopathy focus on characteristics and differential diagnosis. *Asian Spine J.* 2020;14(6):921–930. PMID: 33373515 doi:10.31616/asj.2020.0647
80. Leffert RD. Clinical diagnosis, testing, and electromyographic study in brachial plexus traction injuries. *Clin Orthop Relat Res.* 1988(237):24–31. PMID: 3191635
81. Zaneteas PD. Brachial plexus injuries and the electrodiagnostic examination. *Curr Sports Med Rep.* 2003;2(1):7–14. PMID: 12831670

82. Conley KM, Bolin DJ, Carek PJ, Konin JG, Neal TL, Violette D. National Athletic Trainers' Association position statement: preparticipation physical examinations and disqualifying conditions. *J Athl Train.* 2014;49(1):102–120. PMID: 24499039
83. Huang P, Anissipour A, McGee W, Lemak L. Return-to-play recommendations after cervical, thoracic, and lumbar spine injuries: a comprehensive review. *Sports Health.* 2016;8(1):19–25. PMID: 26502187
84. Rowson S, McNeely DE, Brolinson PG, Duma SM. Biomechanical analysis of football neck collars. *Clin J Sport Med.* 2008;18(4):316–321. PMID: 18614882
85. Heck JF, Clarke KS, Peterson TR, Torg JS, Weis MP. National Athletic Trainers' Association position statement: head-down contact and spearing in tackle football. *J Athl Train.* 2004;39(1):101–111. PMID: 15085218
86. Jae-Min Park A, Nelson SE, Mesfin A. Klippel-Feil syndrome: clinical presentation and management. *JBJS Rev.* 2022;10(2):e21.00166. doi:10.2106/JBJS.RVW.21.00166
87. Holmes FC. Klippel-Feil syndrome in a cheerleader. *Clin J Sport Med.* 2007;17(2):154–156 PMID: 17414488 10.1097/JSM.0b013e31803202ed
88. Marx RG, Wilson SM, Swiontkowski MF. Updating the assignment of levels of evidence. *J Bone Joint Surg Am.* 2015;97(1):1–2. PMID: 25568387
89. Dubow JS, Kelly JP. Epilepsy in sports and recreation. *Sports Med.* 2003;33(7):499–516. PMID: 12762826
90. Howard GM, Radloff M, Sevier TL. Epilepsy and sports participation. *Curr Sports Med Rep.* 2004;3(1):15–19. PMID: 14728909
91. D'Ambrosio R, Perucca E. Epilepsy after head injury. *Curr Opin Neurol.* 2004;17(6):731–735. PMID: 15542983
92. Hirtz D, Berg A, Bettis D, et al; Quality Standards Subcommittee of the American Academy of Neurology; Practice Committee of the Child Neurology Society. Practice parameter: treatment of the child with a first unprovoked seizure: report of the Quality Standards Subcommittee of the American Academy of Neurology and the Practice Committee of the Child Neurology Society. *Neurology.* 2003;60(2):166–175. PMID: 12552027
93. National Collegiate Athletic Association. *Diagnosis and Management of Sport-Related Concussion Best Practices.* Accessed February 17, 2025. https://www.aan.com/siteassets/home-page/tools-and-resources/practicing-neurologist--administrators/patient-resources/sports-concussion-resources/17ncaaconcussion_tr.pdf
94. Grafe MW, Paul GR, Foster TE. The preparticipation sports examination for high school and college athletes. *Clin Sports Med.* 1997;16(4):569–591. PMID: 9330803
95. Rice SG; American Academy of Pediatrics Council on Sports Medicine and Fitness. Medical conditions affecting sports participation. *Pediatrics.* 2008;121(4):841–848. PMID: 18381550
96. Williams SJ, Nukada H. Sport and exercise headache: Part 1. Prevalence among university students. *Br J Sports Med.* 1994;28(2):90–95. PMID: 7921915
97. Headache Classification Committee of the International Headache Society (IHS). The International Classification of Headache Disorders, 3rd edition (ICHD-3). *Cephalalgia.* 2018;38(1):1–211. doi:10.1177/0333102417738202
98. Lewis DW. Headaches in children and adolescents. *Am Fam Physician.* 2002;65(4):625–632. PMID: 11871680
99. McCrory P. Headaches and exercise. *Sports Med.* 2000;30(3):221–229. PMID: 10999425
100. Mihalik JP, Stump JE, Collins MW, Lovell MR, Field M, Maroon JC. Posttraumatic migraine characteristics in athletes following sports-related concussion. *J Neurosurg.* 2005;102(5):850–855. PMID: 15926709
101. Lau B, Lovell MR, Collins MW, Pardini J. Neurocognitive and symptom predictors of recovery in high school athletes. *Clin J Sport Med.* 2009;19(3):216–221. PMID: 19423974

C: General Medical Conditions

MEDICAL HISTORY

History Form Questions

1. *List past and current medical conditions (including mental health disorders such as attention-deficit/hyperactivity disorder, anxiety, depression).*
2. *Have you ever had surgery? If yes, list all past surgical procedures.*
3. *Medications and supplements: List all current prescriptions, over-the-counter medicines, and supplements (herbal and nutritional).*
4. *Do you have any allergies? If yes, please list all your allergies (eg, medicines, pollens, food, stinging insects).*
5. *Do you have any concerns that you would like to discuss with your provider?*
6. *Has a provider ever denied or restricted your participation in sports for any reason?*
7. *Have you had any recent illness?*
8. *Are you missing a kidney, an eye, a testicle, spleen, or any other organ? Are any of these organs not functioning properly?*
9. *Have you ever become ill while exercising in the heat?*
10. *Do you or does someone in your family have sickle cell trait or disease?*
11. *Have you ever had or do you have any problems with your eyes or vision?*

Secondary Questions

- When, why, and how long were you restricted from participation?
- Have you seen a physician for this?
- Are you receiving any treatments or taking any medications for the condition that resulted in your restrictions?
- Do you have any follow-up medical visits or scheduled appointments for the condition?
- What has changed since you were restricted from participation?
- Do you still have the problem that caused your restriction from sports?
- Have you been restricted from participation for other problems?
- Have you stayed overnight in the hospital?
- Have you had any acute care visits, emergency department visits, or hospitalizations in the past 2 years?

Key Points

- Only 1% to 2% of screened individuals are completely restricted from sports participation.
- The preparticipation evaluation (PPE) may identify chronic medical conditions and other measures of general health status that can warrant more in-depth evaluation and follow-up.
- Based on the presence of any current or prior medical conditions, medical eligibility can be coordinated with appropriate subspecialists to determine the most appropriate participation status and to monitor safe participation.

Reports of chronic medical conditions offer opportunities to determine the potential influences on performance and medical eligibility, as well as an assessment of general health. Individuals with adequate control of a chronic illness can usually participate in most sports without restrictions, but ongoing monitoring and care are essential. Some medications can have adverse effects on performance and safety during sports participation, and some are prohibited by the World Anti-Doping Agency (WADA), National Collegiate Athletic Association (NCAA), or other National Governing Bodies, which is important to know when caring for athletes competing at these levels of competition. Similarly, the use of supplements, vitamins, and nutritional aids may or may not be appropriate and may include substances that are prohibited by the aforementioned governing bodies. While genetic testing is increasingly marketed as a means to improve performance and health or reduce injury risk, its use is not evidence based and does not represent the current standard of care.

WEIGHT CONCERNS

Individuals who are underweight, overweight, or obese may be predisposed to long-term health issues that can influence eligibility and the risk of injury or illness during sport participation. During the PPE, values for height, weight, and body mass index (BMI) can be plotted on age-appropriate growth charts and compared, if possible, with past measurements. The classification of underweight, overweight, and obesity is based on age- and sex-based BMI percentiles (Table 5C-1).[1] It is important to recognize that BMI does not measure body composition directly and may overestimate adiposity in muscular individuals, potentially leading to an inaccurate classification; nonetheless, BMI has acceptable clinical validity for most people and can serve as a useful screening tool during the PPE to help identify potential risks.[2] Guidance regarding individuals with underweight is covered in Chapter 5I.

Table 5C-1. Terminology for Body Mass Index Categories for Children Based on Percentile for Age

Body Mass Index Category for Age	Percentile Range for Age
Underweight	< 5th percentile
Normal or healthy weight	5th–85th percentile
Overweight	85th–95th percentile
Obesity	> 95th percentile

Adapted from Barlow SE; American Academy of Pediatrics Expert Committee. Expert committee recommendations regarding the prevention, assessment, and treatment of child and adolescent overweight and obesity: summary report. *Pediatrics*. 2007;120(suppl 4):S164–S192.

With any patient who has overweight or obesity, regular physical activity should be promoted as a vitally important health intervention, and limiting medical eligibility may be counterproductive. However, some medical and musculoskeletal concerns should be addressed in this population during the PPE and before determining medical eligibility.

- Children who have overweight or obesity are at higher risk for slipped capital femoral epiphysis[2] as well as musculoskeletal injuries.[3,4]
- Individuals who have obesity are at increased risk for heat illness.[5] Fat tissue serves as an insulator, storing metabolic heat and delaying heat transfer to the environment

during exercise. Individuals with overweight or obesity may need additional education about sufficient acclimatization and hydration, as well as potential activity and recovery modifications during competition and training to reduce the risk of exertional heat illnesses.[6]

- Healthy food choices and maintenance of a healthy weight can enhance athletic performance and improve health status (see https://www.healthychildren.org/English/ages-stages/gradeschool/nutrition/Pages/Making-Healthy-Food-Choices.aspx).
- The PPE can serve as an initial conversation with individuals who have overweight or obesity to promote physical activity and sport participation as part of a broader intervention to reduce weight, improve fitness, reduce injury and illness risk, and establish a healthy lifestyle.[7,8]

DIABETES MELLITUS

With individualized counseling and planning, good glucose control, and the absence of organ-specific complications, individuals with DM can participate in most sports without restrictions.

Physical activity is considered an important element of disease treatment in diabetes mellitus (DM), and the overall risk of exercise-related events among individuals with DM is low. Nonetheless, individuals with type 1 or type 2 DM are at risk for disease-related complications.[9] Organ-specific complications of DM, including cardiovascular disease (hypertension and coronary artery disease), peripheral vascular disease, retinopathy, nephropathy, neuropathy (peripheral and autonomic), and gastroparesis can limit participation in some activities.[10]

In addition, individuals with DM may be at an increased risk of developing musculoskeletal conditions such as tendinopathies, tenosynovitis, and adhesive capsulitis. These are more commonly seen in adult patients, but can occur in children.

- For patients with coronary artery or peripheral vascular disease, individualized activity recommendations should be determined by either the primary care physician or the consultant.
- Individuals with moderate to severe nonproliferative or proliferative retinopathy should avoid activities that significantly elevate blood pressure due to the Valsalva maneuver, such as weight lifting, or have repetitive high impact, such as jogging.[9,10]
- Diabetic nephropathy typically does not limit exercise participation, but each patient needs to be evaluated and given individualized guidelines.[10,11]
- Patients with autonomic neuropathy may be unable to participate in certain activities, but recommendations should be individualized. Neuropathy can cause muscle weakness, foot deformities, and balance impairments, which may increase the risk of falls and injuries. These individuals may also be at an increased risk of hypothermia or exertional heat illness because of thermoregulatory dysfunction, as well as postural hypotension during activity.[11]
- Significant peripheral neuropathy may limit weight-bearing exercise, given the risk for fractures and ulcer formation.[10]
- Diabetic gastroparesis can influence fluid, nutrient, and electrolyte absorption, potentially limiting participation in strenuous or prolonged exercise, especially in higher temperatures.

Before participation, instruction in appropriate blood glucose concentrations and blood glucose monitoring, dietary choices (particularly carbohydrate intake), hydration, and insulin therapy before, during, and after activity will improve safety and performance. Hyperglycemia and hypoglycemia can occur during exercise, particularly among individuals with type 1 DM. Each individual needs to be educated regarding the potential signs and symptoms of hyperglycemia and hypoglycemia and have an emergency action plan for athletic activity. Continuous glucose monitoring may help reduce the fear of hypoglycemic events during activity, aid in preactivity insulin dosing, and help identify blood glucose responses to different physical activity modes, intensities, and durations.[12,13] With individualized counseling and planning, good glucose control, and the absence of organ-specific complications, individuals with DM can participate in most sports without restrictions.[14,15]

Because of the potentially serious or even fatal implications of hypoglycemia during exercise, certain sports such as rock climbing, skydiving, and scuba diving are considered high-risk for individuals who have diabetes. The process of training for and participating in solo endurance or ultra-endurance events, such as ultramarathons, triathlons, or open-water swimming, requires individualized support and monitoring during training and competition. Training and competition partners can improve response time in the event of hypoglycemic incidents and reduce the risk of serious events.

Different modes, intensities, and durations of activity can have different effects on individual insulin needs. When possible each individual should identify their typical response to exercise and how this interacts with dietary and environmental conditions to guide appropriate insulin modifications. Training regimens that simulate competitive demands can help establish appropriate glucose and insulin dosing before, during, and after exercise.[10]

Many patients with diabetes use insulin pumps, and reductions in basal rates or bolus dosing before exercise may be necessary. If the device is suspended or disconnected during exercise lasting longer than 60 minutes, supplemental insulin should be used.[16] Certain insulin pumps may be able to be used during swimming, and pumps can be used during contact sports provided that the device is properly padded and secured and a backup pump or insulin supply is available if the device is damaged.[16]

Pumps can be used during contact sports provided that the device is properly padded and secured and a backup pump or insulin supply is available if the device is damaged.

Individuals should routinely check their blood glucose level before exercise to guide preactivity glucose intake. Levels above 250 mg/dL require testing of urine or blood for ketone levels. If ketone levels are present, exercise is contraindicated.[16,17]

BLOOD-BORNE PATHOGENS

HIV, hepatitis B virus (HBV), and hepatitis C virus (HCV) are blood-borne pathogens that could theoretically be transmitted during sport participation. While these viruses can potentially spread through contact with body fluids and open wounds, the risk of

Every individual with DM should have an individualized, written action plan for games and practices that is developed collaboratively with the individual (and parents or guardians if the individual is a minor) and medical providers. The school nurses, athletic trainers, coaches, and key activity or sport supervisors should be apprised of the plan and given a written copy.[16] Elements of the care plan should include

- **Guidelines for monitoring and interpreting blood glucose and urine ketone levels, when indicated**
- **Guidelines for insulin therapy, including adjustments for hyperglycemia**
- **Guidelines for rapid treatment of hypoglycemia, including intake of short-acting carbohydrates and use of glucagon**
- **Instructions for changes in glucose intake and monitoring for a given duration or intensity of athletic participation**
- **Guidelines for recognizing hypoglycemia and hyperglycemia, including key signs and symptoms, along with recommended response and treatment options[16]**
- **Medication list**

All individuals who have DM should wear a medication and disease alert tag at all times, and all necessary testing equipment and supplies (including snacks to help rapidly elevate blood glucose) should be in a first aid pack that is readily accessible and fully charged.

transmission during sport participation is believed to be very low. Instead, transmission more commonly occurs through sexual contact, body piercing, tattoos, and the sharing of needles to administer injected anabolic steroids and other drugs.[17]

HIV infections in sports are extremely rare, as there are no well-documented cases of transmission in sports. It was estimated that the theoretical risk of transmission during professional American football was 1 in 85 million game contacts.[18] This risk may be an overestimation, however, as it was extrapolated from data on transmission from needlesticks in health care settings and determined prior to the wide availability of effective antiviral medications.

HBV, on the other hand, is more concentrated in blood than is HIV and more easily transmitted.[19] Research publications from Japan and the United States reported HBV transmission in a high school sumo wrestling club and a college American-rules football team, respectively, and transmission probably occurred because of contact with open wounds in the carrier during sporting activity.[19] In addition, HBV can remain stable on environmental surfaces for up to 1 week, making it potentially transmissible through contact with shared surfaces.[20] HBV immunization reduces this risk. Transmission during professional American football has been estimated at 1 in 850,000 to 4.25 million game contacts. HCV blood concentrations are thought to fall between those of HIV and those of HBV. There are no documented cases of transmission in sports or estimates of transmission risk.

Even in sports in which there is sustained close body contact, the transmission of HIV, HBV, and HCV appears to be very low.[19] Since the risk of transmission is minimal, the NCAA, National Federation of State High School Associations, American Academy of Pediatrics (AAP), and American Medical Society for Sports Medicine (AMSSM) do not view HIV, HBV, or HCV infections as a reason to exclude individuals from participation. Mandatory HIV screening is not recommended by any major sport governing bodies for participation,[17] and for individuals who are known to be living with HIV, participation has not been limited.[14] Confidentiality must be maintained at all times, and the decision to disclose HIV, HBV, or HCV status is up to the individual and family (if the individual is a minor).

Universal precautions are recommended to limit pathogen transmission when handling blood or other body fluids. Education includes both universal precautions and high-risk behaviors such as sharing needles, body piercing or tattoo placement with potentially contaminated equipment, and unprotected sexual activity.

Since the risk of transmission is minimal, the NCAA, National Federation of State High School Associations, American Academy of Pediatrics (AAP), and American Medical Society for Sports Medicine (AMSSM) do not view HIV, HBV, or HCV infections as a reason to exclude individuals from participation.

INFECTIOUS MONONUCLEOSIS

Key Points

- Splenomegaly is almost universally present with infectious mononucleosis (IM).
- Splenic rupture is extremely rare beyond 28 days from the onset of IM symptoms.

IM is a common illness in adolescents and young adults caused by the Epstein-Barr virus (EBV), transmitted through close-contact exposure with saliva or mucous of an infected individual. Cytomegalovirus infection also may be a cause of mononucleosis, although less commonly. A diagnosis of IM may be suggested by the patient's presentation and confirmed with laboratory testing. Symptoms may include the classic triad of fever, exudative pharyngitis, and posterior cervical lymphadenopathy,[21] along with fatigue, headache, and left upper quadrant pain. Clinical manifestations of IM are not specific, however, and physical examination is neither sensitive nor specific. The diagnosis can be confirmed in an individual who has the clinical picture with a combination of a complete blood cell count with at least 50% lymphocytes and 10% atypical lymphocytes,[22] a positive result from a heterophile antibody test (specifically, the monospot test), elevated liver transaminases, and/or elevated EBV immunoglobulin (Ig) M and IgG antibody titers. Diagnosis based on EBV antibody titers is preferred because of decreased sensitivity and specificity of the monospot test in the pediatric population. Supportive care is the foundation for management of IM.

The fatigue associated with IM may limit return to full sport participation for several weeks. In rare cases, fatigue may persist for months after infection, limiting participation in sports. Splenomegaly, and the potential for splenic rupture, is an underlying concern in the first 2 to 4 weeks of the illness while the spleen is enlarging in response to the infection. Splenic rupture can occur during exertion and without trauma. Studies show a 0.1% to 0.2% prevalence of splenic rupture in athletes with IM.[21] The greatest risk for splenic rupture is in the first 21 days after the onset of IM symptoms, and the highest risk is in males younger than 30 years within 4 weeks of symptom onset.[22] Splenic rupture beyond 28 days of symptoms can occur, but it is very rare.[23,24]

Splenic rupture beyond 28 days of symptoms can occur, but it is very rare.

Return to activity and medical eligibility decisions traditionally have been based on resolution of clinical symptoms (mainly fatigue) and the absence of splenomegaly.[22] Physical examination is not sufficiently reliable for quantifying splenic enlargement, although resolution of clinically palpable splenic enlargement during serial monitoring can be helpful in return-to-play decisions.[25] Serial ultrasonography can be used to monitor individual spleen size in IM, to evaluate whether it is trending in the correct direction (ie, decreasing in size). Studies using this modality have shown that spleen size tends to normalize within 28 days.[25] Although normative values for spleen size have been established in a heterogeneous subset of the population, there is considerable variation in normal spleen size between individuals (especially taller athletes), and spleen size alone is not an accurate predictor of the risk of rupture.[26,27] Consequently, the use of ultrasonography is controversial in individual cases and has not been found to be a useful guide for return-to-play decisions.[22,25,27] Serial laboratory testing is also not helpful for return to play decision-making.[22]

Return to play decisions after IM should be individualized for each athlete and family and based on a collaborative, shared decision-making approach. The AMSSM consensus statement recommends no return to sport for 3 to 4 weeks after the onset of IM symptoms, mainly to reduce the risk of splenic rupture.[22,27] Individuals may resume light noncontact activities at 3 to 4 weeks if they are afebrile, they are well hydrated, and their weight and energy levels have been regained. Return to contact or collision activity is more controversial and is not advised for at least 4 weeks after symptom onset, with at least 1 week of noncontact conditioning activities before contact.[22,27] The utility of serial measurement of splenic size to guide return to sport is poorly defined, although decreasing or stable spleen size on serial measurements could be used to inform decision-making for individuals looking to return to contact activity earlier than 4 weeks.[27]

Highly trained individuals and those with significant fatigue during the course of IM may take several months to return to their previous level of fitness. A rapid return to sport may increase the risk of splenic injury and may prolong overall recovery time.[14,22]

Individuals with chronic splenomegaly or hepatomegaly require individual and sport-specific assessment that is based on the degree of organ enlargement and underlying disease states.[14]

SURGICAL HISTORY

History Form Question

1. *Have you ever had surgery? If yes, list all past surgical procedures.*

Secondary Questions

- What type of surgery did you have?
- When and where did you have it?
- Why was the surgery done, and was any treatment tried before the surgery?
- Are you still under the care of the surgeon?

- Are any future surgical procedures being planned?
- Did you gain or lose weight or muscle mass after the surgery?
- Have you been fully cleared by the surgeon to return to sports?
- Do you have any problems from the surgery itself that limit your participation in sports?
- Did you complete a rehabilitation program or see a physical therapist or an athletic trainer after the surgery?

Key Points

- A surgical history may reveal past or current issues that affect medical eligibility for sport participation.
- Complete recovery with no physical activity restrictions that is based on the final evaluation by the surgical team is required for full medical eligibility.

Following surgical procedures, the surgical team should determine readiness for return to physical activity and participation in specific sports. A progressive stepwise return-to-sport program is individualized based on the type of surgery, body parts involved, and general health of the athlete before and after the procedure. An uncomplicated appendectomy or similar procedures typically result in a quick and full recovery in a predictable time frame and with limited impact on future athletic participation. Higher-risk procedures involving the colon, major joints, paired organs, the heart, or the brain may result in longer recovery times, potential restrictions on future participation in specific activities, and/or the use of protective equipment to participate in some activities. Individuals with persistent or easily induced fatigue, continued weight loss, or insufficient rehabilitation (especially following orthopedic procedures) may be at higher risk for new or recurrent injury, and medical eligibility may be deferred until they have fully recovered. Ongoing use of postoperative medications, particularly narcotic pain medications, which may be habit-forming and impair cognitive function, stamina, and reaction time, suggests that an individual is not ready for return to sport.

■ MEDICATIONS

History Form Question

1. *Medications and supplements: List all current prescriptions, over-the-counter medicines, vitamins, and supplements (herbal and nutritional).*

Secondary Questions

- Do you use anything for your skin?
- Are you currently taking any daily or as-needed medications prescribed by your doctor?

Key Points

- Use of medications may reveal medical issues not revealed or recognized in the medical history.
- Any prescription medication, over-the-counter medication, or supplement may affect exercise performance or safety.
- Certain medications may be banned by a sport national governing body or require a WADA therapeutic use exemption.

The PPE is an opportunity to review medications, supplements, and ergogenic aids; counsel individuals on potential risks and benefits; and optimize the frequency and dosing of prescription medications to better control underlying illnesses during exercise. In some cases, participation in sports may require adjustments in the timing and dosing of certain medications, such as using short-acting β-adrenergic agonists before exercise for asthma or adjusting insulin doses depending on the volume and intensity of exercise for individuals who have DM. For athletes who are subject to drug testing (eg, elite athletes, NCAA athletes), information about banned substances can be found at https://www.wada-ama.org/en/prohibited-list and https://www.ncaa.org/sports/2015/6/10/ncaa-banned-substances.aspx. Additional information on supplements is discussed in Chapter 5I.

ALLERGIES AND ANAPHYLAXIS

History Form Question

1. *Do you have any allergies? If yes, please list all your allergies (eg, medicines, pollens, food, stinging insects).*

Secondary Questions

- Have you ever had a severe allergic reaction? If so, to what and what was the reaction?
- Are there certain foods or groups of foods you have been told to avoid because of allergic reactions?
- Did this reaction involve swelling of your lips or tongue, or did it make it difficult for you to swallow, talk, or breathe?
- Have you ever needed medicine, including injected medicine, to treat an allergic reaction?
- Have you ever been taken to an emergency department, been put into the hospital, or had a breathing tube placed because of an allergic reaction?
- Do you carry or have you been told to carry an EpiPen or another epinephrine device (eg, nasal epinephrine)?

Key Points

- Allergic reactions can range from minor rhinitis to life-threatening anaphylaxis.
- Individuals with a history of true anaphylaxis should have immediate on-site access to injected or nasal epinephrine. A history of exercise-associated anaphylaxis requires a thorough evaluation and may require exercise modifications with restricted medical eligibility.
- An emergency action plan involving on-site medical staff, coaches, and other supervising personnel should be created, discussed, and reviewed at the beginning of each season.

An emergency action plan involving on-site medical staff, coaches, and other supervising personnel should be created, discussed, and reviewed at the beginning of each season.

Allergic Reactions and Anaphylaxis

Minor allergic reactions may influence athletic performance and can be associated with asthma, vocal cord dysfunction, and exercise-induced bronchospasm (see Chapter 5D). Improved baseline control of environmental allergies can improve performance, though adverse effects of some antihistamine medications may impair exercise capacity.

True anaphylaxis involves more than one body system and starts with localized erythema and edema before rapidly progressing to generalized urticaria, pruritus, airway obstructions caused by lip or tongue swelling, laryngospasm and laryngeal edema, and progressive hemodynamic instability. Insect envenomation or food allergies (often peanuts or shellfish) are common triggers. Many foods, such as energy bars, contain nuts or are cross-contaminated with nuts during production and may represent a risk for individuals with nut allergies. Past reactions to stinging insects such as Hymenoptera (ie, bees, wasps, and yellow jackets) or fire ants can be a risk for outdoor sport athletes. It is critical to differentiate between localized reactions and systemic urticaria, and life-threatening anaphylaxis. Individuals with local reactions do not require exercise modification or on-site epinephrine.

Any individual with a past history of anaphylaxis should have immediate access to epinephrine on site (or on person for certain events such as distance running or cycling). Academic institutions may restrict students from carrying epinephrine, potentially limiting access and influencing medical eligibility decisions. It is important to have an emergency action plan involving on-site medical staff, coaches, and other supervising personnel that is created, discussed, and reviewed at the beginning of each season. Consultation with an allergist for specific recommendations, potential allergen testing, and immunotherapy (especially with venom-associated anaphylaxis) is highly recommended.[28]

Exercise-Induced Anaphylaxis

Exercise-induced anaphylaxis (EIAn) is a rare form of systemic allergic reaction induced by exercise and characterized by a spectrum of symptoms and signs ranging from a sensation of warmth, pruritus, cutaneous erythema, angioedema, and giant (> 1 cm in diameter) urticaria to hypotension, shock, and death. The underlying mechanism remains poorly defined. In food-dependent forms of EIAn (FDEIAn), exercise may augment the IgE-mediated mast cell degranulation in response to a specific food allergen.[29] Nonsteroidal anti-inflammatory drugs (NSAIDs), including aspirin, before exercise may precipitate EIAn and should be avoided for at least 24 hours before activity in individuals with a history of EIAn triggered by NSAID or aspirin use. In FDEIAn, allergy evaluation may help identify foods that are associated with the reaction, so that these foods can be avoided for at least 3 hours before or after exercise.[28] The diagnosis of EIAn or FDEIAn requires challenge testing with physical exercise alone for EIAn or ingestion of the suspected food followed by physical exercise for FDEIAn. When results are equivocal, a double-blind, placebo-controlled, food-exercise challenge can be performed.[30]

The management of EIAn and of FDEIAn is focused on avoiding identified triggers. Nonsedating antihistamines can be used before activity, but this medication class does not appear to be a reliable prevention strategy.[3] Athletes allowed to exercise with this condition should have immediate access to epinephrine and one or more trained exercise partners who know the signs and symptoms of EIAn to administer epinephrine when needed.

In practice, this may require the availability of 2 EpiPens or 2 nasal epinephrine devices to increase the chance that one is always available—one in the possession of the individual and another in the possession of an athletic trainer or a staff member who would be present during practice and competition. Immunotherapy for FDEIAn has not yet been recommended in consensus documents and is not currently used in clinical practice.[7]

Cholinergic Urticaria

Cholinergic urticaria is an exaggerated response to body warming that is often seen with exercise, especially in hot and humid environments. Cholinergic urticaria can also be triggered by exposure to the heat of a hot tub or sauna. Urticarial papules initially appear on the upper thorax and neck before spreading to the entire body and last from 15 minutes to several hours. There is limited risk for hemodynamic compromise. Second-generation or long-acting antihistamines at double the usual recommended dose are the first-line treatment recommendations.[3]

SOLITARY ORGANS OR ORGAN ABSENCE

History Form Question

1. *Are you missing a kidney, an eye, a testicle, spleen, or any other organ? Are any of these organs not functioning properly?*

Key Points

- Absence of a paired organ may not limit an individual from contact or collision activities.
- Protective equipment may be advised for individuals with only one of usually paired organs.

The absence of one of a paired organ set is not an absolute contraindication to sport participation, but it should prompt shared decision-making with the individual and family based on the risks associated with contact, collision, or limited-contact sports.[14,31]

The absence of one of a paired organ set is not an absolute contraindication to sport participation, but it should involve shared decision-making with the individual and family based on the risks associated with contact, collision, or limited-contact sports.

Protective equipment may sufficiently reduce the risk of injury during collision and contact sports for an individual who is functionally one-eyed or has a solitary kidney to participate safely.[32] Contact or collision sports may pose increased risk for individuals with a single kidney, especially if the remaining kidney is compromised or located in an area at higher risk for injury.[32] The risk of injury leading to loss of a kidney is very small, but not zero, and should be considered when counseling patients with a solitary kidney.[33] A risk classification system for patients with a solitary kidney was developed according to the overall risk of high-grade renal trauma or loss of a renal unit (Box 5C-1).[34]

Box 5C-1. Activity Classification System for Pediatric Patients With Solitary Kidneys

Highest Risk	High Risk (> 1.0%)	Moderate Risk (0.1%–1.0%)	Low Risk (< 0.1%)
• Extreme skiing • Extreme snowboarding • Horse racing • Off-road biking	• Bicycle • Horseback riding	• Football • Ice hockey • Skiing • Sledding • Snowboarding • Soccer	• Baseball • Basketball • Lacrosse • Running • Rollerblading • Skateboarding • Wrestling

Abbreviation: ATV, all-terrain vehicle.

Reproduced from Papagiannopoulos D, Gong E. Revisiting sports precautions in children with solitary kidneys and congenital anomalies of the kidney and urinary tract. *Urology*. 2017;101:9–14

Individuals with a single testicle need to understand the higher risk of injury and loss of fertility in contact, collision, and limited-contact sports. Use of a protective cup is recommended for everyone with a solitary testicle.[14] The injury risk to a single ovary is minimal, and participation need not be restricted.[14]

For consideration of an athlete who has a single eye or what constitutes a functional single eye, please review the Eye Disorders and Vision content later in this chapter.

HEAT-RELATED ILLNESS

History Form Question

1. *Have you ever become ill while exercising in the heat?*

Secondary Questions

- Have you ever had exertional heat stroke?
- When did this occur?
- Did you go to the emergency department?
- How long were you in the hospital?
- Have you had an exercise heat-tolerance test?
- What medications or supplements do you take?
- Have you ever had heat exhaustion?
- Do you have muscle cramping during practices or games?
- What do you drink before, during, and after practices and games?

Key Points

- Exertional heat stroke (EHS) is the third leading cause of death among high school athletes.
- EHS can be fatal. It is most often seen during preseason football in the summer but can occur during other sports and in cooler climates.
- Major EHS risk factors include hot, humid conditions; inadequate heat acclimatization; poor aerobic fitness; high body mass index (> 30 kg/m^2); and the use of protective equipment.

- Maintaining hydration may slow the onset of EHS.
- Gradually acclimatizing to hot conditions over 7 to 14 days, avoiding medications that increase the risk of heat illness, and educating on adequate nutrition, sleep, and hydration are key to preventing heat illness.

Exertional Heat Illness

Exertional heat illness refers to a spectrum of conditions (exercise-associated muscle cramps, heat exhaustion, heat injury, heat stroke) that occur when the body's thermoregulatory capacity is overwhelmed by environmental heat and intense physical exertion. All exertional heat illnesses are associated with an elevation of core body temperature. Exertional heat illness adversely affects athletic performance and can be associated with severe morbidity and even death.[35] Heat illness is a particular concern for unacclimatized individuals practicing and competing in hot environments, especially with occlusive equipment such as helmets and pads. During the PPE, it is important to ask specific questions regarding possible risk factors, including prior heat illness, environmental conditions, acclimatization status, equipment and uniforms, fluid intake, obesity, current viral or bacterial infection, high training loads, medications, and alcohol and supplement use.[36,37] The PPE is an opportunity to significantly reduce the risk of heat illness by educating individuals about risk factors and preventive strategies, which is key to decreasing the incidence of heat illness.

Exercise-Associated Muscle Cramps

Exercise-associated muscle cramps (EAMCs) are common when the workloads are higher than the level of muscle training. Cramping can occur in training or competition. Muscle cramps seem to occur more frequently in hot conditions, but they can also happen in cool to cold conditions. The cause of EAMC is not well understood, even though it occurs regularly in athletes. The 2 competing explanations are (1) altered neuromuscular control and (2) a combination of electrolyte depletion and dehydration. Gradual increases in training load and attention to fluid replacement during exercise may reduce EAMC risk, especially for those known to be prone to cramps. Cramping can also be a presenting concern or part of the clinical constellation of symptoms associated with EHS, exertional rhabdomyolysis, exercise-associated hyponatremia, and exercise collapse associated with sickle cell trait.[38]

Heat Exhaustion

Heat exhaustion is defined by an inadequate cardiac output to maintain exercise performance in hot environments, without central nervous system (CNS) involvement. It usually occurs during high workloads, often in hot conditions, and is a cause of collapse that is primarily the result of extensive cutaneous vasodilation in response to rising core temperatures to increase skin blood flow for heat transfer. This shunts cardiac output to the extremities and reduces the proportion of blood flow to vital organs, which can be compounded by dehydration. If cardiac output is insufficient to maintain blood pressure in the face of cutaneous vasodilatation (and possibly reduced intravascular volume due to dehydration), individuals may become hypotensive and collapse. Body temperature is not always elevated to dangerous levels and is usually less than 40°C (104°F) by rectal measurement. Individuals generally improve with rest and fluid replacement within 24 to 48 hours and often return to play within a few days. Heat exhaustion may be on the pathway to EHS for some, but most individuals collapse before their body temperature rises to EHS levels.

Heat Injury and Exertional Heat Stroke

Heat injury is a moderate to severe heat illness that does not involve the CNS and is characterized by organ and tissue injury associated with sustained high body temperature, potentially resulting in metabolic acidosis, rhabdomyolysis, acute kidney injury, and liver damage. The lack of CNS involvement is what distinguishes heat injury from EHS.

EHS is a multisystem illness defined as an elevated core body temperature (rectal temperature: > 40°C [104°F], usually > 41°C [106°F]) with CNS changes. CNS dysfunction may present as headache, disorientation, irrational behavior, aggression, altered consciousness, coma, or death. Patients may be tachycardic and hypotensive, and other associated symptoms can include dizziness, vomiting, muscle cramps, ataxia, and profuse sweating. Risk factors for EHS are outlined in Box 5C-2. A history of previous EHS, sickle cell disease or trait (see Chapter 5H), a lack of acclimatization, a febrile illness, and high relative humidity in hot temperatures (wet bulb globe temperature [WBGT] greater than usual for the setting) are the most significant risk factors for EHS in athletes.[39] Young age had previously been considered a risk factor, but studies show that children and adolescents are at similar, if not lower, risk for heat stroke as adults.[39] Children can adapt to temperature extremes as effectively as adults when exposed to high climatic heat stress when hydration and other factors are similarly controlled.[39] Children tend to underestimate body water loss, however, and need encouragement to replace their sweat losses. A Centers for Disease Control and Prevention report published in 2010 showed that heat illness was most prominent in the month of August in football players who were overweight or obese.[40] Individuals should be informed of the increased heat intolerance caused by some medications and supplements.[41] The use of alcohol, diuretics, caffeine, antihistamines, or stimulants increases the risk of heat illness.[36,37,41] Stimulants such as ephedra or methamphetamines also increase the risk of heat injury.

Individuals should be informed of the increased heat intolerance caused by some medications and supplements. The use of alcohol, diuretics, caffeine, antihistamines, or stimulants increases the risk of heat illness. Stimulants such as ephedra or methamphetamines also increase the risk of heat injury.

Box 5C-2. Risk Factors for Exertional Heat Stroke

Extrinsic
- Environment (hot, humid, sun exposure, minimal wind)
- Clothing and equipment (multiple layers, pads)
- Delayed recognition/lack of emergency action plan
- Limited access to shade or sufficient breaks in activity
- Medications (eg, stimulants, anticholinergic medications, nonsteroidal anti-inflammatory drugs, diuretics, psychotropic medications)
- Recreational drugs and supplements (alcohol, stimulants)

Intrinsic
- Prior history of heat stroke
- Sickle cell disease or trait
- Inadequate acclimatization
- Febrile condition or recent respiratory or gastrointestinal tract viral illness
- Overexertion
- Dehydration or inadequate access to fluids
- Poor aerobic fitness
- Excess adiposity
- Large body size

Exertional Heat Illness Prevention

Exertional heat illness is best prevented by identifying individual risk factors, modifying equipment, changing the time of practice, increasing hydration breaks, modifying activity intensity in hot conditions, and gradually increasing the workload over several days in hot conditions to facilitate acclimatization (see Box 5C-3). Heat dissipation is compromised by vapor barrier uniforms and protective equipment such as shoulder pads and helmets, and gradual introduction of equipment should be factored into acclimatization.[41] Adjusting physical activity by increasing rest breaks, ensuring access to fluids, and decreasing workload on the basis of the environment using WBGT is essential to reduce the risk of EHS. Poor physical conditioning, high BMI, and wearing dark, heavy clothing or equipment that inhibits heat dissipation are also EHS risk factors.[42] Some individuals (eg, those with a history of an EHS episode) may require exercise testing in a heat chamber to determine heat tolerance. Some medications and dietary supplements can exacerbate hyperthermia and dehydration. Alcohol use can promote dehydration. Individuals with a documented history of heat stroke or heat-related rhabdomyolysis merit further investigation. For more detailed information regarding the management of heat and heat illness in individuals, see Box 5C-3.

Box 5C-3. Resources for Management of Heat and Heat Illness in Athletes

- Armstrong LE, Casa DJ, Millard-Stafford M, Moran DS, Pyne SW, Roberts WO; American College of Sports Medicine. External heat illness during training and competition. *Med Sci Sports Exerc.* 2007;39(3):556–572. doi:10.1249/MSS.0b013e31802fa199uary 22, 2019
- Casa DJ, DeMartini JK, Bergeron MF, et al. National Athletic Trainers' Association position statement: exertional heat illnesses. *J Athl Train.* 2015;50(9):986–1000. doi:10.4085/1062-6050-50.9.07
- McDermott BP, Anderson SA, Armstrong LE, et al. National Athletic Trainers' Association position statement: fluid replacement for the physically active. *J Athl Train.* 2017;52(9):877–895. doi:10.4085/1062-6050-52.9.02
- Sawka MN, Burke LM, Eichner ER, Maughan RJ, Montain SJ, Stachenfeld NS; American College of Sports Medicine. Exercise and fluid replacement. *Med Sci Sports Exerc.* 2007;39(2):377–390. doi:10.1249/mss.0b013e31802ca597

EYE DISORDERS AND VISION

History Form Question

1. *Have you ever had or do you have any problems with your eyes or vision?*

Secondary Questions

- Have you had any eye injuries?
- Do you wear glasses or contact lenses?
- Do you wear protective eyewear, such as safety goggles or a face shield?
- Why don't you wear eye protection (if applicable)?
- When was your last eye examination?
- Have you had eye surgery (eg, photorefractive keratectomy [PRK], laser-assisted in-situ keratomileusis [LASIK])?

Key Points

- It is recommended that all individuals have their visual acuity checked at the PPE.
- If vision is worse than 20/40 at the time of the examination, referral to an optometrist or ophthalmologist for further evaluation is recommended.
- If best corrected vision is worse than 20/40 in one eye, then eye protection of the eye with normal vision should be strongly considered, since injury to the better eye could cause significant disability.
- Eye injury and loss of vision are always a concern in sports.
- Eye protection is recommended for moderate- to high-risk sports.
- Eye injuries may have long-term sequelae such as glaucoma, cataract, retinal detachment, and inflammation, for which patients need continued monitoring.[43]

Visual acuity should be assessed and documented at the time of the PPE.[44] Abnormal visual acuity is among the most frequently reported findings during the PPE,[44] and individuals who are identified should be evaluated and treated by an ophthalmologist. The AAP recommends vision screening at all health supervision visits to detect vision changes early, including those that affect one eye, which may otherwise be asymptomatic.[45] Poor vision can lead to poor sport performance and more injuries.

Eye injury, and the potential for loss of vision, is always a concern in sports. Risk for injury in a particular sport is categorized into high-risk, moderate-risk, low-risk, and "eye safe."[46,47] Certain sports such as basketball, baseball, softball, ice hockey, field hockey, and lacrosse are classified as high-risk because of the number of eye injuries reported and the increased potential for sufficient eye impact to cause injury.[46] For example, the sports with the highest incidence of eye injury are baseball and basketball, while track and gymnastics are considered eye safe sports. Box 5C-4 provides the eye injury risk classification for a variety of sports.

Box 5C-4. Categories of Sports-Related Eye Injury Risk for an Unprotected Player

High-Risk

- Small, fast projectiles
  - Air rifle use
  - BB gun use
  - Paintball
- Hard projectiles, "sticks," and close contact
  - Baseball and softball
  - Basketball
  - Cricket
  - Fencing
  - Hockey (field and ice)
  - Lacrosse (men's and women's)
  - Racquetball
  - Squash
- Intentional injury
  - Boxing
  - Full-contact martial arts

Moderate-Risk

- Badminton
- Fishing
- Football
- Golf
- Soccer
- Tennis
- Volleyball
- Water polo

Low-Risk

- Bicycling
- Diving
- Noncontact martial arts
- Skiing (snow and water)
- Swimming
- Wrestling

Minimal-Risk

- Gymnastics
- Track and field[a]

[a]Javelin and discus have a small but definite potential for injury. However, good field supervision can reduce the extremely low risk of injury to nearly negligible.

Adapted with permission from Vinger PF. A practical guide for sports eye protection. *Phys Sportsmed.* 2000;28(6):49–69.

In the United States, it is estimated that sports-related eye injuries account for more than 100,000 physician visits per year, including more than 30,000 emergency department visits.[48] Although most injuries resulting from sports-related activities were superficial, more than 20% of baseball-related eye injuries were blow-out fractures of the orbit.[48] **Eye protection** is key to reducing eye injuries. Protective devices can significantly reduce the risk of eye injury, so it is important that all participants and their parents or guardians are made aware of the types of eye protection available and the risks of each sport. The AAP and the American Academy of Ophthalmology (AAO) strongly recommend protective eyewear for all participants in sports with a risk of eye injury.[49] To review current National Operating Committee on Standards for Athletic Equipment (NOCSAE) and ASTM eye safety sports requirements, visit https://nocsae.org/standards-library/ and www.astm.org/COMMIT/SUBCOMMIT/F0857.htm, respectively. USA Lacrosse mandates the use of protective eyewear for girls' lacrosse, and a full-face shield is required in boys' lacrosse.[50] USA Hockey requires Hockey Equipment Certification Council (HECC)–approved face masks for eye protection.[51] The AAO reports that significant eye injury can be reduced at least 90% when properly fitted, appropriate eye protectors are used.[52,53]

Significant eye injury can be reduced at least 90% when properly fitted, appropriate eye protectors are used.

Lenses made of polycarbonate are recommended for eye protection. The AAP recommends that even in sports classified as low risk for eye injury, individuals use at least approved frames that meet American National Standards Institute standard Z87.1 with polycarbonate lenses. A strap must secure the frame to the head and must be fitted by an experienced optician. A list of specific sports and recommendations for eyewear are presented in Table 5C-2. It is important to caution athletes that contact lenses do not confer any protection from injury and are not considered eye protectors. Similarly, prescription glasses could represent a secondary hazard during sport participation to the wearer and other competitors as a result of lens or frame fracture.

Table 5C-2. Eye Protection Based on Sport

Sport	Minimal Eye Protector	Comment
Baseball/softball (youth batter and base runner)	ASTM standard F910	Face guard attached to helmet
Baseball/softball (fielder)	ASTM standard F803 for baseball	ASTM specifies age ranges
Basketball	ASTM standard F803 for basketball	ASTM specifies age ranges
Bicycling	Helmet plus sunglasses meeting ANSI Z80.3 standards	—
Boxing	None available; not permitted in the sport	Contraindicated for functionally 1-eyed athletes
Fencing	Protector with neck bib	—
Field hockey (men and women)	ASTM standard F803 for women's lacrosse (goalie: full face mask)	Protectors that pass for women's lacrosse also pass for field hockey
Football	Polycarbonate eye shield attached to helmet-mounted wire face mask	—

Table 5C-2. Eye Protection Based on Sport *(continued)*

Sport	Minimal Eye Protector	Comment
Full-contact martial arts	None available; not permitted in the sport	Contraindicated for functionally 1-eyed athletes
Ice hockey	ASTM standard F513 face mask on helmet (goaltenders: ASTM standard F1587)	HECC- or CSA-certified full-face shield
Lacrosse (men)	Face mask attached to lacrosse helmet	—
Lacrosse (women)	ASTM standard F803 for women's lacrosse	Option to wear helmet
Paintball	ASTM standard F1776 for paintball	—
Racquet sports (badminton, tennis, paddle tennis, handball, squash, and racquetball)	ASTM standard F803 for selected sport	—
Soccer	ASTM standard F803 for selected sport	—
Street hockey	ASTM standard 513 face mask on helmet	Must be HECC or CSA certified
Track and field	Sunglasses meeting ANSI Z80.3 standards[a]	—
Water polo/swimming	Swim goggles with polycarbonate lenses	—
Wrestling	None available; not permitted in the sport	Contraindicated for functionally one-eyed athletes

Abbreviation: HECC, Hockey Equipment Certification Council.

[a]Eyewear that passes ASTM standard F803 is safer than streetwear eyewear for all sports activities with impact potential.

Adapted from American Academy of Pediatrics; American Academy of Ophthalmology, Academy Communications Advisory Board, Academy Board of Trustees. Protective eyewear for young athletes–2013. https://www.aao.org/education/clinical-statement/protective-eyewear-young-athletes. © 2013 American Academy of Ophthalmology.

It is essential to consider eye protection for individuals whose vision is already impaired in one eye, and the AAO and AAP recommend mandatory protective eyewear for all functionally one-eyed individuals, regardless of sport. A visual acuity of 20/40 or better in at least one eye is considered to provide good vision, and as such an individual with a best corrected vision in one eye of less than 20/40 is considered functionally one-eyed.[54] Individuals who have had an eye injury or surgery may have a globe that is weakened and therefore more susceptible to injury. Individuals with eye conditions, including a high degree of myopia, surgical aphakia (missing lens), retinal detachment, corneal dystrophies, keratoconus, and a history of eye surgery, injury, or infection, may be at increased risk for eye injury.[55] Such individuals should be referred to an ophthalmologist for complete evaluation and medical eligibility determination. Functionally one-eyed individuals should not participate in sports during which eye protection cannot be effectively worn. As such, the AAO states that individuals with globe injury or who are functionally one-eyed must not participate in boxing, wrestling, or full-contact martial arts, as these sports do not permit the use of protective eyewear (see Table 5C-2).

The AAO and AAP recommend mandatory protective eyewear for all functionally one-eyed individuals, regardless of sport. Individuals with globe injury or who are functionally one-eyed must not participate in boxing, wrestling, or full-contact martial arts, as these sports do not permit the use of protective eyewear.

An athlete, parents or guardians, the coach, and school administrators, if necessary, should be educated regarding the risk of injury (with and without protection), the level of protection available, and the long-term consequences of injury to the better eye.

If, after this discussion, a functionally one-eyed individual still wishes to participate in a given sport, appropriate protective eyewear should be used during participation.

REFERENCES

1. Barlow SE; Expert Committee. Expert committee recommendations regarding the prevention, assessment, and treatment of child and adolescent overweight and obesity: summary report. *Pediatrics.* 2007;120(suppl 4):S164–S192. PMID: 18055651 doi:10.1542/peds.2007-2329C
2. Manoff EM, Banffy MB, Winell JJ. Relationship between Body Mass Index and slipped capital femoral epiphysis. *J Pediatr Orthop.* 2005;25(6):744–746. PMID: 16294129 doi:10.1097/01.bpo.0000184651.34475.8e
3. Taylor ED, Theim KR, Mirch MC, et al. Orthopedic complications of overweight in children and adolescents. *Pediatrics.* 2006;117(6):2167–2174. PMID: 16740861 doi:10.1542/peds.2005-1832
4. Krul M, van der Wouden JC, Schellevis FG, van Suijlekom-Smit LW, Koes BW. Acute non-traumatic hip pathology in children: incidence and presentation in family practice. *Fam Pract.* 2010;27(2):166–170. PMID: 20026553 doi:10.1093/fampra/cmp092
5. Tripp BL, Eberman LE, Smith MS. Exertional heat illnesses and environmental conditions during high school football practices. *Am J Sports Med.* 2015;43(10):2490–2495. PMID: 26264766 doi:10.1177/0363546515593947
6. Council on Sports Medicine and Fitness; Council on School Health. Active healthy living: prevention of childhood obesity through increased physical activity. *Pediatrics.* 2006;117(5):1834–1842. PMID: 16651347 doi:10.1542/peds.2006-0472
7. Fajardo EJ. Deliz YD, Rice SG. Concerns among obese and overweight athletes. In: Koutures CG, Wong VYM, eds. *Pediatric Sports Medicine: Essentials for Office Evaluation.* SLACK Inc; 2014:124–129
8. Confroy K, Miles C, Kaplan S, Skelton JA. Pediatric obesity and sports medicine: a narrative review and clinical recommendations. *Clin J Sport Med.* 2021;31(6):e484–e498. PMID: 32852300 doi:10.1097/JSM.0000000000000839
9. Shugart C, Jackson J, Fields KB. Diabetes in sports. *Sports Health.* 2010;2(1):29–38. PMID: 23015921 doi:10.1177/1941738109347974
10. Wang D. Achar SK, Achar S. Diabetes issues. In: Koutures CG, Wong VYM, eds. *Pediatric Sports Medicine: Essentials for Office Evaluation.* SLACK Inc; 2014:92–102
11. Colberg SR, Sigal RJ, Yardley JE, et al. Physical activity/exercise and diabetes: a position statement of the American Diabetes Association. *Diabetes Care.* 2016;39(11):2065–2079. PMID: 27926890 doi:10.2337/dc16-1728

12. Moser O, Riddell MC, Eckstein ML, et al. Glucose management for exercise using continuous glucose monitoring (CGM) and intermittently scanned CGM (isCGM) systems in type 1 diabetes: position statement of the European Association for the Study of Diabetes (EASD) and of the International Society for Pediatric and Adolescent Diabetes (ISPAD) endorsed by JDRF and supported by the American Diabetes Association (ADA). *Pediatr Diabetes.* 2020;21(8):1375–1393. PMID: 33047481 doi:10.1111/pedi.13105
13. Brar G, Carmody S, Lumb A, Shafik A, Bright C, Andrews RC. Practical considerations for continuous glucose monitoring in elite athletes with type 1 diabetes mellitus: a narrative review. *J Physiol.* 2024;602(10):2169–2177. PMID: 38680058 doi:10.1113/JP285836
14. Rice SG; American Academy of Pediatrics Council on Sports Medicine and Fitness. Medical conditions affecting sports participation. *Pediatrics.* 2008;121(4):841–848. PMID: 18381550 doi:10.1542/peds.2008-0080
15. American Diabetes Association. Diabetes mellitus and exercise. *Diabetes Care.* 2002;25(suppl 1):S64–S68
16. Jimenez CC, Corcoran MH, Crawley JT, et al. National Athletic Trainers' Association position statement: management of the athlete with type 1 diabetes mellitus. *J Athl Train.* 2007;42(4):536–545. PMID: 18176622
17. Committee on Sports Medicine and Fitness. American Academy of Pediatrics. Human immunodeficiency virus and other blood-borne viral pathogens in the athletic setting. *Pediatrics.* 1999;104(6):1400–1403. PMID: 10585997 doi:10.1542/peds.104.6.1400
18. Brown LS Jr, Drotman DP, Chu A, Brown CL Jr, Knowlan D. Bleeding injuries in professional football: estimating the risk for HIV transmission. *Ann Intern Med.* 1995;122(4):273–274. PMID: 7825762 doi:10.7326/0003-4819-122-4-199502150-00005
19. Kordi R, Wallace WA. Blood borne infections in sport: risks of transmission, methods of prevention, and recommendations for hepatitis B vaccination. *Br J Sports Med.* 2004;38(6):678–684. PMID: 15562159 doi:10.1136/bjsm.2004.011643
20. Beltrami EM, Williams IT, Shapiro CN, Chamberland ME. Risk and management of blood-borne infections in health care workers. *Clin Microbiol Rev.* 2000;13(3):385–407. PMID: 10885983 doi:10.1128/CMR.13.3.385
21. Miller MG. Monaco R. Acute illness. In: Koutures C, Wong V, eds. *Pediatric Sports Medicine: Essentials for Office Evaluation.* SLACK Inc; 2014:43–45
22. Putukian M, O'Connor FG, Stricker P, et al. Mononucleosis and athletic participation: an evidence-based subject review. *Clin J Sport Med.* 2008;18(4):309–315. PMID: 18614881 doi:10.1097/JSM.0b013e31817e34f8
23. Johnson MA, Cooperberg PL, Boisvert J, Stoller JL, Winrob H. Spontaneous splenic rupture in infectious mononucleosis: sonographic diagnosis and follow-up. *AJR Am J Roentgenol.* 1981;136(1):111–114. PMID: 6779555 doi:10.2214/ajr.136.1.111
24. Maki DG, Reich RM. Infectious mononucleosis in the athlete. Diagnosis, complications, and management. *Am J Sports Med.* 1982;10(3):162–173. PMID: 7114352 doi:10.1177/036354658201000308
25. Dommerby H, Stangerup SE, Stangerup M, Hancke S. Hepatosplenomegaly in infectious mononucleosis, assessed by ultrasonic scanning. *J Laryngol Otol.* 1986;100(5):573–579. PMID: 3517206 doi:10.1017/S0022215100099680
26. McCorkle R, Thomas B, Suffaletto H, Jehle D. Normative spleen size in tall healthy athletes: implications for safe return to contact sports after infectious mononucleosis. *Clin J Sport Med.* 2010;20(6):413–415. PMID: 21079435 doi:10.1097/JSM.0b013e3181f35fe5
27. Putukian M, McGrew CA, Benjamin HJ, et al. American Medical Society of Sports Medicine position statement: mononucleosis and athletic participation. *Clin J Sport Med.* 2023; 33(4):359 1/N 367. PMID: 37186809 doi:10.1097/JSM.0000000000001161
28. Waibel N. Roberts WO. Environmental factors: heat, cold, altitude, humidity, and anaphylaxis. In: Koutures C, Wong V, eds. *Pediatric Sports Medicine: Essentials for Office Evaluation.* SLACK Inc; 2014:60–65
29. Christensen MJ, Eller E, Mortz CG, Brockow K, Bindslev-Jensen C. Exercise lowers threshold and increases severity, but wheat-dependent, exercise-induced anaphylaxis can be elicited at rest. *J Allergy Clin Immunol Pract.* 2018;6(2):514–520. PMID: 29524997 doi:10.1016/j.jaip.2017.12.023
30. Pravettoni V, Incorvaia C. Diagnosis of exercise-induced anaphylaxis: current insights. *J Asthma Allergy.* 2016;9:191–198. PMID: 27822074 doi:10.2147/JAA.S109105
31. Brydon PD. Wang D, Taylor KS. Preparticipation physical evaluation. In: Koutures C, Wong V, eds. *Pediatric Sports Medicine: Essentials for Office Evaluation.* SLACK Inc; 2014:14–20
32. Gomez J. E. Paired organ loss. In: DeLee JC, Drez D Jr, Miller MD, eds. *DeLee and Drez's Orthopaedic Sports Medicine: Principles and Practice.* 2nd ed. Saunders; 2003:264–271

33. Styn NR, Wan J. Urologic sports injuries in children. *Curr Urol Rep.* 2010;11(2):114–121. PMID: 20425099 doi:10.1007/s11934-010-0098-4
34. Papagiannopoulos D, Gong E. Revisiting sports precautions in children with solitary kidneys and congenital anomalies of the kidney and urinary tract. *Urology.* 2017;101:9–14. PMID: 27890687 doi:10.1016/j.urology.2016.11.025
35. Coris EE, Ramirez AM, Van Durme DJ. Heat illness in athletes: the dangerous combination of heat, humidity and exercise. *Sports Med.* 2004;34(1):9–16. PMID: 14715036
36. Casa DJ, DeMartini JK, Bergeron MF, et al. National Athletic Trainers' Association Position Statement: Exertional Heat Illnesses. *J Athl Train.* 2015;50(9):986–1000. doi:10.4085/1062-6050-50.9.07
37. Guideline 4b. Exertional heat illness. In: *NCAA Sports Medicine Handbook.* 26th ed. National Collegiate Athletic Association; 2025:65–67
38. Schwellnus MP. Cause of exercise associated muscle cramps (EAMC)—altered neuromuscular control, dehydration or electrolyte depletion? *Br J Sports Med.* 2009;43(6):401–408. PMID: 18981039 doi:10.1136/bjsm.2008.050401
39. American Academy of Pediatrics. Committee on Sports Medicine and Fitness. Climatic heat stress and the exercising child and adolescent. *Pediatrics.* 2000;106(1 Pt 1):158–159. PMID: 10878169
40. Gilchrist J. Murphy M, Comstock RD, Collins C, Yard E; Centers for Disease Control and Prevention. Heat illness among high school athletes—United States, 2005–2009. *MMWR Morb Mortal Wkly Rep.* 2010;59(32):1009–1013. https://www.cdc.gov/mmwr/preview/mmwrhtml/mm5932a1.htm.
41. Casa DJ, DeMartini JK, Bergeron MF, et al. National Athletic Trainers' Association position statement: exertional heat illnesses. *J Athl Train.* 2015;50(9):986–1000. PMID: 26381473 doi:10.4085/1062-6050-50.9.07
42. Kulka TJ, Kenney WL. Heat balance limits in football uniforms how different uniform ensembles alter the equation. *Phys Sportsmed.* 2002;30(7):29–39. PMID: 20086533 doi:10.3810/psm.2002.07.377
43. Bojikian KD, Stein AL, Slabaugh MA, Chen PP. Incidence and risk factors for traumatic intraocular pressure elevation and traumatic glaucoma after open-globe injury. *Eye (Lond).* 2015;29(12):1579–1584. PMID: 26381097 doi:10.1038/eye.2015.173
44. American Optometric Association (AOA) Sports Vision Section. National Athletic Trainers' Association (NATA) vision screening protocols. https://my.usskiandsnowboard.org/sites/default/files/documents/athletics/freestyle/2014-15/documents/sports-vision-section-NATA-vision-screening-protocols-august-2011.pdf Accessed June 8, 2026
45. American Academy of Pediatrics Committee on Practice and Ambulatory Medicine, Section on Ophthalmology; American Association of Certified Orthoptists; American Association for Pediatric Ophthalmology and Strabismus; American Academy of Ophthalmology. Eye examination in infants, children, and young adults by pediatricians. *Pediatrics.* 2003;111(4 Pt 1):902–907. PMID: 12671132. doi:10.1542/peds.111.4.902
46. American Academy of Pediatrics Committee on Sports Medicine and Fitness. Protective eyewear for young athletes. *Pediatrics.* 2004;113(3 Pt 1):619–622. PMID: 14993558
47. Strahlman E, Sommer A. The epidemiology of sports-related ocular trauma. *Int Ophthalmol Clin.* 1988;28(3):199–202. PMID: 3042659 doi:10.1097/00004397-198802830-00003
48. Haring RS, Sheffield ID, Canner JK, Schneider EB. Epidemiology of sports-related eye injuries in the United States. *JAMA Ophthalmol.* 2016;134(12):1382–1390. PMID: 27812702
49. American Academy of Pediatrics, American Academy of Ophthalmology (AAO) Communications Advisory Board. Protective eyewear for young athletes - 2013. April 2013. Accessed February 22, 2019. https://www.aao.org/clinical-statement/protective-eyewear-young-athletes
50. USA Lacrosse. USA Lacrosse Equipment Guide for the 2026 Boys, Girls, and Box/Indoor Seasons. https://www.usalacrosse.com/sites/default/files/documents/Safety/USAL-equipment-guide-2025b.pdf Accessed June 9, 2026
51. USA Hockey. *Official Rules and Casebook 2025–2029.* USA Hockey; 2017. https://www.usahockey rulebook.com/page/7463/official-rules-casebook-2025-2029. Accessed June 9, 2026
52. Jeffers JB. An on going tragedy: pediatric sports-related eye injuries. *Semin Ophthalmol.* 1990;5(4):216–223. doi:10.3109/08820539009060173
53. Larrison WI, Hersh PS, Kunzweiler T, Shingleton BJ. Sports-related ocular trauma. *Ophthalmology.* 1990;97(10):1265–1269. PMID: 2243676 doi:10.1016/S0161-6420(90)32421-1
54. Napier SM, Baker RS, Sanford DG, Easterbrook M. Eye injuries in athletics and recreation. *Surv Ophthalmol.* 1996;41(3):229–244. PMID: 8970237 doi:10.1016/S0039-6257(96)80025-7
55. Rodriguez JO, Lavina AM, Agarwal A. Prevention and treatment of common eye injuries in sports. *Am Fam Physician.* 2003;67(7):1481–1488. PMID: 12722848

D: Respiratory System

■ HISTORY FORM QUESTION

1. *Do you cough, wheeze, or have difficulty breathing during or after physical activity?*

■ SECONDARY QUESTIONS

- If you have difficulty breathing during or after physical activity, is it:
  - —When breathing in (inspiratory) or out (expiratory)?
  - —Do these symptoms occur during or after exercise?
  - —How long does it take for symptoms to resolve (seconds, minutes, or hours)?
- Have you been diagnosed with a respiratory condition, such as asthma?
  - —If yes, have you ever been hospitalized for this condition?
  - —Have you used an inhaler?
    - ▪ If yes, what kind?
    - ▪ If you used an inhaler, does it help with your symptoms?
- Do you have any environmental allergies?
- If you have respiratory symptoms, do you have any triggers that make these symptoms worse (eg, allergies, cold air, illness, anxiety)?

■ KEY POINTS

- Exercise-induced bronchoconstriction (EIB) may be suggested by symptoms, but definitive diagnosis can only be made via spirometry, with and without a bronchodilator.
- EIB is treated with short-acting β-2 agonists 15 to 20 minutes before activity.
- Frequent episodes of EIB can be a feature of poorly treated asthma. Reassessment of the individual's asthma action plan is recommended in these cases to optimize care.
- Continuous laryngoscopy during exercise (CLE) is the "gold-standard" test to diagnose exercise induced laryngeal obstruction (EILO).
- Cardiopulmonary exercise testing may help identify cardiorespiratory pathology, breathing pattern disorder (BPD), or deconditioning.
- Comorbidities are common with exercise-induced respiratory conditions, and these also need to be treated to optimize care.

INTRODUCTION

The immediate and long-term benefits of physical activity on a person's overall well-being and quality of life have been well-documented. Although participation in physical activity is strongly encouraged, some individuals may experience respiratory symptoms that can significantly reduce their ability to participate in or enjoy these activities. Respiratory symptoms, such as wheezing, cough, and dyspnea, are the most common symptoms reported by active individuals.[1]

Dyspnea during physical activity is a subjective feeling that is very common, and it can be difficult to ascertain its true cause. It has been estimated that at least 1 in 4 individuals report exercise-related respiratory issues, with asthma being the most prevalent medical cause.[2]

Among those with asthma, physical activity can exacerbate symptoms, resulting in exercise-induced bronchoconstriction with asthma (EIBa). Other common respiratory issues seen in active individuals include exercise-induced bronchoconstriction without asthma (EIB), EILO—formerly known as vocal cord dysfunction—and breathing pattern disorder (BPD).

Acute respiratory tract infections are the most common acute illnesses in athletes.[3] These respiratory conditions can impact any population, and although the evaluation is important regardless of whether the individuals are athletes, some of these conditions are more common in certain environments.

ASSESSMENT OF RESPIRATORY SYMPTOMS

For someone experiencing respiratory symptoms during activity, it can be challenging to determine whether these symptoms are due to a respiratory issue or are simply a normal response to increased physical exertion. The initial assessment of an individual with respiratory symptoms is the same regardless of activity level. During a thorough history, red flag symptoms need to be evaluated further, and any symptoms occurring during exercise need to be clarified (Figure 5D-1).[2]

If an individual experiences symptoms during or immediately following increased physical activity, then EIBa, EIB, EILO, and BPD should be in the differential diagnosis. Since the physical examination results are usually normal at rest, it is important to focus on the timing of symptoms (Figure 5D-2).[4] By taking into account symptoms, their timing, and response to β-2 agonists, along with an individual's medical history (eg, asthma, atopy, anxiety, reflux), a more accurate diagnosis can be made.

EXERCISE-INDUCED RESPIRATORY CONDITIONS

Exercise-Induced Bronchoconstriction

The most prevalent respiratory issue for participants is asthma. Among elite athletes, asthma affects about 1 in 5 individuals, a rate that has not changed over 40 years.[5] Among individuals with asthma, about 40% to 90% have exercise-induced asthma.[6] Individuals with a confirmed history of asthma via spirometry, whose symptoms are exacerbated with exercise, have EIBa. Those who do not have asthma and experience symptoms only during exercise have EIB. While EIBa and EIB both result in acute reversible airway narrowing, distinguishing between the 2 is vital to provide the best management.

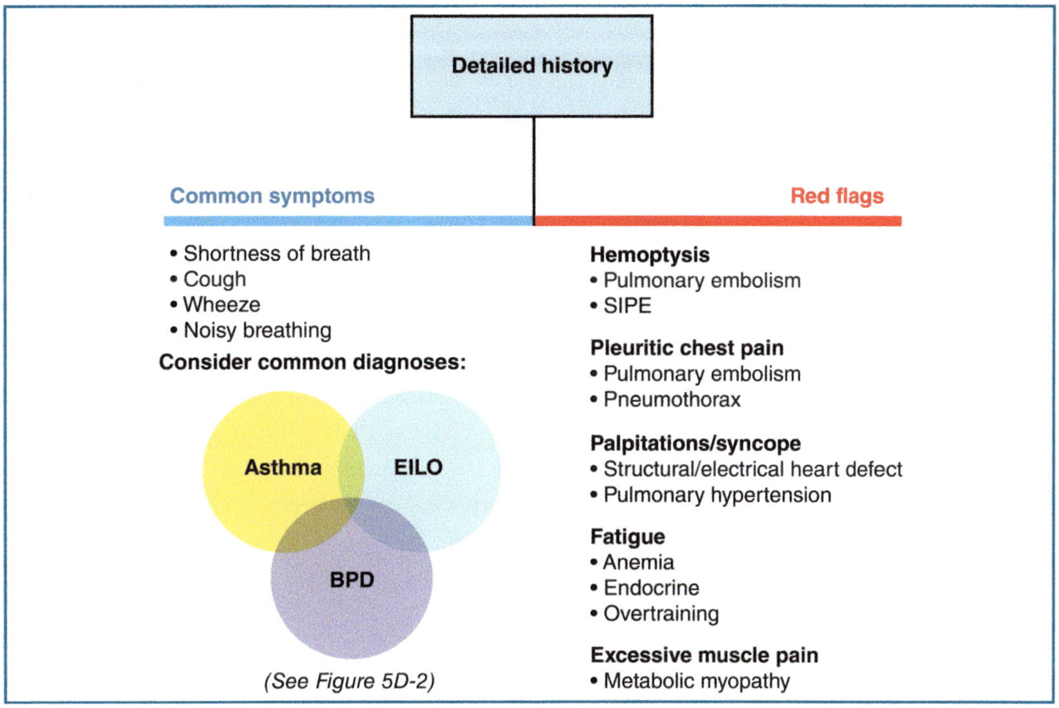

Figure 5D-1. Initial Approach to Exercise-Associated Respiratory Symptoms in the Athlete

Abbreviations: BPD, breathing pattern disorder; EILO, exercise-induced laryngeal obstruction; SIPE, swimming-induced pulmonary edema.

From Hull JH, Burns P, Carre J, et al. BTS clinical statement for the assessment and management of respiratory problems in athletic individuals. *Thorax.* 2022;77:540–551. doi:10.1136/thoraxjnl-2021–217904

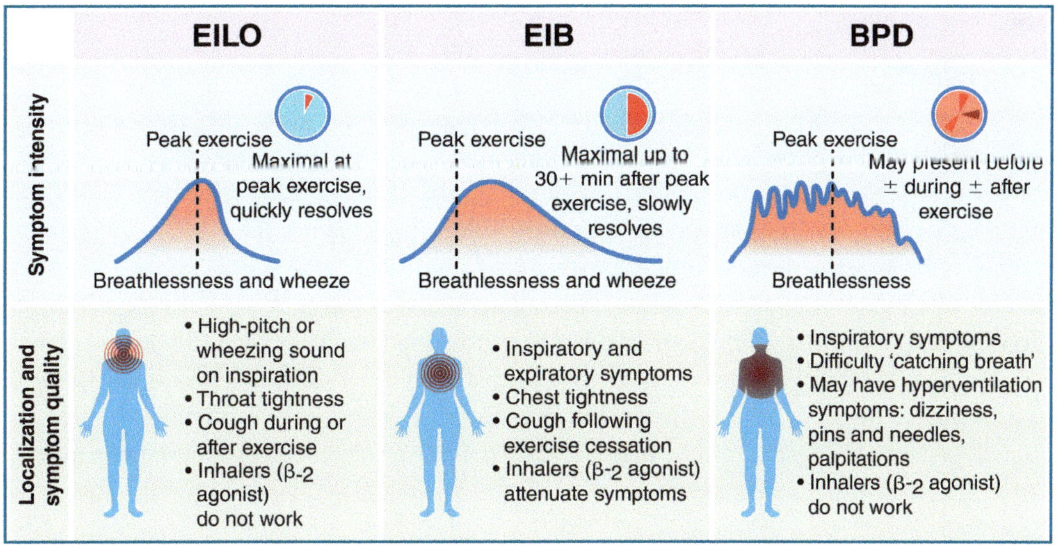

Figure 5D-2. Clinical Features of the Key Differential Diagnoses for Breathlessness ± Wheeze in Athletic Individuals

Abbreviations: BPD, breathing pattern disorder; EIB, exercise-induced bronchoconstriction; EILO, exercise-induced laryngeal obstruction.

Reproduced from Hull JH, Burns P, Carre J, et al. BTS clinical statement for the assessment and management of respiratory problems in athletic individuals. *Thorax.* 2022;77:540–551. doi:10.1136/thoraxjnl-2021–217904

Pathogenesis

Although the exact cause of EIB is not known, the osmotic theory is currently proposed. This theory suggests that increased ventilation during exercise results in water loss and dehydration of the airway. This osmotic change then induces an inflammatory response resulting in bronchoconstriction.[7]

Prevalence

The prevalence of EIB in children has been reported to be between 10% and 20%, with a higher likelihood in girls and in those from urban environments.[8] The prevalence of EIB in adolescent athletes ranged from 2.1% to 6.1%, with a higher prevalence seen in low-income areas.[9] The prevalence of EIB is directly correlated with the type of activity being performed. Individuals participating in sports that require a longer duration of effort and are conducted in a dry or cold environment have a higher prevalence of EIB (Table 5D-1).[8] Various environmental exposures also increase the prevalence of EIB (eg, swimmers exposed to high chlorine levels, individuals using ice rinks exposed to ice resurfacers' byproducts, and outdoor participants exposed to aeroallergens and pollution).[10]

Symptoms

Individuals with EIB usually present with cough, wheezing, chest tightness, and/or shortness of breath. These symptoms typically occur within 15 minutes after at least 5 to 8 minutes of intense aerobic activity, and last from 30 to 90 minutes.[8,11,12] It has been well-documented that symptoms are not a sensitive predictor of EIB.[13] Studies have shown that there is often a poor correlation between subjective symptoms and objective measures of bronchoconstriction. Simpson et al[14] found that self-reported respiratory symptoms did not correlate well with changes in airway caliber in athletes with EIB, indicating that it is best not to rely on subjective ratings as the sole diagnostic tool.

Diagnosis

The diagnosis of EIBa or EIB is confirmed by changes seen on spirometry before and after exercise or via bronchoprovocation testing. Spirometry should be the initial diagnostic test performed to evaluate an individual with symptoms of EIB or EIBa. Since some athletes may have higher baseline forced expiratory volume in 1 second (FEV_1), it is important that spirometry testing be administered with a bronchodilator to establish reversibility. An increase in FEV_1 of 12% from baseline is considered a positive test result. Because of the variability of spirometry in children, a lower threshold has been suggested (8%), as well as considering not using a spirometry cutoff value at all as a criterion for diagnosis.[8] If spirometry results are negative or inconclusive but EIB diagnosis is still on the differential, then bronchoprovocation testing can be performed. If the test results are negative, then an alternative diagnosis should be considered.

Management

Individuals with EIB or EIBa can participate in activities if their symptoms are controlled. The approach to managing EIBa or EIB involves both pharmacologic and nonpharmacologic strategies. Frequent episodes of EIB often indicate poorly controlled asthma; therefore, optimizing asthma medication is essential. Nonpharmacologic management focuses on

Table 5D-1. Examples of Sports and Their Potential Risk of EIBa/EIB

Low-Risk Sports	Medium-Risk Sports	High-Risk Sports
All sports in which the athlete performs a <5–8 min effort	Team sports in general, in which the continuous effort rarely lasts more than 5–8 min	All sports in which the athlete performs a >5–8 min effort and/or in a dry/cold air environment
Track and field: • Sprint (100, 200, and 400 m) • Middle distance (800 and 1,500 m) • Hurdles (100, 110, and 400 m) • Jumps • Throws • Decathlon • Heptathlon Tennis Fencing Gymnastics Downhill skiing Boxing Golf Body building Weightlifting Martial arts	Soccer Rugby American football Basketball Volleyball Handball Baseball Cricket Field hockey	Track and field: • Long distance (5,000 and 10,000 m) • 3,000 m steeplechase • Pentathlon (mixed) • Walks (20 and 50 km) • Marathon • High-altitude sports Cycling Cross-country skiing Ice hockey Ice skating Biathlon
Swimming, water polo		

Abbreviations: EIB, exercise-induced bronchoconstriction; EIBa, exercise-induced bronchoconstriction with asthma.

Reproduced from Del Giacco SR, Firinu D, Bjermer L, Carlsen KH. Exercise and asthma: an overview. *Eu Clin Respir J.* 2015;2(1):27984.

reducing environmental exposure to aeroallergens and warming and humidifying inhaled air using a face covering. Warming up before activity is another strategy used to induce a refractory period. Performing high-intensity intervals or a combination of high- and low-intensity warm-ups for 10 to 15 minutes is theorized to lead to a release of protective prostaglandins, resulting in decreased airway constriction after exercise for about 2 hours.[8,15]

The goal of pharmacologic management is to decrease airway inflammation and reduce bronchoconstriction. Short-acting β-2 agonists (SABAs) with their rapid onset of action are the mainstay of treatment for EIB when given 15 to 20 minutes before activities. Daily long-acting β-2 agonists, with or without inhaled corticosteroids, should not be used for EIB, unless treating asthma, since, as with SABAs, tachyphylaxis may develop with frequent use.[8] The use of leukotriene receptor antagonists (LTRAs), such as montelukast, can be used in those with EIB and EIBa. Daily prophylactic use of LTRAs has been shown to prevent EIB for up to 12 to 24 hours, without development of tolerance.[8,16–20]

Return to Activity Criteria

Well-controlled exercise-induced bronchoconstriction is defined as an individual experiencing minimal to no symptoms during or after exercise and a post-exercise FEV_1 decrease of less than 10%.[7] Since spirometry availability can be limited, most clinicians will rely on an individual's self-reporting of symptoms. For those with EIBa, similar to those with asthma, "well-controlled" is defined as outlined in Table 5D-2.

Exercise-Induced Laryngeal Obstruction

Exercise-induced laryngeal obstruction (EILO), sometimes used interchangeably with vocal cord dysfunction (VCD), is a common cause of respiratory symptoms in young individuals. However, EILO specifically occurs in the setting of exercise. EILO is frequently misdiagnosed as asthma or EIB. EILO is a transient, reversible narrowing at the glottic or supraglottic level (most commonly), precipitated by high-intensity activity. This transient obstruction results in exertional dyspnea and audible stridor, peaking during maximum exertion and quickly resolving within minutes after cessation of activity.

Table 5D-2. Components of Well-Controlled Asthma or EIB

Components of Control		Well-Controlled		
		Ages 0–4 years	Ages 5–11 years	Ages ≥ 12 years
Impairment	Symptoms	≤2 days/week	≤2 days/week but not more than once on each day	≤2 days/week
	Nighttime awakenings	≤1×/month		2×/month
	Interference with normal activity	None		
	SABA use for symptom control (not to prevent EIB)	≤2 days/week		
	Lung function —FEV_1 (% *predicted*) or peak flow (% *personal best*) —FEV_1/FVC	Not applicable	>80% >80%	>80% Not applicable

Abbreviations: EIB, exercise-induced bronchoconstriction; FEV_1, forced expiratory volume in 1 second; FVC, forced vital capacity; SABA, short-acting β-2 agonist.

Reproduced from National Heart, Lung, and Blood Institute, National Institutes of Health. *Asthma Care Quick Reference: Diagnosing and Managing Asthma;* 2012. https://www.nhlbi.nih.gov/files/docs/guidelines/asthma_qrg.pdf

Pathogenesis

The exact cause and mechanism of EILO are poorly understood. Several risk factors associated with EILO are asthma, gastroesophageal reflux disease, rhinosinusitis, and genetic predisposition.[21,22] Although psychological conditions, such as anxiety, have been suggested as a contributor to EILO, recent studies demonstrated that anxiety symptoms in patients with EILO were comparable to those in baseline populations.[23]

Prevalence

The prevalence data for EILO are poor, although studies show that the prevalence is similar to that of EIB. In the adolescent population, the prevalence rate of EILO ranges from 5% to 8%.[22,24–26] Most studies show a higher prevalence in females.[25–27] Since the prevalence rates for EILO are similar at a prepubertal age, it is hypothesized that the higher prevalence seen in pubertal females can be attributed to having smaller upper airways than those in males, leading to an increased chance of laryngeal obstruction.[28]

Symptoms

An array of symptoms have been described with EILO that are often confused with asthma or EIB. EILO and asthma/EIB also frequently coexist, complicating the clinical diagnosis. Dyspnea and stridor are the most common symptoms reported,[28] along with dysphonia, throat tightness, chest tightness, wheezing, and cough. These symptoms occur during peak exertion, are more noticeable during the inspiratory phase, and typically subside within minutes after stopping exercise.

Diagnosis

Obtaining a thorough history, focusing on when symptoms occur and resolve during physical activity, response to β-2 agonists, and a video of the episode can help with diagnosis. However, CLE testing, which entails visualization of the larynx during intense physical activity, is the gold standard for diagnosing EILO. With the high prevalence of coexisting asthma/EIB, spirometry testing should also be considered.

Management

Although many management strategies have been suggested for EILO, there is a lack of randomized controlled studies to recommend a specific evidence-based approach. After an accurate diagnosis is obtained, EILO is usually addressed with education about the condition and conservative management (Figure 5D-3).[22] Management is tailored to the individual and usually involves learning different breathing techniques to manage symptoms, which can be learned from physical therapists specifically trained in managing EILO and treating comorbidities.

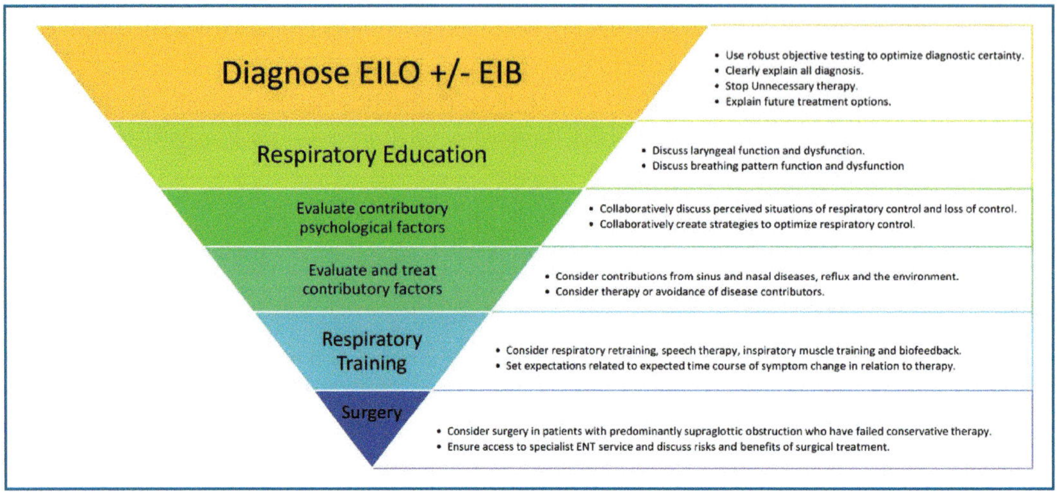

Figure 5D-3. Suggested Treatment Strategies for Athletes With EILO

Abbreviations: EIB, exercised-induced bronchoconstriction; EILO, exercise-induced laryngeal obstruction; ENT, ear, nose, and throat.

Reproduced from Clemm HH, Olin JT, McIntosh C, et al. Exercise-induced laryngeal obstruction (EILO) in athletes: a narrative review by a subgroup of the IOC Consensus on 'acute respiratory illness in the athlete'. *Br J Sports Med.* 2022;56(11):622–629.

Breathing Pattern Disorder

Breathing pattern disorder (BPD), also known as dysfunctional breathing or hyperventilation syndrome, is an increasingly recognized cause of breathlessness in young athletes. BPD represents an alteration in the normal breathing pattern, resulting in symptoms (Table 5D-3). Since BPD can coexist with the other conditions previously mentioned, it is important to treat any comorbidities before diagnosing BPD.

Table 5D-3. Signs and Symptoms of Breathing Pattern Disorder or Dysfunctional Breathing During Exercise

1	Bias toward chest breathing (rather than diaphragm breathing)
2	Rapid, shallow breathing pattern during exercise, and possibly also at rest (breathing pattern can be regular or irregular)
3	Inability to synchronize breathing to movement cadence with a consistent rhythm
4	Blunted ventilatory compensation for metabolic acidosis (supralactate threshold VE/VO_2 ratio < 5 units)
5	Inappropriate ventilatory distress, especially during high-intensity exercise

Reproduced from Dickinson J, McConnell A, Ross E, Brown P, Hull J. The BASES expert statement on assessment and management of non-asthma related breathing problems in athletes. *Sport Exerc Sci.* 2015;45. https://www.bases.org.uk/imgs/tses_autumn_2015_p8_9__pages__breathing_problems369.pdf

Pathogenesis

BPD can result in symptoms without a known cause; however, there are a variety of medical, physiological, and psychological triggers that can result in BPD. There has been a correlation between BPD and poor posture,[29] neck[30] and back pain,[31] anxiety, and depression.[32]

Prevalence

Because there is no formal definition or gold standard diagnostic test for BPD, determining an accurate prevalence is challenging. In the general population, studies have shown that BPD exists in 2% of males and 14% of females[33] and in up to 20% of elite athletes.[34,35] BPD has been reported in 29%[33] to 64%[36] of individuals with asthma. In children and adolescents, the prevalence of BPD and asthma is between 5% and 25%.[37] BPD has been shown in up to 41% of individuals with anxiety and 44% with depression.[38]

Symptoms

BPD symptoms can be nonspecific but are usually out of proportion to the level of exertion. The most commonly reported symptoms are hyperventilation, breathlessness, chest pain/tightness, dizziness, anxiety, lightheadedness, and fatigue.[39] Symptoms usually occur at the peak of exercise intensity but may also occur before or after exercise.[2]

Diagnosis

Since there is no gold standard diagnostic test and symptoms can be nonspecific, BPD can be difficult for clinicians to diagnose. A thorough history and comprehensive physical examination, including assessing poor posture and poor core strength, which can impede diaphragmatic recruitment, can be helpful for diagnosis.

A video of the episode that shows the above symptoms, specifically the breathlessness out of proportion to activity, can help lead to the diagnosis. A multidisciplinary approach with supplementary testing, such as spirometry, CLE testing, and cardiopulmonary exercise testing, is usually needed to rule out cardiopulmonary pathology if suspected. The British Thoracic Society clinical statement on Assessment and Management of Respiratory Problems in Athletic Individuals outlines such an approach.[2]

Management

There is little research to recommend specific treatments for BPD. Education on BPD and breathing pattern retraining, with a focus on diaphragmatic breathing, are the most common treatment modalities and result in improvements in both physical health and quality of life.[40–42]

Treatment of any comorbidities is important to optimize care; these include any associated anxiety and depression because they can greatly impact BPD.

OTHER RESPIRATORY CONDITIONS

Respiratory Tract Infections

Other respiratory conditions that affect athletes are acute conditions, which are less likely to impact long-term medical clearance. Respiratory tract infections (RTI) are the most common acute illness. Management of RTI in athletes and physically active individuals is usually the same as it is in the general population. Since the most common etiology is viral, supportive care is needed most. There are no standardized studies addressing the return to physical activity following an RTI. However, the most commonly used guidance is once fever free for at least 24 hours off antipyretic treatment, an individual can return to physical activity if the symptoms are confined to the upper respiratory tract (neck and up) and are improving.

Pneumothorax

A pneumothorax in a young, tall individual with a low body mass index is usually spontaneous and not due to underlying lung disease. Traumatic pneumothorax can occur in contact sports, such as football, soccer, and ice hockey.[43] There is an increased risk of pneumothorax in scuba diving and breath-hold diving because of barotrauma during ascent. Returning to physical activity after pneumothorax usually entails full radiographic resolution and normal lung function. Return to scuba or breath-hold diving after a spontaneous pneumothorax is usually not recommended unless there has been surgical intervention and clearance.

KEY RECOMMENDATIONS FOR PRACTICE

Exercise-Induced Respiratory Conditions	Symptoms	Diagnosis	Evidence Rating	Management	Evidence Rating	Return to Activity Criteria
Exercise-induced bronchoconstriction (EIB)	Inspiratory/expiratory, wheeze; peaks after exercise; occurs within 15 min of exercise, resolves within 30 min	Spirometry with documented bronchodilator reversibility (with a history consistent with EIB)[7]	B	*Pharmacologic* Short-acting β-2 agonists[7] Consider daily leukotriene inhibitor[7]	A A	Well-controlled symptoms (minimal to no symptoms during or after exercise, and a post-exercise FEV_1 decrease of less than 10%)[7]
		If spirometry negative but EIB suspected: bronchoprovocation testing[7]	A	*Nonpharmacologic* Warming up air[44] Warm-up before exercise[7]	C A	
Exercise-induced laryngeal obstruction	Inspiratory, stridor, wheeze; peak during maximum effort; resolve after stopping exercise	Continuous laryngoscopy during exercise (CLE) test[22]	C	Education, breathing retraining[22]	C	No restrictions
Breathing pattern disorder	Can occur before, during, or after activity	No "gold standard" testing[38] Multidisciplinary approach Consider: Spirometry CLE Cardiopulmonary exercise testing[7]	C	Education, breathing pattern retraining (focus on diaphragmatic breathing)[38,39]	C	No restrictions

EVALUATING RESPIRATORY SYMPTOMS DURING ACTIVITY ALGORITHM

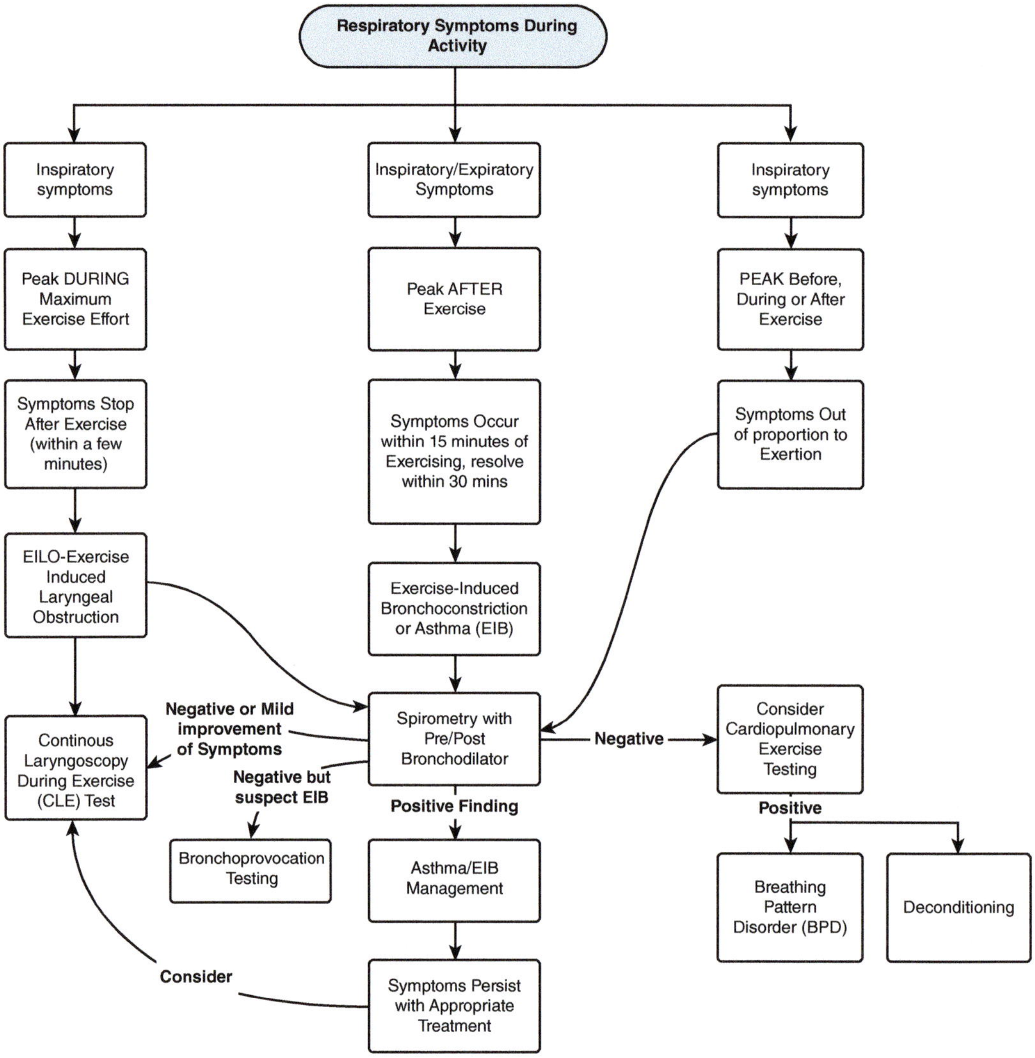

REFERENCES

1. Turcotte H, Langdeau JB, Thibault G, Boulet LP. Prevalence of respiratory symptoms in an athlete population. *Respir Med.* 2003;97(8):955–963. PMID: 12924524
2. Hull JH, Burns P, Carre J, et al. BTS clinical statement for the assessment and management of respiratory problems in athletic individuals. *Thorax.* Published online April 11, 2022. doi:10.1136/thoraxjnl-2021–217904
3. Derman W, Badenhorst M, Eken MM, et al. Incidence of acute respiratory illnesses in athletes: a systematic review and meta-analysis by a subgroup of the IOC consensus on "acute respiratory illness in the athlete." *Br J Sports Med.* Published online March 8, 2022. doi:10.1136/bjsports-2021-104737
4. Griffin SA, Walsted ES, Hull JH. Breathless athlete: exercise-induced laryngeal obstruction. *Br J Sports Med.* 2018;52(18):1211–1212. PMID: 29669719
5. Hull JH, Clemm H, Backer V, et al. Protecting respiratory health of athletes: an Olympic challenge. *Lancet Respir Med.* 2024;12(7):509–510. PMID: 38851194
6. Goldin J, Bruner PJ. Exercise-induced bronchoconstriction. In: *StatPearls* [Internet]. StatPearls Publishing. Updated June 2, 2025. https://www.ncbi.nlm.nih.gov/books/NBK557554/

7. Weiler JM, Brannan JD, Randolph CC, et al. Exercise-induced bronchoconstriction update-2016. *J Allergy Clin Immunol.* 2016;138(5):1292–1295.e36. PMID: 27665489
8. Greiwe J, Cooke A, Nanda A, et al. Work Group Report: perspectives in diagnosis and management of exercise-induced bronchoconstriction in athletes. *J Allergy Clin Immunol Pract.* 2020;8(8):2542–2555. PMID: 32636147
9. Hashim SH, Alenezi MI, Alenezi RM, et al. Exercise-induced bronchoconstriction among adolescent athletes with asthma: a systematic review. *Cureus.* 2023;15(6):e40643. PMID: 37476118 doi:10.7759/cureus.40643
10. Del Giacco SR, Firinu D, Bjermer L, Carlsen KH. Exercise and asthma: an overview. *Eur Clin Respir J.* 2015;2(1):27984. PMID: 26672959
11. Bonini M, Silvers W. Exercise-induced bronchoconstriction: background, prevalence, and sport considerations. *Immunol Allergy Clin North Am.* 2018;38(2):205–214. PMID: 29631730 doi:10.1016/j.iac.2018.01.007
12. Parsons JP, Hallstrand TS, Mastronarde JG, et al; American Thoracic Society Subcommittee on Exercise-induced Bronchoconstriction. An official American Thoracic Society clinical practice guideline: exercise-induced bronchoconstriction. *Am J Respir Crit Care Med.* 2013;187(9):1016–1027. PMID: 23634861 doi:10.1164/rccm.201303-0437ST
13. Weiler JM, Hallstrand TS, Parsons JP, et al. Improving screening and diagnosis of exercise-induced bronchoconstriction: a call to action. *J Allergy Clin Immunol Pract.* 2014;2(3):275–280.e7. PMID: 24811017 doi:10.1016/j.jaip.2013.11.001
14. Simpson AJ, Romer LM, Kippelen P. Self-reported symptoms after induced and inhibited bronchoconstriction in athletes. *Med Sci Sports Exerc.* 2015;47(10):2005–2013. PMID: 25710876 doi:10.1249/MSS.0000000000000646
15. Stickland MK, Rowe BH, Spooner CH, Vandermeer B, Dryden DM. Effect of warm-up exercise on exercise-induced bronchoconstriction. *Med Sci Sports Exerc.* 2012;44(3):383–391. PMID: 21811185 doi:10.1249/MSS.0b013e31822fb73a
16. de Benedictis FM, del Giudice MM, Forenza N, Decimo F, de Benedictis D, Capristo A. lack of tolerance to the protective effect of montelukast in exercise-induced bronchoconstriction in children. *Eur Respir J.* 2006;28(2):291–295. PMID: 16641126 doi:10.1183/09031936.06.00020606
17. Leff JA, Busse WW, Pearlman D, et al. Montelukast, a leukotriene-receptor antagonist, for the treatment of mild asthma and exercise-induced bronchoconstriction. *N Engl J Med.* 1998;339(3):147–152. PMID: 9664090 doi:10.1056/nejm199807163390302
18. Duong M, Amin R, Baatjes AJ, et al. The effect of montelukast, budesonide alone, and in combination on exercise-induced bronchoconstriction. *J Allergy Clin Immunol.* 2012;130(2):535–539.e3. PMID: 22534533 doi:10.1016/j.jaci.2012.02.051
19. Pearlman DS, van Adelsberg J, Philip G, et al. Onset and duration of protection against exercise-induced bronchoconstriction by a single oral dose of montelukast. *Ann Allergy Asthma Immunol.* 2006;97(1):98–104. PMID: 16892789 doi:10.1016/s1081-1206(10)61377-4
20. Philip G, Pearlman DS, Villarán C, et al. Single-dose montelukast or salmeterol as protection against exercise-induced bronchoconstriction. *Chest.* 2007;132(3):875–883. PMID: 17573489 doi:10.1378/chest.07-0550
21. Walsted ES, Hvedstrup J, Eiberg H, Backer V. Heredity of supraglottic exercise-induced laryngeal obstruction. *Eur Respir J.* 2017;50(2):1700423. PMID: 28818875 doi:10.1183/13993003.00423-2017
22. Clemm HH, Olin JT, McIntosh C, et al. Exercise-induced laryngeal obstruction (EILO) in athletes: a narrative review by a subgroup of the IOC Consensus on 'acute respiratory illness in the athlete'. *Br J Sports Med.* 2022;56(11):622–629. PMID: 35193856 doi:10.1136/bjsports-2021-104704
23. Benestad MR, Drageset J, Clemm H, et al. Self-reported health in adolescents with exercise-induced laryngeal obstruction; a cross-sectional study. *Front Pediatr.* 2021;9:617759. PMID: 34307244 doi:10.3389/fped.2021.617759
24. Johansson H, Norlander K, Berglund L, et al. Prevalence of exercise-induced bronchoconstriction and exercise-induced laryngeal obstruction in a general adolescent population. *Thorax.* 2015;70(1):57–63. PMID: 25380758 doi:10.1136/thoraxjnl-2014-205738
25. Christensen PM, Thomsen SF, Rasmussen N, Backer V. Exercise-induced laryngeal obstructions: prevalence and symptoms in the general public. *Eur Arch Otorhinolaryngol.* 2011;268(9):1313–1319. PMID: 21528411 doi:10.1007/s00405-011-1612-0
26. Ersson K, Mallmin E, Malinovschi A, Norlander K, Johansson H, Nordang L. Prevalence of exercise-induced bronchoconstriction and laryngeal obstruction in adolescent athletes. *Pediatr Pulmonol.* 2020;55(12):3509–3516. PMID: 33002318 doi:10.1002/ppul.25104

27. Walsted ES, Famokunwa B, Andersen L, et al. Characteristics and impact of exercise-induced laryngeal obstruction: an international perspective. *ERJ Open Res.* 2021;7(2):00195-2021. PMID: 34195253 doi:10.1183/23120541.00195-2021
28. Liyanagedera S, McLeod R, Elhassan HA. Exercise induced laryngeal obstruction: a review of diagnosis and management. *Eur Arch Otorhinolaryngol.* 2017;274(4):1781–1789. PMID: 27730324 doi:10.1007/s00405-016-4338-1
29. Lewit K. Relation of faulty respiration to posture, with clinical implications. *J Am Osteopath Assoc.* 1980;79(8):525–529. PMID: 7364597
30. Dimitriadis Z, Kapreli E, Strimpakos N, Oldham J. Respiratory weakness in patients with chronic neck pain. *Man Ther.* 2013;18(3):248–253. PMID: 23199797 doi:10.1016/j.math.2012.10.014
31. Smith MD, Russell A, Hodges PW. Disorders of breathing and continence have a stronger association with back pain than obesity and physical activity. *Aust J Physiother.* 2006;52(1):11–16. PMID: 16515418 doi:10.1016/s0004-9514(06)70057-5
32. Han JN, Stegen K, De Valck C, Clément J, Van de Woestijne KP. Influence of breathing therapy on complaints, anxiety and breathing pattern in patients with hyperventilation syndrome and anxiety disorders. *J Psychosom Res.* 1996;41(5):481–493. PMID: 9032712 doi:10.1016/s0022-3999(96)00220-6
33. Thomas M, McKinley RK, Freeman E, Foy C. Prevalence of dysfunctional breathing in patients treated for asthma in primary care: cross sectional survey. *BMJ.* 2001;322(7294):1098–1100. PMID: 11337441 doi:10.1136/bmj.322.7294.1098
34. Hull JH, Jackson AR, Ranson C, Brown F, Wootten M, Loosemore M. The benefits of a systematic assessment of respiratory health in illness-susceptible athletes. *Eur Respir J.* 2021;57(6):2003722. PMID: 33334943 doi:10.1183/13993003.03722-2020
35. Smyth CME, Winter SL, Dickinson JW. Breathing pattern disorders distinguished from healthy breathing patterns using oxptoelectronic plethysmography. *Transl Sports Med.* 2022;2022:2816781. doi:10.1155/2022/2816781
36. Stanton AE, Vaughn P, Carter R, Bucknall CE. An observational investigation of dysfunctional breathing and breathing control therapy in a problem asthma clinic. *J Asthma.* 2008;45(9):758–765. PMID: 18972291 doi:10.1080/02770900802252093
37. Vahlkvist S, Jürgensen L, Hell TD, Petersen TH, Kofoed PE. Dysfunctional breathing and its impact on asthma control in children and adolescents. *Pediatr Allergy Immunol.* 2023;34(1):e13909. PMID: 36705034 doi:10.1111/pai.13909
38. Denton E, Bondarenko J, Tay T, et al. Factors associated with dysfunctional breathing in patients with difficult to treat asthma. *J Allergy Clin Immunol Pract.* 2019;7(5):1471–1476. https://doi.org/10.1016/j.jaip.2018.11.037
39. Trompenaars AMP, Roest APJ, Vaessen-Verberne AAPH. Dysfunctional breathing in children. *J Pulmonol Respir Res.* 2020;4:001–005. doi:10.29328/journal.jprr.1001013
40. Karkouli G, Douros K, Moriki D, et al. Dysfunctional breathing in children: a literature review. *Children (Basel).* 2024;11(5):556. PMID: 38790551 doi:10.3390/children11050556
41. Barker NJ, Elphick H, Everard ML. The impact of a dedicated physiotherapist clinic for children with dysfunctional breathing. *ERJ Open Res.* 2016;2(3):00103–2015. PMID: 27957485 doi:10.1183/23120541.00103-2015
42. Niggemann B, Lehmann C, Pfeiffer-Kascha D, Weiss C. Therapeutic options for dysfunctional breathing in children and adolescents. *Acta Paediatr.* 2017;106(7):1067–1069. PMID: 28316098 doi:10.1111/apa.13838
43. Partridge RA, Coley A, Bowie R, Woolard RH. Sports-related pneumothorax. *Ann Emerg Med.* 1997;30(4):539–541. PMID: 9326870 doi:10.1016/s0196-0644(97)70018-0
44. Dickinson J, Amirav I, Hostrup M. Nonpharmacologic strategies to manage exercise-induced bronchoconstriction. *Immunol Allergy Clin North Am.* 2018;38(2):245–258. PMID: 29631733 doi:10.1016/j.iac.2018.01.012

E: Gastrointestinal and Urogenital Systems

HISTORY FORM QUESTIONS

1. *Are you missing a kidney, a testicle (males), your spleen, or any other organ?*
2. *Have you ever noticed blood in your urine?*

SECONDARY QUESTIONS

- Do you have groin or testicle pain or a bulge or hernia in the groin area?
- Does it limit your activity?
- Does it become red, swollen, or tender to touch?
- Is it a solid or hard lump?
- Do you have gastrointestinal (GI) symptoms with exercise?

KEY POINTS

- Palpate the abdomen supine for masses or enlarged organs (enlarged spleen, liver, or kidney, or gravid uterus).
- A solitary kidney may not limit participation in contact or collision sports, and each person should receive individual counseling.[1–4]
- Sports participation in individuals with GI tubes (gastrotomy, jejunostomy, or naso-enteric) is allowed in noncontact sports if they are secured with an abdominal binder, compression wrap, or tight-fitting shirt to decrease the risk of injury.[5]
- A solitary testicle may not limit participation in contact or collision sports, and each person should receive individual counseling. A protective cup should be considered for high-risk sports, although there are limited data on their effectiveness.[1,6,7]
- The preparticipation evaluation (PPE) allows the individual a chance to ask questions regarding the urogenital system.
- The presence of an **asymptomatic** hernia in the abdomen or groin is not a reason to limit participation. **Symptomatic** hernias may limit a person's ability to participate and need to be evaluated for surgical intervention.
- Many individuals engaged in endurance sports experience GI symptoms and need to be screened for symptoms that may indicate a serious medical problem.[3,8,9]

BACKGROUND

Problems identified in the GI and urogenital systems seldom limit medical eligibility for physical activity and sports, and acute, life-threatening problems are rarely uncovered during the PPE. However, blunt trauma to the abdomen and fixed organs can be catastrophic, and organ loss may influence future participation. Chronic nausea, vomiting, or diarrhea can interfere with hydration and reduce heat tolerance, alter electrolyte balance, and reduce performance. Some symptoms such as severe abdominal pain and bloody diarrhea may be a sign of more serious medical conditions such as hemorrhagic gastritis and ischemic or inflammatory bowel disease (Table 5E-1).

Table 5E-1. Summary of Potential Health Issues of Gastrointestinal and Urogenital Systems

Anatomy	Function	Health Issues
Teeth, tongue, lips, jaw	Mastication, deglutition, initiating digestion	Trauma, laceration, dental caries
Esophagus, stomach	Digestion, absorption	GI upset, GERD, trauma, hemorrhagic gastritis
Liver, spleen, gallbladder	Digestion, detoxification	Hepatitis, infection, mononucleosis, hematoma, drug toxicity
Small and large intestines	Digestion, absorption	Inflammatory bowel disease, including Crohn disease and ulcerative colitis; absorptive deficiency; mesenteric ischemia; ischemic colitis
Kidney	Fluid excretion, detoxification	Solitary kidney; kidney stone, pyelonephritis; drug toxicity
Ureter, bladder, urethra	Fluid excretion	UTI, kidney stone, bladder contusion, urethral disruption
Groin pain	Stabilizing core	Inguinal hernia, athletic pubalgia; adductor muscle strain; osteitis pubis; stress fracture
Testicle, penis	Hormonal, reproduction	Traumatic orchitis; contusion; infection; solitary organ; dermatitis
Ovary, uterus, vagina, vulva	Hormonal, reproduction	Primary and secondary amenorrhea; infection; solitary organ; dermatitis

Abbreviations: GERD, gastrointestinal esophageal reflux disease; GI, gastrointestinal; UTI, urinary tract infection.

In children and young adults, 10% of abdominal injuries are sports related.[10] Combining injuries to the abdomen and those to the thorax, there are approximately 5 sports-related injuries per 100,000 athlete exposures at the high school level.[11] Injury surveillance at the high school and college levels shows that the highest rates of internal organ injury were among male players in contact sports, with incidence rates per 1,000,000 athlete exposures at 12 for high school football, 10 for high school lacrosse, and 8 for college football and ice hockey.[12] Blunt abdominal trauma can result in organ contusion, bleeding, and hematoma, especially for those with organomegaly from acute and chronic diseases. The spleen and liver are fixed organs and vulnerable to high-speed contact injury in collision sports.

Splenic enlargement is a common complication of mononucleosis, generally developing 3 days after onset of symptoms and peaking at approximately day 12.[13] Among college students, mononucleosis is present in up to 4% of the population.[14,15] However, physical examination of an enlarged spleen is difficult, and sensitivity in detecting enlargement is poor. The increased use of point-of-care ultrasonography may improve the ability to detect splenic enlargement. Normative data for spleen size have been established for both adult and pediatric patients.[16,17] Normative data for splenic size should be interpreted cautiously in males taller than 74 inches and females taller than 67 inches.[18] A recent study found that normal splenic size in adults is significantly influenced by body height and sex, with over 6% of women and 26% of men having a splenic length greater than 12 cm.[16] The use of ultrasonography is controversial for individual cases because of the variation in normal spleen size and lack of accuracy in predicting the risk of rupture.[8,16,19–21] Serial ultrasonographic imaging rather than single-point ultrasonography is more effective in determining the trending size of the spleen, as splenic rupture generally occurs when splenic size is increasing.[22] Serial ultrasonographic imaging should be considered when an asymptomatic individual with mononucleosis desires an early return to activity (prior to 3 to 4 weeks) to confirm that the spleen size is stable or decreasing.[19] Splenic rupture risk is greatest during the first 21 days after symptom onset and in males younger than 25 years. See Chapter 5C for further guidance on return-to-play decisions for infectious mononucleosis.

Individuals with underlying medical conditions may require the use of GI tubes or implanted devices such as baclofen pumps or pacemakers. The North American Society for Pediatric Gastroenterology encourages participation in noncontact sports with the appropriate binding of the tubes, either with an abdominal binder, tape, a compression wrap, or a tight-fitting shirt or pants to stabilize tubes close to the body and decrease the risk of injury. These individuals need to be encouraged to notify the medical team if there are signs of excessive moisture or rash surrounding the site secondary to sweating.[5] Individuals with other abdominal medical devices (eg, pacemakers, baclofen pumps) need to consult with the specialist prescribing these to determine any limitations or adjustments for sports participation.

Hematuria can be painless or painful and indicates disease of the kidney or collecting systems, either acute or chronic. Evaluation is warranted. **Athletic individuals with hematuria should be held from participation until the cause is determined and treated before a final medical eligibility decision is made.** Individuals with renal trauma should not return to sports until microscopic hematuria has resolved. This rest period can vary depending on the degree of trauma (mild to moderate 2 to 6 weeks to major 6 to 12 months); some urologists recommend a minimum of 12 weeks' rest from sports for resolution of hematuria.[23,24]

A history of organ loss in the GI or urogenital system (eg, kidney, testicle) does not always limit medical eligibility, but it does require a discussion of risk to the remaining paired organ and shared decision-making on return to sport, as well as use of appropriate protective equipment. Reproductive and sexual concerns can be addressed during the evaluation, and athletes should be given the opportunity to ask questions about the urogenital system that they have not addressed in the past. When possible, discussion of sexually transmitted infections and safe-sex practices should be included. Primary amenorrhea and secondary amenorrhea, including pregnancy, are discussed in Chapter 5J.

PHYSICAL EXAMINATION

Abdomen

The abdominal examination is performed with the individual supine. The anterior superior iliac spine is exposed for adequate inspection and palpation of all 4 quadrants. Abdominal masses, abdominal or flank tenderness, rigidity, or enlargement of the liver, spleen, or kidneys requires further evaluation before determining medical eligibility. Detection of a palpable (gravid) uterus in a female will require additional evaluation. Medical eligibility for pregnant athletes is discussed in Chapter 5J.

Genitalia

The indication to perform a male genitourinary (GU) examination is based on the history of a possible undescended testicle, testicular lump, inguinal bulge, or groin pain. A male GU examination should be performed in a private setting and begin with a brief description and reason for the examination. A chaperone is recommended as part of best practices; however, the individual can decline the chaperone.[25] The testicular examination is commonly done with the patient standing. If testes are not palpated, the examination should be repeated with the individual supine to assess for an undescended testicle. Testicular irregularities or masses suggestive of cancer, testicular size abnormalities (eg, steroid use, genetic syndromes), inguinal canal hernias, or athletic pubalgia (previously called sports hernia) may be detected. If a hernia is detected, the athlete (and parents or guardians if a minor) needs to be educated regarding symptoms requiring surgical repair.

A GU examination of female athletes is not part of the PPE (see Chapter 5J).

Assessing physical maturity with Tanner staging has not been useful in determining medical eligibility and is not recommended as a routine part of the PPE.[26] However, Tanner staging may be used as a guide to counseling on growth and development, sport safety, and anabolic steroid use. It is easy to do as part of the physical examination, and a discrepancy between an individual's age and their Tanner staging may lead to an investigation of endocrine issues or discussion of physically immature athletes competing against more physically mature opponents in contact or collision sports. Studies looking at self-reported Tanner staging have demonstrated that individuals are able to distinguish prepubertal from pubertal but have difficulty with accurately grading later Tanner stages.[27]

MEDICAL ELIGIBILITY FOR PARTICIPATION

Organomegaly

An enlarged liver or spleen is at risk for rupture, and the underlying cause needs to be determined. The spleen is discussed in detail in Chapter 5C, in relation to infectious mononucleosis. Hepatomegaly may signal the presence of infection (eg, hepatitis, infectious mononucleosis) or malignant disease (eg, hepatocellular carcinoma, lymphoma). Even though the incidence of hepatic rupture among patients with acute hepatomegaly is low, **participation in all sports should be avoided until the hepatomegaly has stabilized or is diminishing in size and after the team physician, athlete, parents or guardians (if a minor), and medical team have come to a shared decision on return to sport or other physical activities.** For individuals with chronic hepatomegaly, participation in sports should be assessed individually and decisions based on the degree of enlargement, the associated disease state, and the risk of the sport.

Inguinal Hernia

An individual with an **asymptomatic** inguinal canal hernia may participate in all sports and other physical activities. The individual should be counseled regarding red flag symptoms for strangulated hernia—sudden pain, nausea, and vomiting—or change in symptoms, such as heaviness, swelling, and tugging, or burning sensation in the area. Males may have a mass within the scrotum and females may have a bulge in their labia. Symptomatic inguinal hernias may limit a person's ability to participate and should be evaluated individually for surgical intervention.

Kidney Abnormalities

Individuals with a single functioning kidney need to be counseled regarding the potential for kidney injuries ranging from contusion to complete rupture, and shared decision-making is recommended to determine medical eligibility. Some experts believe that an individual with a pelvic, iliac, or polycystic kidney, or evidence of hydronephrosis or a ureteropelvic junction abnormality, should not participate in contact or collision sports.[3,26,28–31] Although the risk is small, the consequences of the loss of a single functioning kidney (eg, transplantation or dialysis) may warrant disqualification from collision sports.[2,28–31] Restricting medical eligibility of athletes with a solitary kidney from participation in contact/collision sports is not universally accepted by experts.[2,28–32] Individuals with evidence of impairment in the solitary kidney, as demonstrated by reduced creatinine clearance, elevated serum creatinine levels, proteinuria, and renal hypertension, should avoid contact sports.[3] The leading causes of pediatric kidney injuries are not in contact/collision sports but rather bicycling, sledding, downhill skiing, snowboarding, horseback riding, and riding all-terrain vehicles[4] (Box 5E-1). Evaluation by a urologist or nephrologist may be prudent before determining medical eligibility.

Box 5E-1. Leading Causes of Pediatric Kidney Injuries

- Bicycling
- Downhill skiing
- Horseback riding
- Sledding
- Snowboarding
- All-terrain vehicles

The leading causes of pediatric kidney injuries are not in contact/collision sports but rather bicycling, sledding, downhill skiing, snowboarding, horseback riding, and riding all-terrain vehicles.

An individual with a functional solitary kidney who chooses to play in a contact/collision sport or high-risk activity should receive an explanation of the risks of kidney injury, the possible need for dialysis or transplantation, the lack of protective equipment (eg, flak or shock-absorbing jacket) proven to reduce the risk of injury, and the signs and symptoms of renal injuries.[13] Although wearing a protective shock-absorbing jacket may reduce the risk of renal injury, it does not guarantee complete protection.

Testicular Disorders

The incidence of sport-related testicular injury is extremely low.[33,34] Counseling concerning participation in contact or collision sports is recommended for individuals with unpaired or undescended testicles. An individual with a single testicle is usually medically eligible for participation, although the use of a protective cup is suggested for higher-risk sports.[1] In a study using self-reported data of testicular injury in high school and college athletes, the highest prevalence of testicular injuries was in lacrosse, wrestling, baseball, and football (48.5%, 32.8%, 21%, and 17.8%, respectively). Only 12.9% of athletes reported using an athletic cup.[7] Athletes need to be informed of the risk for injury to, or loss of, the remaining testicle. Although wearing a protective cup may reduce the incidence of injury, it does not guarantee complete protection.[33]

If an athlete has an undescended testicle that has not been thoroughly evaluated, the examining physician should make a referral to a urology specialist for evaluation and to inform the athlete of the increased risk of testicular cancer and infertility associated with this condition. Medical eligibility determination for an athlete who has an undescended testicle is the same as that for an athlete with a single testicle.

REFERENCES

1. Rice SG; American Academy of Pediatrics Council on Sports Medicine and Fitness. Medical conditions affecting sports participation. *Pediatrics.* 2008;121(4):841–848. PMID: 18381550 doi:10.1542/peds.2008-0080
2. Grinsell MM, Showalter S, Gordon KA, Norwood VF. Single kidney and sports participation: perception versus reality. *Pediatrics.* 2006;118(3):1019–1027. PMID: 16950993 doi:10.1542/peds.2006-0663
3. Coghlan K, McDermott J, Molloy M, Nason G, Carton P, O'Kelly F. A narrative review of contact sports participation in children and young athletes with a solitary (functioning) kidney. *Am J Sports Med.* 2024;52(11):2939–2947. PMID: 38348484
4. Kin JK, Koyle MA, Lee MJ, Nason GJ, Ren LY, O'Kelly F. A systematic review of genitourinary injuries arising from rugby and football. *J Pediatr Urol.* 2020;16(2):130–148. PMID: 32029358
5. Wendel D, Mezoff EA, Raghu VK, et al. Management of central venous access in children with intestinal failure: a position paper from the NASPGHAN Intestinal Rehabilitation Special Interest Group. *J Pediatr Gastroenterol Nutr.* 2021;72(3):474–486. PMID: 33399327 doi:10.1097/MPG.0000000000003036
6. Jain R, Nadella M, Byrne R, Jayachandran N, Quinn M, Owens BD. Epidemiology of testicular trauma in sports: analysis of the National Electronic Injury Surveillance System database. *J Emerg Med.* 2024;67(6):e544–e552. PMID: 39277497
7. Bieniek JM, Sumfest JM. Sports-related testicular injuries and the use of protective equipment among young male athletes. *Urology.* 2014;84(6):1485–1489. PMID: 25432843

8. de Oliveira EP, Burini RC, Jeukendrup A. Gastrointestinal complaints during exercise: prevalence, etiology, and nutritional recommendations. *Sports Med.* 2014;44(suppl 1):S79–S85. PMID: 24791919
9. Pugh JN, Fearn R, Morton JP, Close GL. Gastrointestinal symptoms in elite athletes: time to recognise the problem? *Br J Sports Med.* 2018;52(8):487–488. PMID: 29018062
10. Bergqvist D, Hedelin H, Karlsson G, Lindblad B, Mätzsch T. Abdominal trauma during thirty years: analysis of a large case series. *Injury.* 1981;13(2):93–99. PMID: 7327735 doi:10.1016/0020-1383(81)90041-3
11. Johnson BK, Comstock RD. Epidemiology of chest, rib, thoracic spine, and abdomen injuries among United States high school athletes, 2005/06 to 2013/14. *Clin J Sport.* 2017;27(4):388–393. PMID: 274286
12. Kucera KL, Currie DW, Wasserman EB, et al. Incidence of sport-related internal organ injuries due to direct-contact mechanisms among high school and collegiate athletes across 3 national surveillance systems. *J Athl Train.* 2019;54(2):152–164. doi:10.4085/1062-6050-271-17
13. Shephard RJ. Exercise and the athlete with infectious mononucleosis. *Clin J Sport Med.* 2017;27(2):168–178. PMID: 27347865
14. Van Cauwenberge PB, Vander Mijnsbrugge A. Pharyngitis: a survey of the microbiologic etiology. *Pediatr Infect Dis J.* 1991;10(10 suppl):S39–S42. PMID: 1945595
15. Candy B, Chalder T, Cleare AJ, Wessely S, White PD, Hotopf M. Recovery from infectious mononucleosis: a case for more than symptomatic therapy? A systematic review. *Br J Gen Pract.* 2002;52(483):844–851. PMID: 12392128
16. Chow KU, Luxembourg B, Seifried E, Bonig H. Spleen size is significantly influenced by body height and sex: establishment of normal values for spleen size at US with a cohort of 1200 healthy individuals. *Radiology.* 2016;279(1):306–313. PMID: 26509293
17. Nemati M, Hajalioghli P, Jahed S, Behzadmehr R, Rafeey M, Fouladi DF. Normal values of spleen length and volume: an ultrasonographic study in children. *Ultrasound Med Biol.* 2016;42(8):1771–1778. PMID: 27108037
18. McCorkle R, Thomas B, Suffaletto H, Jehle D. Normative spleen size in tall healthy athletes: implications for safe return to contact sports after infectious mononucleosis. *Clin J Sport Med.* 2010;20(6):413–415. PMID: 21079435
19. Putukian M, McGrew CA, Benjamin HJ, et al. American Medical Society of Sports Medicine Position Statement: mononucleosis and athletic participation. *Clin J Sport Med.* 2023;33(4):359–367. PMID: 37186809
20. Putukian M, O'Connor FG, Stricker P, et al. Mononucleosis and athletic participation: an evidence-based subject review. *Clin J Sport Med.* 2008;18(4):309–315. PMID: 18614881 doi:10.1097/jsm.0b013e31817e34f8
21. Dommerby H, Stangerup SE, Stangerup M, Hancke S. Hepatosplenomegaly in infectious mononucleosis, assessed by ultrasonic scanning. *J Laryngol Otol.* 1986;100(5):573–579. PMID: 3517206 doi:10.1017/S0022215100099680
22. Ceraulo AS, Bytomski JR. Infectious mononucleosis management in athletes. *Clin Sports Med.* 2019;38(4):555–561. PMID: 31472766 doi:10.1016/j.csm.2019.06.002
23. Hoen LA, O'Kelly F, Lammers RJM, et al. Mobility and sporting activity after renal trauma: a survey regarding best clinical practice during the recovery stage. *Urology.* 2024;183:199–203. PMID: 37806456
24. Coccolini F, Moore EE, Kluger Y, Biffl W, et al; WSES-AAST Expert Panel. Kidney and uro-trauma: WSES-AAST guidelines. *World J Emerg Surg.* 2019;14:54. PMID: 31827593 doi:10.1186/s13017-019-0274-x
25. Berhane A, Hackell J, Wallace S; Committee on Practice and Ambulatory Medicine; Committee on Adolescence. Use of chaperones for the pediatric and adolescent encounter: policy statement. *Pediatrics.* 2025;155(6):e2025071810. doi:10.1542/peds.2025-071810
26. Carek PJ, Mainous A III. The preparticipation physical examination for athletics: a systematic review of current recommendations. *BMJ.* 2003;327:e170. doi:10.1136/bmjusa.02120003
27. Ebo C, McCray J, Bowers K, Rose SR, Jones N-H Y. Self-puberty staging in endocrine encounters during the COVID pandemic. *Front Endocrinol (Lausanne).* 2024;15:1487329. PMID: 39530119 https://www.frontiersin.org/journals/endocrinology/articles/10.3389/fendo.2024.1487329/full
28. Sharp DS, Ross JH, Kay R. Attitudes of pediatric urologists regarding sports participation by children with a solitary kidney. *J Urol.* 2002;168(4 Pt 2):1811–1814. PMID: 12352366
29. Johnson B, Christensen C, Dirusso S, Choudhury M, Franco I. A need for reevaluation of sports participation recommendations for children with a solitary kidney. *J Urol.* 2005;174(2):686–689. PMID: 16006949 doi:10.1097/01.ju.0000164719.91332.42
30. Gerstenbluth RE, Spirnak JP, Elder JS. Sports participation and high grade renal injuries in children. *J Urol.* 2002;168(6):2575–2578. PMID: 12441987 doi:10.1016/S0022-5347(05)64219-X

31. Psooy K. Sports and the solitary kidney: how to counsel parents. *Can J Urol.* 2006;13(3):3120–3126. PMID: 16813703
32. Grinsell MM, Butz K, Gurka MJ, Gurka KK, Norwood V. Sport-related kidney injury among high school athletes. *Pediatrics.* 2012;130(1):e40–e45. PMID: 22711726
33. McAleer IM, Kaplan GW, LoSasso BE. Renal and testis injuries in team sports. *J Urol.* 2002;168(4 Pt 2):1805–1807. PMID: 12352364
34. Wan J, Corvino TF, Greenfield SP, DiScala C. Kidney and testicle injuries in team and individual sports: data from the National Pediatric Trauma Registry. *J Urol.* 2003;170(4 Pt 2):1528–1533. PMID: 14501652 doi:10.1097/01.ju.0000083999.16060.ff

F: Dermatologic Conditions

■ HISTORY FORM QUESTION

Medical Question

1. *Do you have any recurring skin rashes including herpes or* Staphylococcus aureus *infection?*

Secondary Questions

- Do you use medication for your skin problem (oral or topical)?
- Have you ever missed practices or games because of your skin problem?

■ KEY POINTS

- Skin infections are common reasons to temporarily restrict participation in sports with skin-to-skin contact to reduce the risk of transmission.
- Herpes simplex, staphylococcal infections (including community-acquired methicillin-resistant *Staphylococcus aureus* [CA MRSA] infection), molluscum contagiosum, and tinea (fungal) are common skin infections that require treatment before participation is allowed.
- Contact, collision, and shared-equipment sports pose the greatest risk of transmission of skin infections.
- Proper diagnosis, documentation, and appropriate treatment are critical in determining return to play.

The American Academy of Pediatrics has a policy statement on infectious diseases in athletes that includes skin infection identification and care.[1] A standard approach to skin infections used by the National Federation of State High School Associations (NFHS) can be found in the NFHS *Sports-Related Skin Infections Position Statement and Guidelines*.[2] A return to play form can be found at www.nfhs.org. Similar guidelines by the National Collegiate Athletic Association (NCAA) for wrestling can be found in the *NCAA Wrestling Rules* book.[3]

The ability to safely compete with other athletes can be compromised by various common skin conditions that may be transmissible to other athletes. Participation by athletes with active infections may lead to outbreaks among teammates and opponents. Participation must be restricted if the infections are communicable by themselves or if the conditions increase the risk of transmission of blood-borne pathogens.

In a national survey of high school athletes, skin infections occurred at a reported rate of 2.27 cases per 100,000 athlete exposures. Wrestling (73%) and football (18%) accounted for the majority of infections, with bacterial (60%) and fungal (28%) infections being the most common.[4] A 5-year surveillance study of NCAA wrestling from 2009 to 2014 found a skin infection rate of 14.23 cases per 10,000 athlete exposures, with 74% resulting in at least 24 hours of time loss from practice/competition.[5] It accounted for almost 9% of reported practice injuries and the largest percentage of time loss injuries (17%).[5] Skin infections are most easily transmitted during sports by skin-to-skin contact, but they can also be spread by using shared equipment, towels, or razors. Anderson[6] found the incidence of skin infections to be 8% and 20% among high school wrestlers and collegiate wrestlers, respectively, with more than half of the infections involving the head, face, and neck. Researchers in one study reported a 33% likelihood of contracting herpes simplex virus (HSV) when wrestling with an infected opponent.[6]

Data analysis from the National High School Sports-Related Injury Surveillance Study showed that more than 60% of skin infections were bacterial, with tinea and herpes representing 28% and 5%, respectively.[4] NCAA surveillance found that herpetic infections represented more than 45% of skin infections, with fungal and bacterial infections representing 22% and 14%, respectively.[5] These conditions and the timing of their treatment can affect whether athletes will be declared eligible according to the rules of their sport at the time of practice or competition. Both the NCAA and the NFHS have very specific policies on the identification of, treatment of, and return to play for players with skin infections.

A 5-year surveillance study of NCAA wrestling found that most skin infections (67.9%) occurred during the regular season. The majority were reported during practices (89.3%), and this resulted in a minimum of 24 hours of time loss. Data were captured via the NCAA Injury Surveillance Program. The most common skin infections were viral, herpes simplex, bacterial, fungal, tinea versicolor, and impetigo. Fungal skin infections typically result in more time loss. The rate of recurrent skin infections was 22.3%.[5]

The NCAA recommends "... that qualified personnel, including a knowledgeable, experienced physician examine the skin of all wrestlers before any participation."[3] Restriction from participation because of dermatologic conditions ranges from 6% to 8%, making this one of the more common reasons to restrict participation.[7]

PHYSICAL EXAMINATION

The physical examination includes a thorough skin survey with particular attention to exposed areas and any areas that might potentially come into contact with another competitor or equipment (eg, wrestling mats, batting helmets). The principal objective in the dermatologic examination is to identify skin infections that might limit participation, including fungal rashes (tinea), viral conditions (herpes simplex, molluscum contagiosum, and warts), infestations (scabies and lice), and bacterial conditions (impetigo, CA MRSA, carbuncles, furuncles, and folliculitis) (Table 5F-1). The examination includes looking for signs of trauma, atypical bruising, acne, sun damage, and dermatitis (contact dermatitis, eczema, psoriasis, or urticarial dermatitis), as well as marks of illicit drug use or evidence of scarring, which may raise concerns for behaviors of self-harm such as cutting or burning.[8–10]

While a thorough search for abnormal nevi is not possible within the limits of the preparticipation evaluation, individuals with suspicious nevi noted during the examination should be referred for further evaluation or treatment. These lesions should not preclude medical eligibility for participation.

Skin conditions manifest differently on different skin tones. Skin diseases and conditions, such as rosacea, skin cancer, sarcoidosis, melanoma, acne keloidalis nuchae, keloids, vitiligo, and seborrheic dermatitis, can present differently in darker skin tones. Melanoma is one of the most serious types of skin cancer. People of African or Asian descent commonly develop melanoma in the hands and feet.[5] Vitiligo is an autoimmune disorder that causes skin to lose its natural pigment or color. It is more evident in darker skin tones. Seborrheic dermatitis manifests on lighter skin tones as scaly patches and red rash. However, on darker skin tones, the rash can present as pink, purplish, or white.[5] Accurate diagnosis of skin conditions is essential for proper treatment. It is important to distinguish these skin conditions (which do not preclude participation) from skin infections (which do preclude participation).

HSV (Figure 5F-1) is widespread and has the potential for epidemic outbreaks among wrestlers (**herpes gladiatorum**). Herpes simplex also causes perioral lesions—"cold sores"—that are spread by contact. Athletes can be infectious before the actual skin outbreak is visible. Typical lesions are vesicular, generally clustered on an erythematous base, and can progress to shallow ulcers with surrounding erythema. They are mostly seen around the face, neck, and arms, often on the right side because most wrestlers "lock up" on their right side. During the initial outbreak, systemic symptoms may be present, including fever and adenopathy, sore throat, general malaise, and headache.

Table 5F-1. Categorization and Appearance of Common Skin Infections in Athletes

Skin Infections	Category	Appearance
Herpes simplex infection	Viral	Clustered lesions; shallow ulcers
Tinea	Fungal	Lesions with flaking, raised border, and central clearing
Impetigo	Bacterial	"Honey" crusted vesicles and pustules or rash
Molluscum contagiosum	Viral	Flesh-colored, small (3–5 mm) papules with central indentation
Warts	Viral	Firm, skin-colored papules
Community-acquired methicillin-resistant *Staphylococcus aureus*	Bacterial	Cellulitis or bulla; abscess
Cellulitis	Bacterial	Swelling; red, hot, and tender skin
Boils (Furuncles)	Bacterial	Reddish or purplish, tender bumps
Carbuncle	Bacterial	Cluster of boils

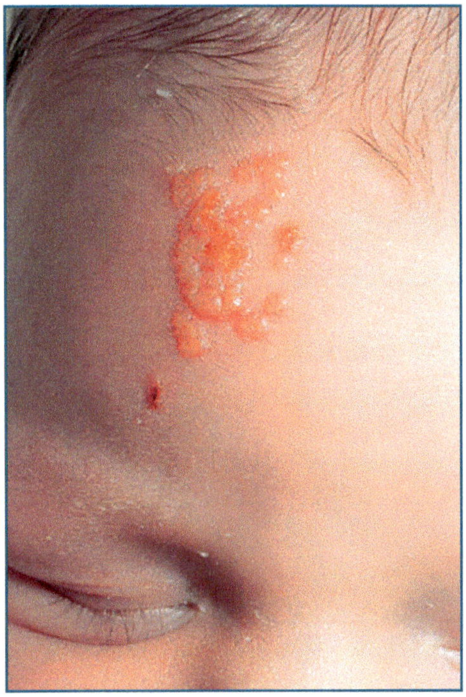

Figure 5F-1. Herpes Simplex

Reproduced from American Academy of Pediatrics Section on Dermatology. Approach to the patient with a rash. In: Krowchuk DP, Mancini AJ, eds. *Pediatric Dermatology: A Quick Reference Guide*. 5th ed. American Academy of Pediatrics; 2025:1–13.

Tinea is a fungal infection of the skin (tinea corporis) (Figure 5F-2) or scalp (tinea capitis) and has been reported to occur in up to 42% of wrestlers (**tinea gladiatorum**).[10] It can also be found across all sports because of shared facilities. Typically, these lesions are erythematous plaques with flaking, a raised border, and central clearing. Scalp lesions may be accompanied by hair loss. Diagnosis can be confirmed with potassium hydroxide (KOH) microscopy, a fungal culture, or both. The skin change can last far longer than the infectious period of the rash.

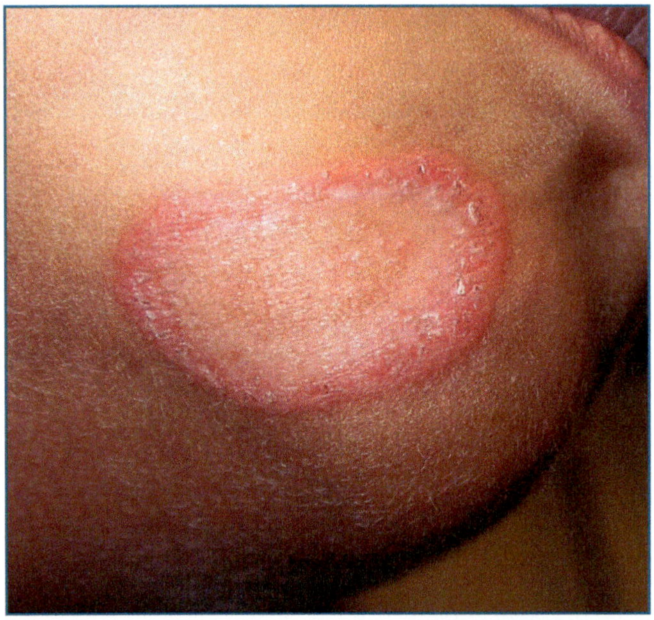

Figure 5F-2. Tinea Corporis

Reproduced from American Academy of Pediatrics Section on Dermatology. Approach to the patient with a rash. In: Krowchuk DP, Mancini AJ, eds. *Pediatric Dermatology: A Quick Reference Guide*. 5th ed. American Academy of Pediatrics; 2025:1–13.

Impetigo (Figure 5F-3) is a bacterial infection caused by *Staphylococcus* or *Streptococcus* species that is highly contagious. It can appear as classic "honey"-crusted vesicles and pustules or as a bullous rash (Figure 5F-4) that may be accompanied by adenopathy; however, systemic symptoms are unusual.[11] The rash can be confused with herpes gladiatorum.

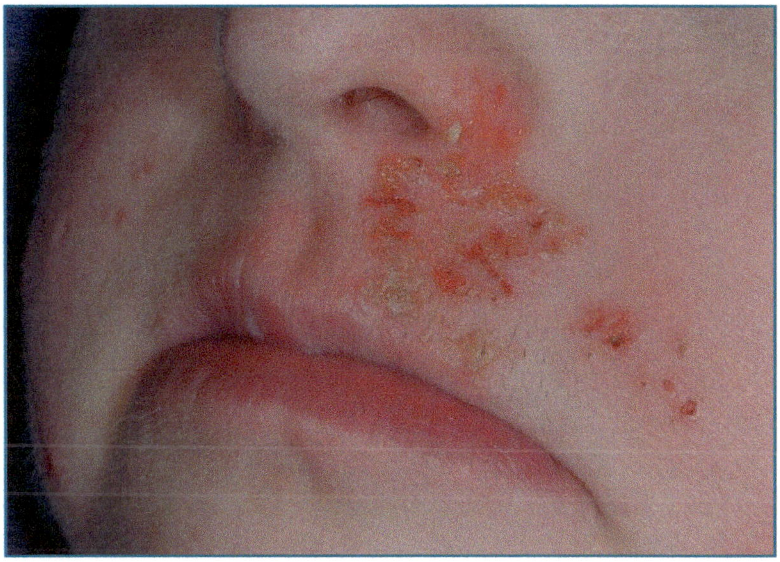

Figure 5F-3. Nonbullous Impetigo

Reproduced from American Academy of Pediatrics Section on Dermatology. Impetigo. In: Krowchuk DP, Mancini AJ, eds. *Pediatric Dermatology: A Quick Reference Guide.* 5th ed. American Academy of Pediatrics; 2025:191–196.

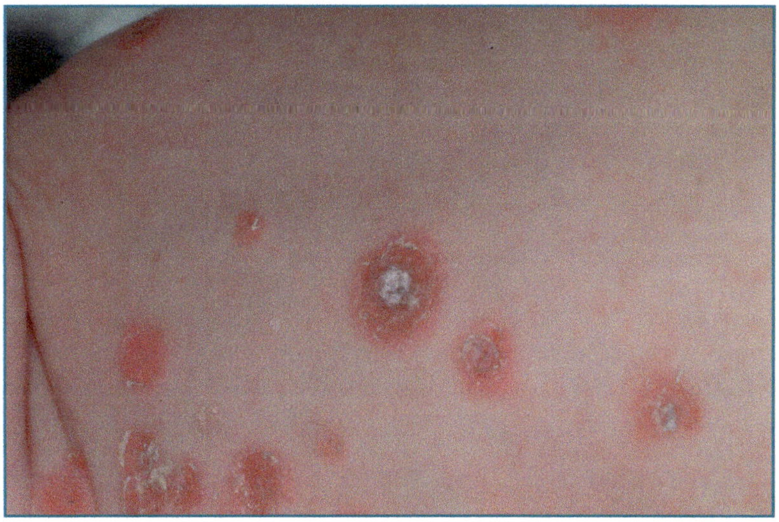

Figure 5F-4. Bullous Impetigo

Reproduced from American Academy of Pediatrics Section on Dermatology. Impetigo. In: Krowchuk DP, Mancini AJ, eds. *Pediatric Dermatology: A Quick Reference Guide.* 5th ed. American Academy of Pediatrics; 2025:191–196.

Molluscum contagiosum (Figure 5F-5) appears as flesh-colored, small (3- to 5-mm) papules with a central indentation, giving it the classic umbilicated appearance. It is reportedly more common in swimmers, gymnasts, and wrestlers. Although athletes who have these lesions are usually asymptomatic, some lesions may develop erythema and pruritus.[12]

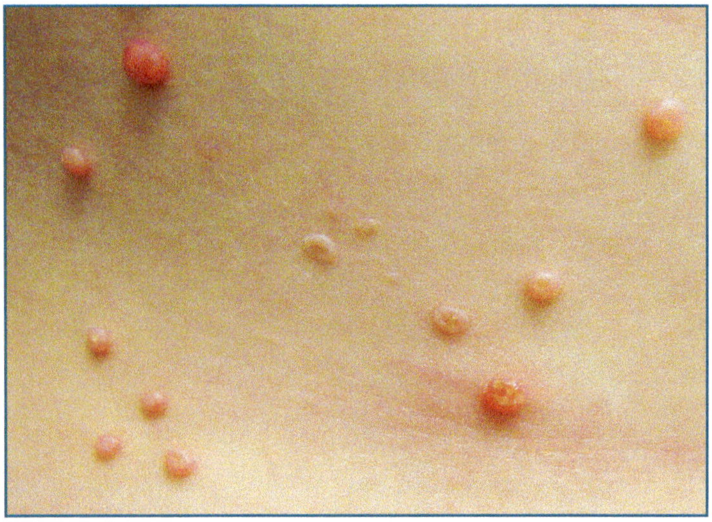

Figure 5F-5. Molluscum Contagiosum

Reproduced from American Academy of Pediatrics Section on Dermatology. Approach to the patient with a rash. In: Krowchuk DP, Mancini AJ, eds. *Pediatric Dermatology: A Quick Reference Guide*. 5th ed. American Academy of Pediatrics; 2025:1–13.

Warts (Figures 5F-6 and 5F-7) appear as firm, skin-colored, hyperkeratotic papules and are not typically painful. They may be present anywhere on the body but typically affect the fingers and hands. Plantar warts may have a flat, skin-colored, hyperkeratotic appearance, and can be painful. Diagnosis is typically made by simple visual inspection.[13]

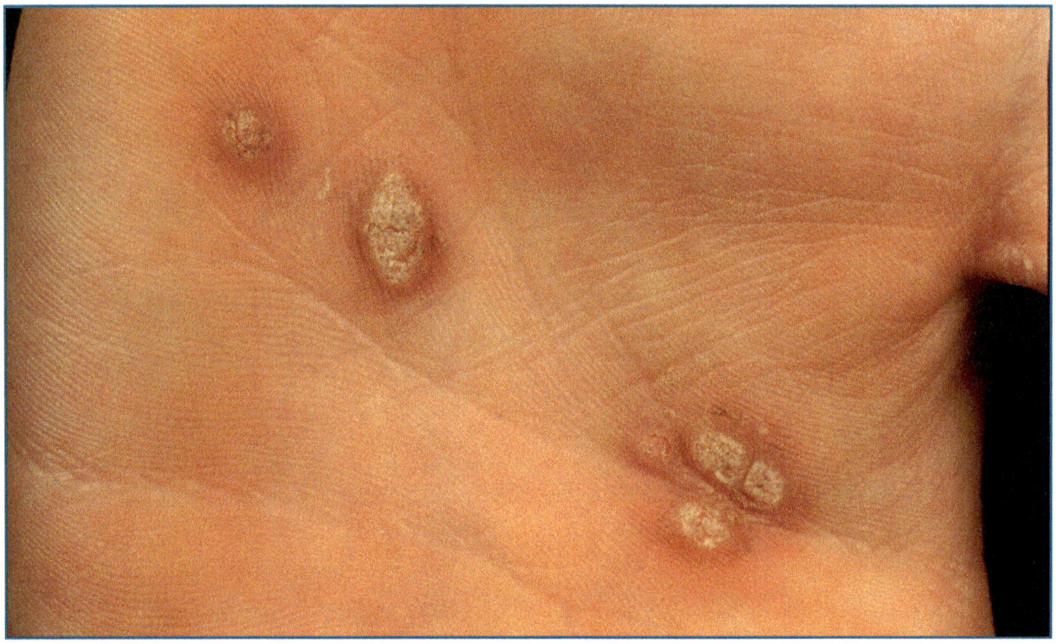

Figure 5F-6. Common Warts

Reproduced from American Academy of Pediatrics Section on Dermatology. Warts. In: Krowchuk DP, Mancini AJ, eds. *Pediatric Dermatology: A Quick Reference Guide*. 5th ed. American Academy of Pediatrics; 2025:111–118.

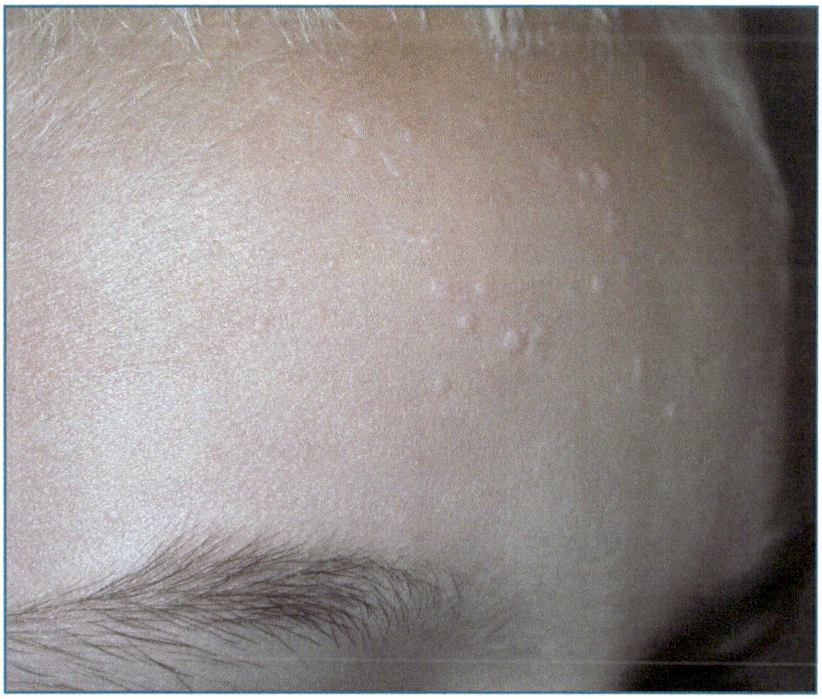

Figure 5F-7. Flat Warts

Reproduced from American Academy of Pediatrics Section on Dermatology. Warts. In: Krowchuk DP, Mancini AJ, eds. *Pediatric Dermatology: A Quick Reference Guide.* 5th ed. American Academy of Pediatrics; 2025:111–118.

CA MRSA is an increasing problem that seems to have a disproportionate prevalence in athletes.[14] CA MRSA infections are often a complication of a skin laceration or an abrasion and may present as cellulitis or bulla, but often develop into an abscess.[14,15] Fever and chills may be present if bacteremia complicates the infection. All abscesses and any superficial skin infections that do not respond to standard antibiotics should be cultured and treated empirically as CA MRSA (strength of recommendation [SOR] C).[14]

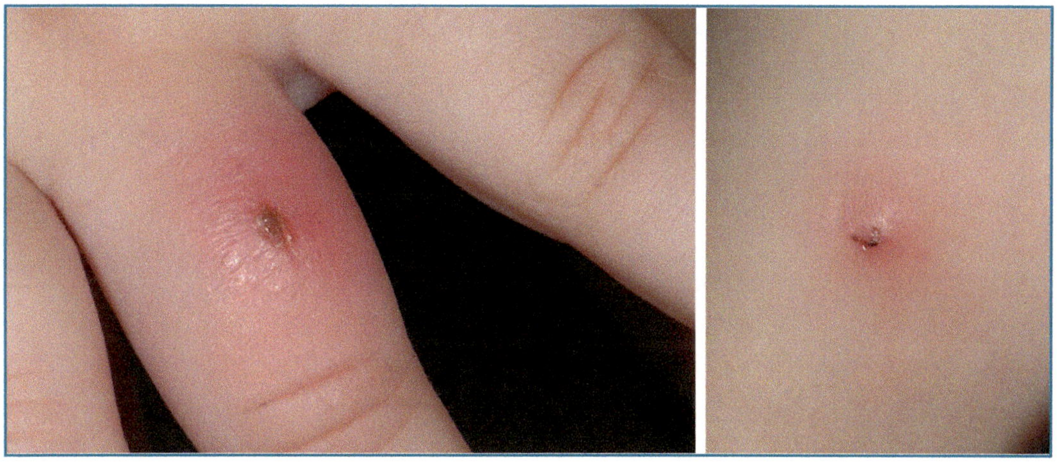

Figure 5F-8. Furuncles

Reproduced from American Academy of Pediatrics Section on Dermatology. Folliculitis/furunculosis/carbunculosis. In: Krowchuk DP, Mancini AJ, eds. *Pediatric Dermatology: A Quick Reference Guide.* 5th ed. American Academy of Pediatrics; 2025:185–190.

MEDICAL ELIGIBILITY FOR PARTICIPATION

The presence of any open wound or infectious skin condition that cannot be protected warrants exclusion from competition that involves close contact with another player or shared equipment until the wound is healed. Merely covering the rash without treatment is not acceptable for return to close-contact sports. Examples include open wounds that cannot be adequately covered and infections, including herpes simplex, scabies, louse infestation, molluscum contagiosum, tinea corporis, cellulitis, impetigo, and furuncles (Figure 5F-8) or carbuncles.

Restricting participation is especially important for sports that involve close physical contact, such as wrestling, rugby, and martial arts, and for sports during which equipment (eg, mats, helmets) is shared. Recent studies suggest that prompt identification and treatment of athletes who have been infected is essential to reduce the spread of the infection to teammates and opponents.[16] Participation may resume when the condition has been adequately treated, is no longer contagious, and the appropriate guidelines (eg, NCAA, NFHS) have been met. For athletes with recurrent herpes gladiatorum, prophylactic treatment during the entire season with a nucleoside analogue (eg, acyclovir, famciclovir, or valacyclovir) is recommended.[17] Similarly, fluconazole has been demonstrated to be a reasonably effective prophylactic for recurrent tineal infections.[18]

The NFHS and NCAA wrestling regulations for skin disorders are similar, although there are some differences in the specific requirements for return to participation for wrestlers with skin infections. The NCAA requires that wrestlers be checked by a qualified examiner before and during each day of a meet or tournament and that written documentation be provided regarding diagnosis, type, and time of treatment and communicability.[3] Both NCAA and NFHS regulations require treatment for a specific period and the ability to cover the lesion adequately. The requirements are based on case series, expert consensus, and disease-oriented evidence. The guidelines and recommended form for return to high school sports with skin infections can be obtained through the NFHS *Sports-Related Skin Infections Position Statement and Guidelines*[2] (www.nfhs.org) and in Appendix C of the *NCAA Wrestling Rules*[3] (www.ncaa.org) (SOR C).

For an initial outbreak of **herpes gladiatorum**, wrestlers should be treated and not allowed to practice or compete for a minimum of 10 days. If general body signs and symptoms such as fever and swollen lymph nodes are present, the minimum period of treatment should be extended to 14 days. If antivirals are not used, the infected participant may return to full contact wrestling only after all lesions are well healed with well-adhered scabs, there has been no new vesicle formation in the preceding 72 hours, and there are no swollen lymph nodes near the affected area. For a recurrent HSV infection, athletes must be free of systemic symptoms, have had no new lesions for 72 hours, and have been receiving oral antiviral treatment for 120 hours to return to competition. Questionable cases can be laboratory confirmed with viral culture, serology, immunofluorescence, or polymerase chain reaction testing.[2,3]

Tinea corporis requires treatment with a topical fungicide for a minimum of 72 hours, while **tinea capitis** requires a minimum of 2 weeks of treatment with an oral antifungal medication. Treatment failure is common for tinea capitis, with one study showing only a

70% cure rate.[19] **Molluscum and warts** require treatment (topical or surgical) and covering.[13] **Bacterial dermatoses** (CA MRSA infection, impetigo, furuncle, carbuncle, cellulitis, folliculitis, and skin abscess) require no new lesions for 48 hours, no moist or draining lesions (active lesions may not be covered to participate), and completion of at least 72 hours of oral antibiotic treatment.[11]

Restriction of athletes with infectious skin conditions from practice and competition is recommended until appropriate intervention, including guideline-based treatment with appropriate medications, and, when necessary and appropriate, barrier protection is used. Occlusive coverage of the lesion must be with a nonpermeable membrane and a securely attached bandage or patch. Most sports require that competitors completely cover open wounds and infectious skin conditions to prevent exposure to other competitors.[16] Standard precautions are recommended by the Centers for Disease Control and Prevention for wounds that are open or bleeding.

Prevention strategies for skin infections are varied and not standardized.[16] Recommended approaches include close surveillance of all athletes, sanitizing the mats and equipment daily, cleaning practice clothing daily, immediate showering with soap after practices, and implementing pharmacologic intervention to reduce the risk of new and recurrent skin infections.[19]

Although the primary mode of skin infection transmission is through skin-to-skin contact, most support the recommendation that mats and equipment (headgear) be cleaned using a solution of 1 part bleach in 9 parts water made daily. Season-long prophylactic treatment of HSV with antiviral agents for individuals, as well as for entire teams, has been demonstrated to be effective and is increasingly being implemented to prevent widespread infection.[13,20]

Controlling MRSA transmission includes handwashing, showering with soap, covering cuts and abrasions, laundering personal items such as towels and athletic supporters, and refraining from sharing razors and towels (SOR C). Carriage rates have been reported in the range of 5% to 27% and are generally higher among athletes than among the general population. One study demonstrated a 75% reduction in MRSA cases after implementing an athlete educational program on hygiene[21] (SOR B). Guidelines from the Infectious Diseases Society of America suggest that efforts to eradicate carriers with recurrent infections can be considered, but this is controversial (SOR C).[22]

Other skin conditions such as acne and conditions that might be worsened by exercise or possibly affect performance (eg, urticaria, angioedema, cold-induced conditions such as Raynaud syndrome)[23] should be noted. While not typical reasons to restrict athlete medical eligibility, these conditions may, at times, limit participation.[13,24] Atopic and allergic skin ailments can often be managed effectively. Acne can be difficult to control, even among the athletes being treated, because sweat and constrictive uniforms and equipment may exacerbate the condition. Although acne should not affect eligibility or performance, it may have adverse social and emotional consequences for an athlete, may be confused with other skin conditions, and may be a break in the protective skin barrier and a portal for secondary infection. Spironolactone use is becoming widespread for the treatment of acne, but it is listed on the NCAA banned substance list.

REFERENCES

1. Davies HD, Jackson MA, Rice SG; COMMITTEE ON INFECTIOUS DISEASES; COUNCIL ON SPORTS MEDICINE AND FITNESS. Infectious diseases associated with organized sports and outbreak control. *Pediatrics.* 2017;140(4):e20172477. PMID: 28947608 doi:10.1542/peds.2017-2477
2. National Federation of State High School Associations (NFHS) Sports Medicine Advisory Committee (SMAC). *Sports-Related Skin Infections Position Statement and Guidelines.* National Federation of State High School Associations; 2022. Accessed April 18, 2025. https://www.nfhs.org/media/5546437/2022-nfhs-sports-related-skin-infections-position-statement-and-guidelines-final-3-8-22.pdf
3. NCAA Publishing. *2025–26 and 2026–27 NCAA Wrestling Rules.* https://ncaapublications.com/products/2025-26-and-2026-27-ncaa-mens-wrestling-rules-online-pdf
4. Ashack KA, Burton KA, Johnson TR, Currie DW, Comstock RD, Dellavalle RP. Skin infections among US high school athletes: a national survey. *J Am Acad Dermatol.* 2016;74(4):679–684.e1. PMID: 26850656
5. Herzog MM, Fraser MA, Register-Mihalik JK, Kerr ZY. Epidemiology of skin infections in men's wrestling: analysis of 2009–2010 through 2013–2014 National Collegiate Athletic Association surveillance data. *J Athl Train.* 2017;52(5):457–463. PMID: 28362160 doi:10.4085/1062-6050-52.2.16
6. Anderson BJ. The epidemiology and clinical analysis of several outbreaks of herpes gladiatorum. *Med Sci Sports Exerc.* 2003;35(11):1809–1814. PMID: 14600542 doi:10.1249/01.MSS.0000093759.79673.3C
7. Bender TW III. Cutaneous manifestations of disease in athletes. *Skinmed.* 2003;2(1):34–40. PMID: 14673322 doi:10.1111/j.1540-9740.2003.01968.x
8. Brooks C, Kujawska A, Patel D. Cutaneous allergic reactions induced by sporting activities. *Sports Med.* 2003;33(9):699–708. PMID: 12846592 doi:10.2165/00007256-200333090-00005
9. Metelitsa A, Barankin B, Lin AN. Diagnosis of sports-related dermatoses. *Int J Dermatol.* 2004;43(2):113–119. PMID: 15125501 doi:10.1111/j.1365-4632.2004.02101.x
10. Kohl TD, Lisney M. Tinea gladiatorum: wrestling's emerging foe. *Sports Med.* 2000;29(6):439–447. PMID: 10870869 doi:10.2165/00007256-200029060-00006
11. Sedgwick PE, Dexter WW, Smith CT. Bacterial dermatoses in sports. *Clin Sports Med.* 2007;26(3):383–396. PMID: 17826190 doi:10.1016/j.csm.2007.04.008
12. Cyr PR, Dexter W. Viral skin infection: preventing outbreaks in sports settings. *Phys Sportsmed.* 2004;32(7):33–38. PMID: 20086420 doi:10.3810/psm.2004.07.444
13. Pleacher MD, Dexter WW. Cutaneous fungal and viral infections in athletes. *Clin Sports Med.* 2007;26(3):397–411. PMID: 17826191 doi:10.1016/j.csm.2007.04.004
14. Benjamin HJ, Nikore V, Takagishi J. Practical management: community-associated methicillin-resistant *Staphylococcus aureus* (CA-MRSA): the latest sports epidemic. *Clin J Sport Med.* 2007;17(5):393–397. PMID: 17873553 doi:10.1097/JSM.0b013e31814be92b
15. Barrett TW, Moran GJ. Update on emerging infections: news from the Centers for Disease Control and Prevention. Methicillin-resistant *Staphylococcus aureus* infections among competitive sports participants—Colorado, Indiana, Pennsylvania, and Los Angeles County, 2000-2003. *Ann Emerg Med.* 2004;43(1):43–45. PMID: 14707939 https://doi.org/10.1016/j.annemergmed.2003.10.007
16. Rifat SF, Ruffin MT IV, Gorenflo DW. Disqualifying criteria in a preparticipation sports evaluation. *J Fam Pract.* 1995;41(1):42–50. PMID: 7798065
17. Anderson BJ. The effectiveness of valacyclovir in preventing reactivation of herpes gladiatorum in wrestlers. *Clin J Sport Med.* 1999;9(2):86–90. PMID: 10442623 doi:10.1097/00042752-199904000-00008
18. Brickman K, Einstein E, Sinha S, Ryno J, Guiness M. Fluconazole as a prophylactic measure for tinea gladiatorum in high school wrestlers. *Clin J Sport Med.* 2009;19(5):412–414. PMID: 19741315 doi:10.1097/JSM.0b013e3181b2f397
19. Adams BB. Tinea corporis gladiatorum. *J Am Acad Dermatol.* 2002;47(2):286–290. PMID: 12140477 doi:10.1067/mjd.2002.120603
20. Howe WB, Harmon KG, Rubin A. Preventing infectious disease in sports. *Phys Sportsmed.* 2003;31(2):23–29. PMID: 20086454 doi:10.3810/psm.2003.02.186
21. Sanders JC. Reducing MRSA infections in college student athletes: implementation of a prevention program. *J Community Health Nurs.* 2009;26(4):161–172. PMID: 19866384 doi:10.1080/07370010903259162

22. Farhadian JA, Tlougan BE, Adams BB, Leventhal JS, Sanchez MR. Skin conditions of baseball, cricket, and softball players. *Sports Med.* 2013;43(7):575–589. PMID: 23456491 https://doi.org/10.1007/s40279-013-0022-4
23. Tlougan BE, Mancini AJ, Mandell JA, Cohen DE, Sanchez MR. Skin conditions in figure skaters, ice-hockey players and speed skaters: part II—cold-induced, infectious and inflammatory dermatoses. *Sports Med.* 2011;41(11):967–984. PMID: 21985216 doi:10.2165/11592190-000000000-00000
24. Katelaris CH. Exercise and skin-related allergies: diagnosis and management: review article. *Int SportsMed J.* 2002;3(2):1–5

G: Musculoskeletal Concerns

HISTORY FORM QUESTIONS

1. *Have you ever had a fracture or an injury to a bone, muscle, ligament, joint, or tendon that caused you to miss a practice or game?*
2. *Do you have a bone, muscle, ligament, or joint injury that currently bothers you?*

SECONDARY QUESTIONS

- Have you ever had any surgeries on bones, joints, ligaments, muscles, as well as associated injury mechanisms?
- Have you ever had any musculoskeletal injury that resulted in time loss (missed practice and/or games)? How much time was lost?
- Have you ever had any physical therapy or rehabilitation?
- Have you ever had swelling of a joint not related to an injury?
- Have you ever been diagnosed with chronic arthritis (juvenile idiopathic arthritis) or juvenile rheumatoid arthritis?
- Have you ever had a referral to a specialist such as an orthopedist, a physiatrist, a neurologist, or a rheumatologist?
- Were you ever "cleared to play" by a treating physician, and do you consider yourself "back to normal"?

KEY POINTS

- A general musculoskeletal screening examination is reasonable for individuals with no symptoms and no previous injury.
- Individuals with unresolved musculoskeletal pain require additional evaluation and management before sports participation.
- Stress fractures, overuse injuries, and recurrent soft-tissue injuries can be associated with nutritional deficiencies, training errors, poor neuromuscular control, and abnormal biomechanics.

Musculoskeletal injuries and concerns are the most common problems that team physicians and health care professionals see in the office, in the athletic training facility, and during the preparticipation evaluation (PPE). Musculoskeletal injuries include fractures, stress fractures, and other injuries to bone, muscles, tendons, ligaments, and joints. A thorough review of the musculoskeletal history and targeted physical examination of previously injured areas may improve detection of musculoskeletal conditions during the PPE.

The first and most important step in the evaluation of the musculoskeletal system to determine medical eligibility is to take a focused musculoskeletal history. Missed practices or games suggest a potentially serious condition impacting the musculoskeletal system. The nature and duration of missed practices or games are important to discuss and document.

The provider needs to understand the mechanism of injury and any subsequent treatment, rehabilitation, or surgical intervention. It is essential to understand whether the individual was fully rehabilitated and able to return to the prior level of competition without disability. Individuals with unresolved musculoskeletal pain, weakness, instability, or loss of joint motion may need additional evaluation and rehabilitation to optimize function and exclude other conditions.

In addition to this history, the examining clinician needs to understand key elements of a general musculoskeletal screening examination, as well as joint and injury-specific examinations. This section addresses the issues for medical eligibility related to the musculoskeletal system.

BONE STRESS INJURIES

One special area of note is bone stress injuries. These are often a result of training errors, overload, nutritional or hormonal deficiency, or other metabolic issues. These injuries result when repetitive, submaximal compression, torsion, or tension forces outpace the bone's ability to remodel and heal. Bone stress injuries range on a continuum from a stress reaction to cortical fracture, with symptoms ranging from broad, low-intensity pain to severe focal pain with associated difficulty with weight-bearing (in the case of lower extremity bone stress injuries) as the fracture progresses. Early identification of bone stress injury is important because delayed diagnosis may result in a higher-grade injury that requires longer healing time or even surgical intervention. The initial management is identifying the cause and limiting painful activity. Common sports where bone stress injuries occur are figure skating, gymnastics, dance, basketball, rowing, baseball, cheerleading, and cross country and distance running.

Risk factors for bone stress injuries include:

- Training errors: either a rapid increase in intensity and/or duration or prolonged high-level training without periodization (including short- and long-term rest breaks) and adequate workout recovery time.[1–4]
- Low energy availability or relative energy deficiency in sport (RED-S) can lead to decreased bone mineral density (BMD) and stress fractures. A dietary history, including daily caloric intake, vitamin D, and calcium, is important. A menstrual history is also very important because of the association of amenorrhea/oligomenorrhea with risk for osteoporosis or osteopenia. For individuals 18 years and older, 3 evidence-based risk assessment tools (LEAF-Q, LEAM-Q, and RED-S CAT) have been shown to be predictive of bone stress injury and impaired bone health.[5–10] See Chapter 5I for more information.

Assessment of BMD by dual-energy x-ray absorptiometry (DXA) is based on the severity and number of triad risk factors.[5] Consensus statements from the Female and Male

Athlete Triad Coalition provide detailed recommendations for DXA testing, summarized in Table 5G-1 and Table 5G-2.[5,11] They recommend BMD Z-Score (and not T-Score) be reported for all children, adolescents, premenopausal women, and men younger than 50 years. For those younger than 20 years, posteroanterior spine and whole body except for the head are the preferred sites of measurement.[5] For adults 20 years and older, they recommend that the weight-bearing sites (posteroanterior spine, total hip, and femoral neck) be evaluated. Follow-up BMD assessment by DXA may be as frequent as every 1 to 2 years and is based on both the initial BMD and the ongoing clinical status of the individual.[5]

Table 5G-1. Indications for Dual-Energy X-ray Absorptiometry Testing to Detect Low Bone Mineral Density in Females

Risk Factors	≥ 1 High-Risk Triad Risk Factors[a]	≥ 2 Moderate-Risk Triad Risk Factors[a]
Eating disorders	• History of a diagnosed eating disorder (See *Diagnostic and Statistical Manual of Mental Disorders, Fifth Edition.*)	• Currently experiencing or history of disordered eating for ≥ 6 mo
BMI[b]	• BMI < 17.5 kg/m^2; < 85% estimated weight; and recent weight loss of > 10% in 1 mo	• BMI between 17.5 kg/m^2 and 18.5 kg/m^2, 85%–90% estimated weight, or recent weight loss of 5%–10% in 1 mo
Menstruation	• Menarche at > 16 years of age • Currently experiencing or history of < 6 menses over 12 mo	• Menarche between 15 years of age and 16 years of age • Currently experiencing or history of 6–8 menses over 12 mo
Fractures	• 2 prior stress reactions/fractures, 1 high-risk stress reaction/fracture,[c] or a low-energy, non-traumatic fracture	• One prior stress reaction/fracture • History of ≥ 1 nonperipheral or ≥ 2 peripheral long-bone traumatic fractures (nonstress) should be considered for DXA testing if there is ≥ 1 moderate- or high-risk triad risk factor
Prior Z value	• Prior Z value <−2.0	• Prior Z value between −1.0 and −2.0 (after at least a 1-y interval from baseline DXA)

Abbreviations: BMI, body mass index; DXA, dual-energy x-ray absorptiometry.

[a] See https://doi.org/10.1136/bjsports-2013-093218 for risk factors.

[b] BMI can be calculated as the weight in kilograms divided by the height in meters squared.

[c] High-risk stress reaction/fracture = femoral neck, sacrum, or pelvis.

Derived from De Souza MJ, Nattiv A, Joy E, et al; Expert Panel. 2014 Female Athlete Triad Coalition Consensus Statement on Treatment and Return to Play of the Female Athlete Triad: 1st International Conference held in San Francisco, California, May 2012 and 2nd International Conference held in Indianapolis, Indiana, May 2013. *Br J Sports Med.* 2014;48(4):289–309.

Table 5G-2. Indications for Dual-Energy X-ray Absorptiometry Testing to Detect Low Bone Mineral Density (BMD) in Males

Athletes With 1 or More High-Risk Factors[a]:
Body mass index (BMI) ≤ 17.5 in adults, *or* % median BMI ≤ 85% in adolescents, *or* ≥ 10% weight loss/month
Two prior bone stress injuries or 1 prior injury in a high-risk location such as the femoral neck, sacrum, or pelvis
A clinical eating disorder
Prior BMD Z-score ≤ −2.0
Athletes With 2 or More Moderate-Risk Factors[a]:
BMI between 17.5 and 18.5 kg/m² in adults, *or* % median BMI 86%–89% in adolescents, *or* weight loss between 5% and 10% of body weight per month
One prior bone stress injury
Some history of disordered eating behaviors
Prior BMD Z-score between −1.0 and −2.0 in athletes involved in weight-bearing sports[b]
Athletes who have been taking a medication that may affect their BMD may need screening

[a] See https://doi.org/10.1097/JSM.0000000000000948 for risk factors.

[b] For athletes in non–weight-bearing sports, a Z-score of −2.0 is used.

Reproduced from Fredericson M, Kussman A, Misra M, et al. The Male Athlete Triad—a consensus statement from the Female and Male Athlete Triad Coalition part II: diagnosis, treatment, and return-to-play. Clin J Sport Med. 2021;31(4):349 -366

PHYSICAL EXAMINATION

The type and extent of the musculoskeletal examination appropriate for the PPE is a much-debated topic, with few studies and little consensus available to guide the clinician. Examiners need to determine which method best suits a given situation, depending on the history of injury, musculoskeletal signs or symptoms, resources and time available, type of sport or activity in which the athlete will participate, level of competition, and experience level of the examining clinician.

General Screening Examination

The yield of musculoskeletal examination is low in asymptomatic athletes who have no history of injury. In addition, history alone has been shown to be 92% sensitive in detecting significant musculoskeletal injuries.[12] **A general screening examination** (Figure 5G-1) may be a reasonable approach for asymptomatic athletes who have no previous injury, despite a sensitivity of 50%.[12] It enables the examiner to identify strength and range-of-motion deficits/asymmetries and limb discrepancies, and assess whether any of the movements elicit pain, which aids in identifying significant injuries and neuromuscular impairments.

The examination may also reveal scars from undisclosed surgery in athletes trying to avoid restrictions of medical eligibility. pGALS (paediatric Gait Arms Legs and Spine) is another resource that can be used as a general musculoskeletal screening examination.[13]

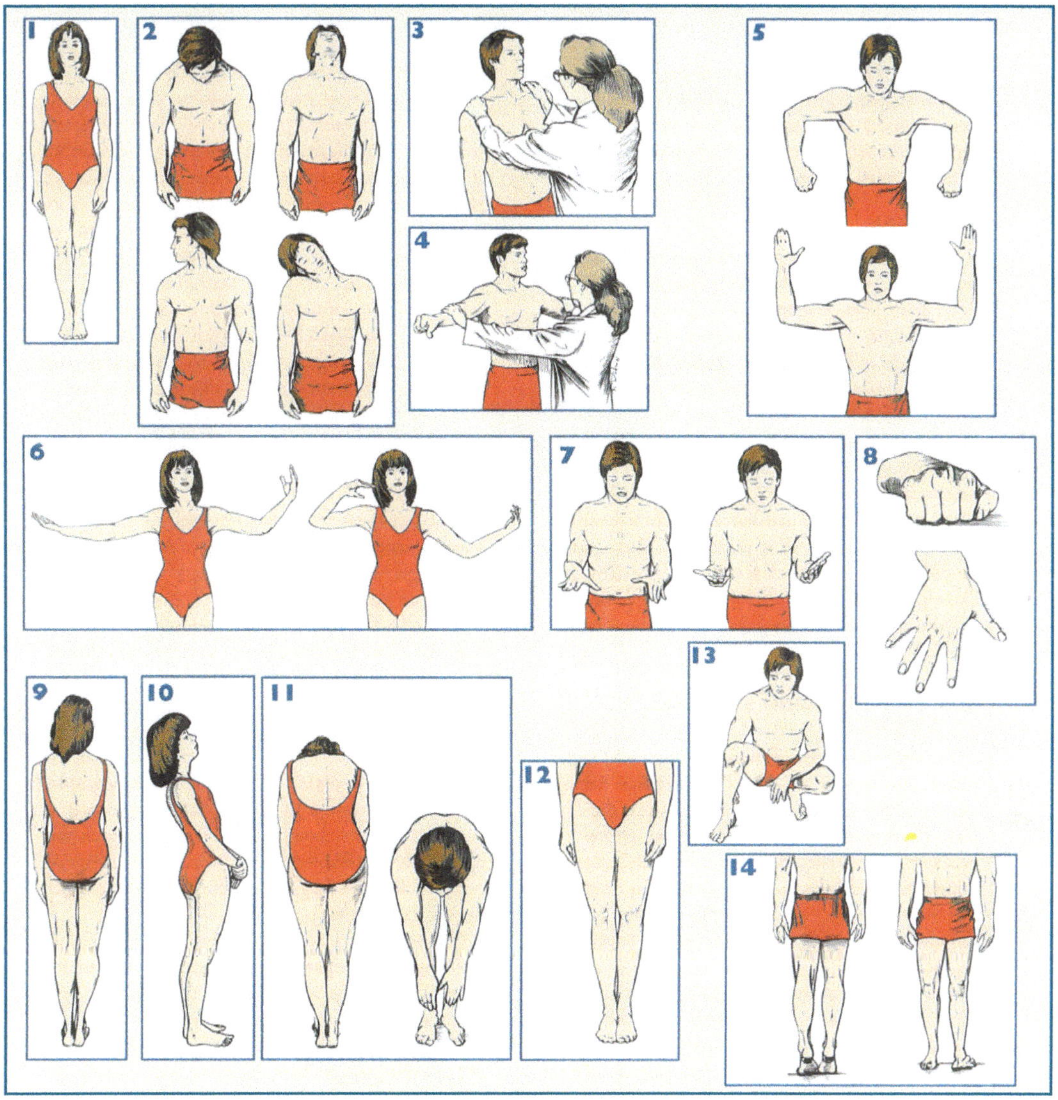

Figure 5G-1. General Musculoskeletal Screening Examination

The general musculoskeletal screening examination consists of (1) inspection, with athlete standing, facing toward examiner (symmetry of trunk, upper extremities); (2) forward flexion, extension, rotation, and lateral flexion of neck (range of motion, cervical spine); (3) resisted shoulder shrug (strength, trapezius); (4) resisted shoulder abduction (strength, deltoid); (5) internal and external rotation of shoulder (range of motion, glenohumeral joint); (6) extension and flexion of elbow (range of motion, elbow); (7) pronation and supination of forearm or wrist (range of motion, elbow and wrist); (8) athlete clenching fist, then spreading fingers (range of motion, hand and fingers); (9) inspection, with athlete facing away from examiner (symmetry of trunk, upper extremities); (10) back extension, with knees straight (spondylolysis or spondylolisthesis); (11) back flexion, with knees straight, facing toward and away from examiner (range of motion, thoracic and lumbosacral spine, spine curvature, hamstring flexibility); (12) inspection of lower extremities, with contraction of quadriceps muscles (alignment, symmetry); (13) "duck walk" 4 steps (motion of hip, knee, and ankle; strength; balance); (14) toe stand and heel walk.

Adding a screening to assess lower extremity neuromuscular control may identify athletes at risk for anterior cruciate ligament (ACL) tears or other lower extremity injuries. If poor neuromuscular control is identified, the examiner can educate the individual on neuromuscular training programs that aim to mitigate injury risk.[14] If the athlete has (1) a previous injury or (2) pain, weakness, atrophy, or other signs or symptoms detected by the general screening examination or the history, the general screening examination is supplemented with relevant elements of the joint-specific examination, or more in-depth evaluation may be required at an additional encounter or with a sports medicine physician.[15]

Joint-Specific Examinations

Assessing individual joints by inspection (scarring, atrophy, asymmetry, swelling), palpation (for tenderness), range of motion, and pain, along with well-established specific maneuvers is more definitive than the general screening examination. If the general screening examination identifies an abnormality, a more thorough and focused joint examination with relevant diagnostic testing may be indicated before determining medical eligibility. However, joint-specific examinations are time-consuming and have a low yield in an asymptomatic athlete without a previous injury. The authoring societies do not consider it necessary to perform an entire joint-specific examination for every individual, but rather to focus the examination using the history or abnormal findings from the general screening. If the setting, time available, and examiner expertise allow, joint-specific examinations can supplement the general screening examination as part of the PPE.

Spine. The cervical spine is inspected for posture and alignment. The ear canal should line up with the middle of the shoulder. Forward flexion of the neck should allow the chin to touch the manubrium; extension should allow a nearly vertical gaze; rotation should enable the chin to almost touch the clavicle in both directions, and the ears should approach the shoulders with lateral flexion. Any asymmetrical or deficient motion should be noted. If the athlete reports any nerve symptoms, the examiner can also include a Spurling test.

Examination of the thoracolumbar spine and back focuses on posture, range of motion, and potential deformities. The scapulae should be level, symmetrical, and flat against the thoracic cage. The presence of scoliosis, kyphosis at the thoracic level, or lordosis at the lumbar level should be noted. As part of the thoracolumbar examination, the athlete bends forward at the waist. The rotary deformities of scoliosis, such as asymmetrical, prominent ribs; curvature of the spine; or an asymmetrical waist, are accentuated in this position (Figure 5G-2). If significant deformity is noted, a referral to a pediatric orthopedic or spine specialist is warranted, as radiographs and treatment may be indicated. Pain or restriction of forward flexion may indicate lumbar disc disease or spondyloarthropathy. If any nerve symptoms are reported, a seated slump test can be performed to assess for nerve root tension (Figure 5G-3). Pain from vertebral body compression fractures is most often midline, is most often worse with flexion of the spine, and may be related to neurological findings. Lumbar extension may increase pain from a facet injury, spondylolysis, spondylolisthesis, or a sprain or strain. If pain is present with lumbar extension in a skeletally immature athlete, further evaluation is warranted to assess for spondylolysis.

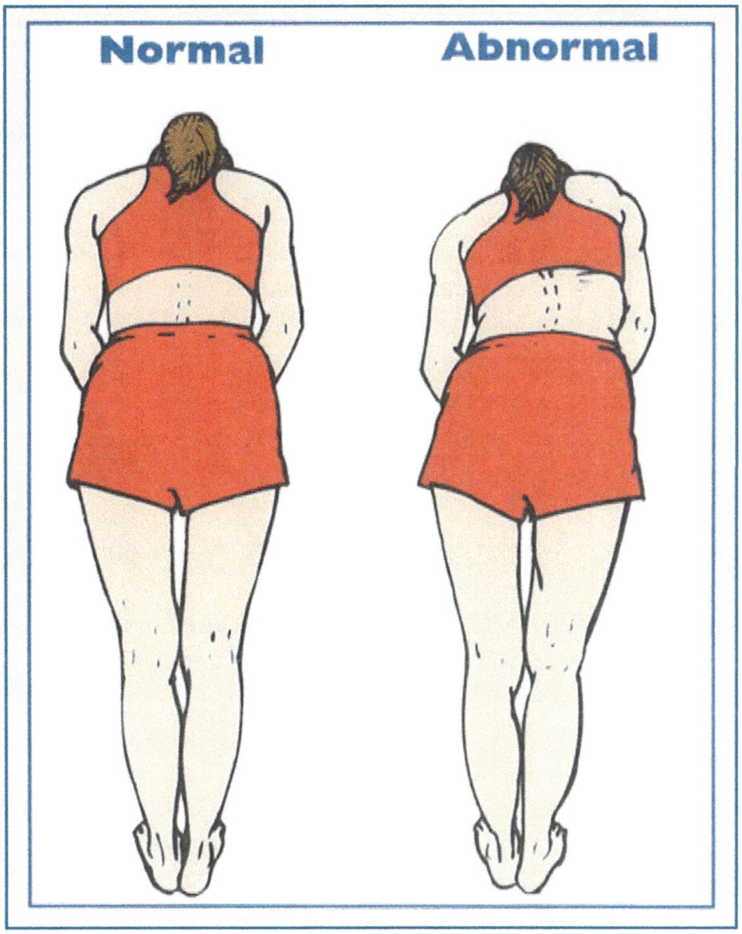

Figure 5G-2. Thoracolumbar Examination for Scoliosis

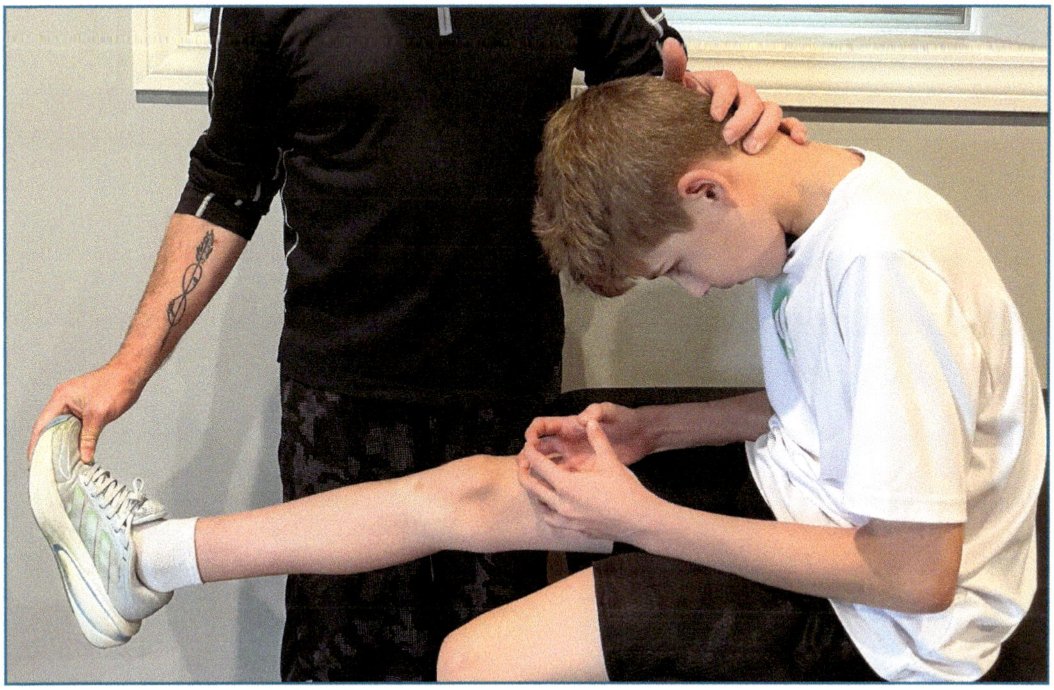

Figure 5G-3. Seated Slump Test
Courtesy of Brian Scott Harvey, DO, FAAP.

Upper Extremity Examination

Shoulder

The shoulder examination begins with inspection for symmetry with the athlete standing. It is important to visualize the posterior and anterior aspects of the shoulder bony and muscular anatomies (for bruising, scapular symmetry, winging, atrophy, acromioclavicular joint prominence, and sternoclavicular joint prominence). Palpate the bilateral sternoclavicular joint, acromioclavicular joint, and bicipital groove. Range of motion in abduction (Figure 5G-4A), flexion (Figure 5G-4B), and internal rotation (Figure 5G-4C) and external rotation (Figure 5G-4D) are then assessed. Some overhead athletes (eg, baseball, tennis, volleyball) can exhibit an increase in external rotation and a decrease in internal rotation in their dominant arm, which can be adaptive in the setting of symmetrical total arc of motion and pathological when there is a loss of total motion compared to the nonthrowing shoulder.

Deltoid strength can be assessed with manual resistance to straight abduction and forward flexion assessments. Shoulder rotator cuff strength can be assessed while the athlete is sitting. The supraspinatus is tested when the shoulder is lifted to 90 degrees into scapular plane abducted to at least 45 degrees and internally rotated (empty can test) (Figure 5G-5A) while the examiner applies resistance to abduction movement over the distal humerus. The infraspinatus and teres minor are tested with the shoulder in adduction, in neutral rotation, and the elbows flexed to 90 degrees, with resistance against external rotation applied to the distal forearm (Figure 5G-5B). The subscapularis is tested with the belly-press test or the lift-off test or with internal rotation strength (Figure 5G-6). For the belly press, the patient's hand is placed flat on their abdomen with the hand, wrist, and elbow in a straight line. The patient is then instructed to press down on their abdomen, and a normal result is the ability to compress the abdomen without flexing at the wrist. The lift-off test is done with the patient's elbow flexed and arm behind the back with their hand at midline and at waist level. The patient is instructed to raise their hand off the back, and a normal result is the ability to do so without pain.[16]

Tests for shoulder impingement signs include the Neer impingement test and the Hawkins test (Figure 5G-7). If there is a history of shoulder instability, the clinician can also assess the shoulder in the supine position with apprehension/relocation maneuvers, as well as anterior and posterior load and shift (Figure 5G-8).

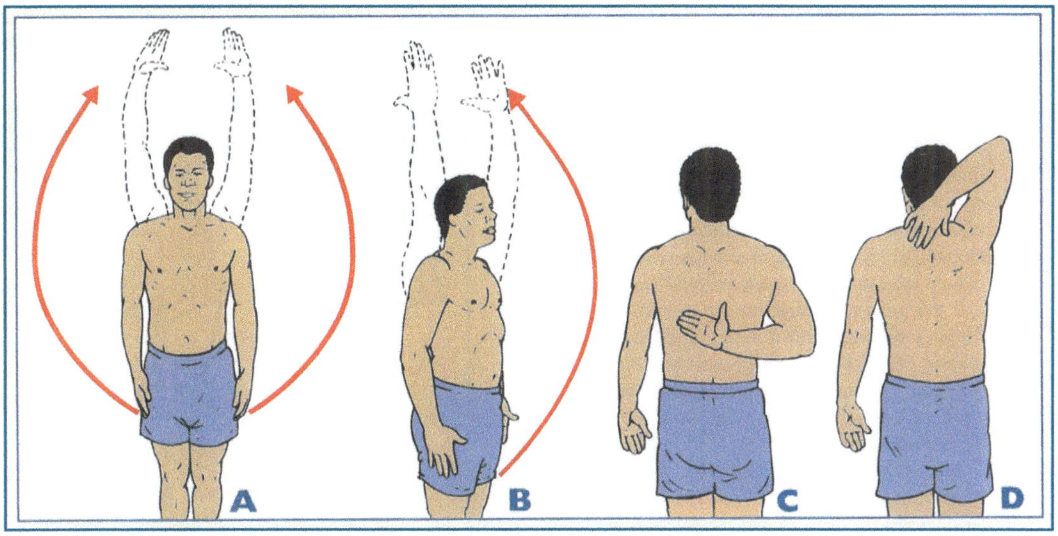

Figure 5G-4. Shoulder Range of Motion

Shoulder range of motion is evaluated in 4 directions. In abduction (A) and forward flexion (B), the athlete should be able to reach completely overhead without excessive or asymmetrical motion of the scapula; in internal rotation (C), the fingertips should reach approximately to the bottom of the opposite scapula; and in external rotation (D), the fingertips should approach the top of the opposite scapula.

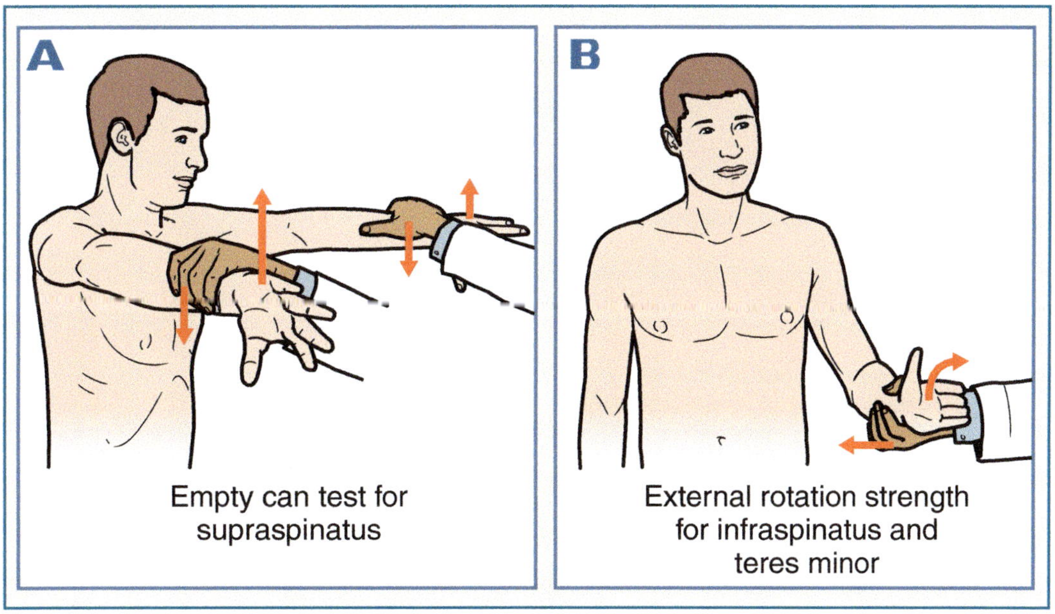

Figure 5G-5. Rotator Cuff Tests

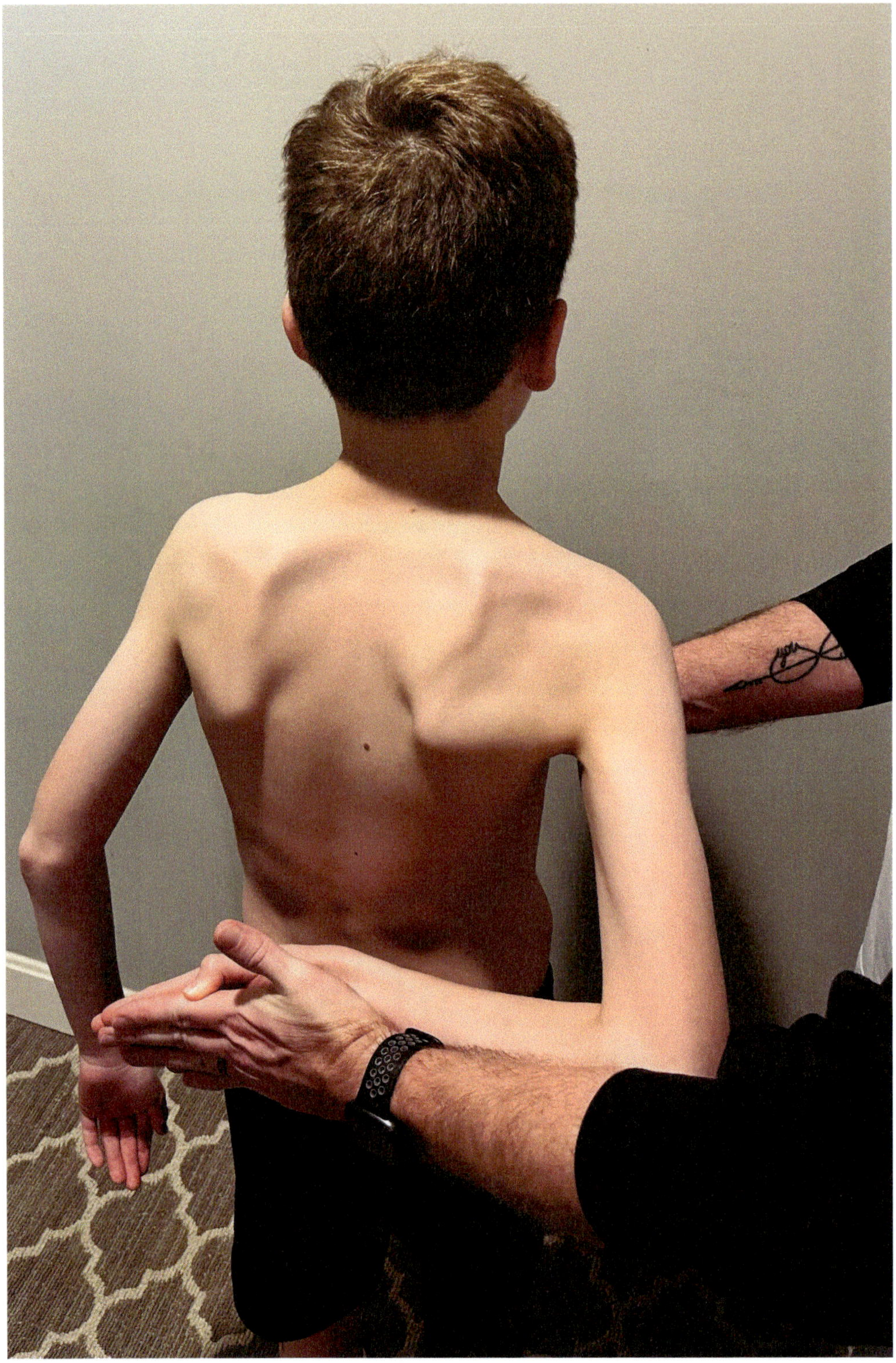

Figure 5G-6. Lift-Off Test
Courtesy of Brian Scott Harvey, DO, FAAP.

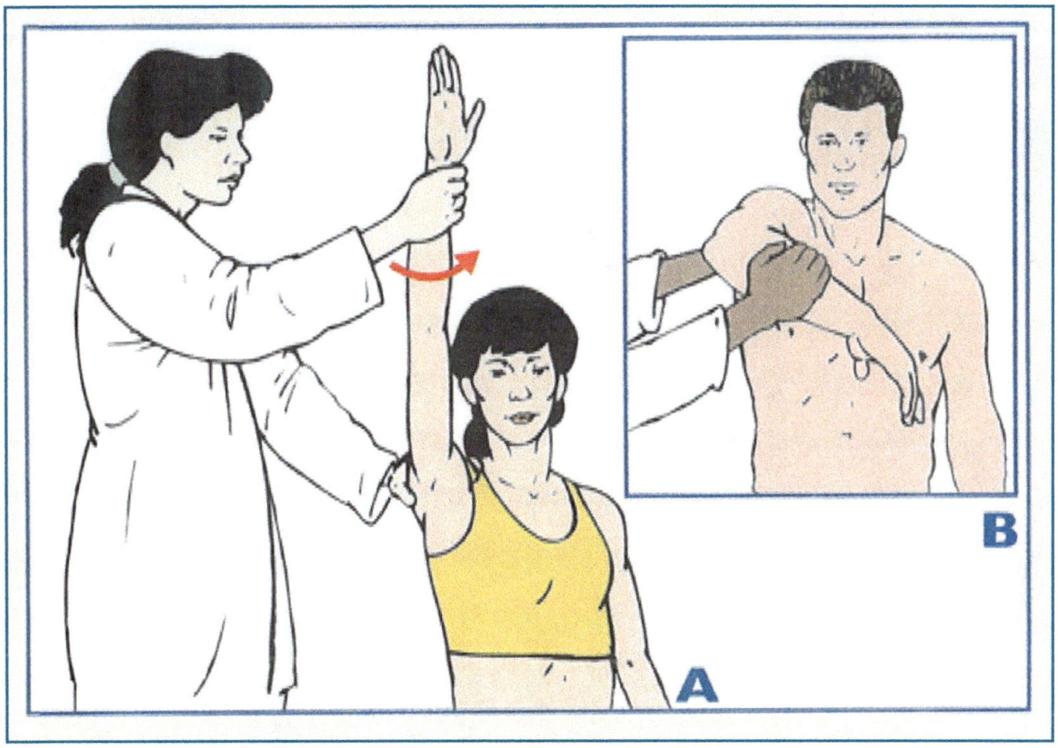

Figure 5G-7. Assessing Rotator Cuff Impingement

The Neer impingement test (A) involves fully abducting and forward flexing the shoulder and arm. An alternative examination for shoulder impingement, the Hawkins test (B), involves forward flexion to 90°, and the shoulder is internally rotated. With internal shoulder rotation, the examiner notes whether there has been an exacerbation of shoulder pain. Localizing the exact site of the pain can help distinguish biceps tendinopathy or acromioclavicular pathology from rotator cuff pathology. If there is true outlet impingement, pain should localize to the anterior acromion of the shoulder and radiate laterally down the arm.

© 2005 Terry Boyles

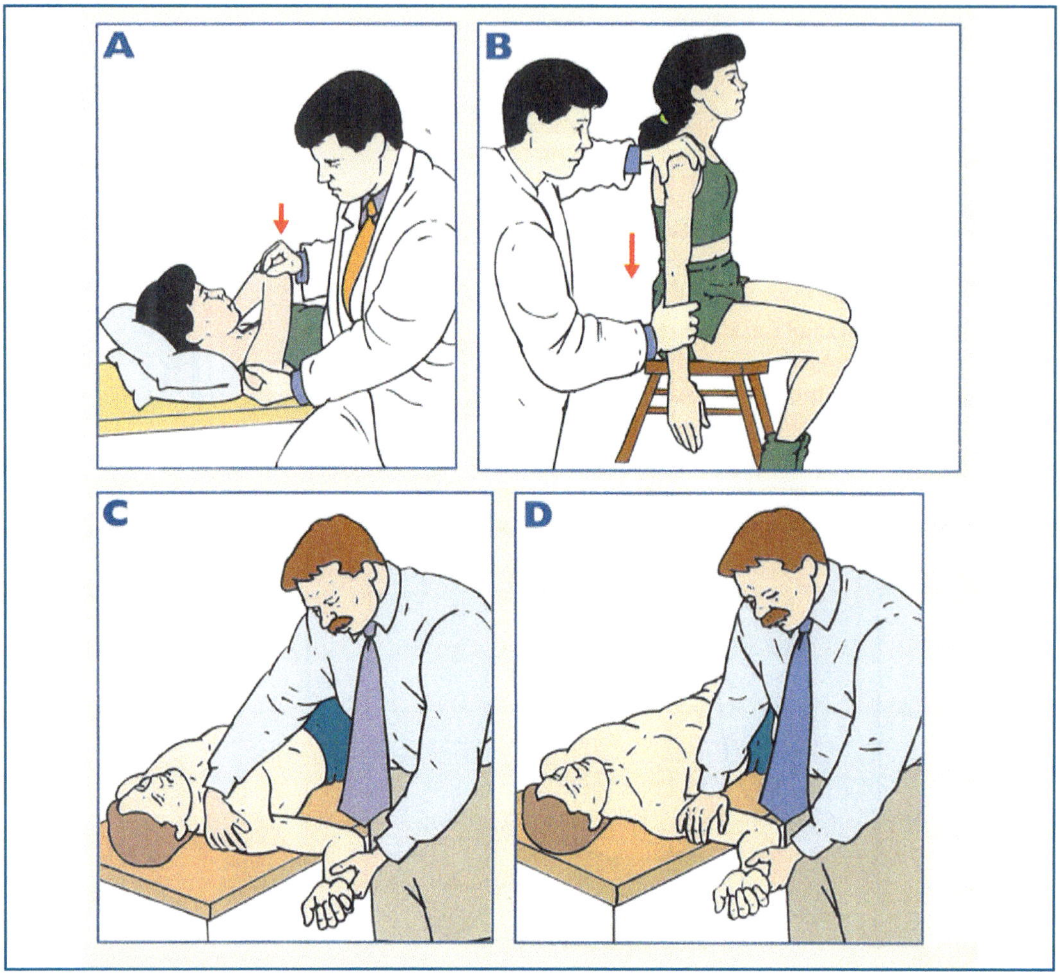

Figure 5G-8. Multidirectional Instability

Multidirectional instability can be gauged by assessing glenohumeral motion in several planes. Posterior instability of the shoulder is assessed with the athlete supine by positioning the arm perpendicular to the table with the elbow bent, then applying pressure along the long axis of the arm (A). The hand supporting the posterior shoulder palpates for excessive motion. When assessing shoulder internal rotation, it is important to stabilize the scapula by placing a hand against the scapular spine in the upright patient; for the supine patient, placing the shoulder firmly against the examination table can achieve the same goal. With the athlete seated (B), inferior subluxation is confirmed by the presence of the sulcus sign—appearance of an indentation beneath the acromion with traction along the axis of the adducted arm. In a normal shoulder, there should be some inferior laxity with the arm at the side. However, as the arm is externally rotated with the arm maintained at the side, this laxity should correct as the rotator interval is placed into tension. Inferior subluxation that persists or is asymmetrical to the opposite side suggests a tear of the rotator interval. During the apprehension test (C), which is used to assess for anterior instability, the examiner abducts the arm in the scapular plane and externally rotates the supine athlete's shoulder. It is important to look at the athlete's face while performing the maneuver to assess for visible signs of apprehension of a dislocation event. If apprehension is observed during the test, the relocation test (D) may be performed in the same position by applying a posteriorly directed force to the humeral head, reducing anterior translation of the humeral head. Relocation of the head will decrease the feeling of apprehension if instability is present. It is important to determine whether there is frank apprehension or pain with this test. If the athlete experiences increasing pain with progressive external rotation of the humeral head, this suggests that the humeral head has anterior subluxation; secondary (internal) impingement of the rotator cuff is occurring, causing pain.[17]

Elbow

The elbow is observed for swelling, discoloration, and carrying angle (cubital valgus) (Figure 5G-9A). The elbow should extend fully and then flex to allow the athlete to touch the ipsilateral shoulder with the hand. Forearm motion is assessed by having the athlete pronate and supinate the forearms with the elbows bent 90 degrees at their sides. The athlete should be able to turn the hand completely palm up and completely palm down.

In a throwing athlete, medial elbow stability can be assessed by applying a valgus force to the elbow (Figure 5G-9B). The modified milking maneuver (Figure 5G-9C) also assesses medial instability. The test result is considered positive if pain is noted over the ulnar collateral ligament or if the joint opens more medially compared to the opposite elbow.

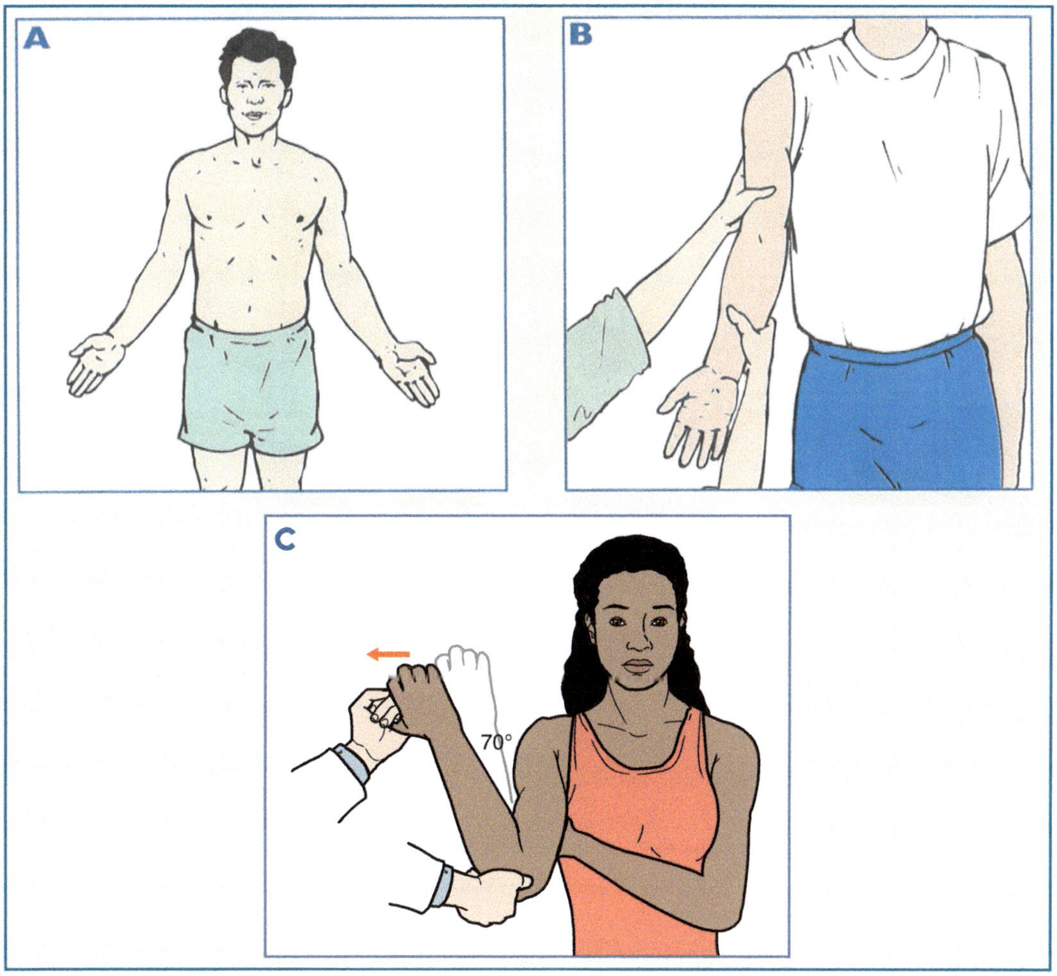

Figure 5G-9. Elbow Examination

Abbreviation: UCL, ulnar collateral ligament.

The normal carrying angle of the elbow is at least 15° valgus with the athlete standing and the palms forward (A). An excessive valgus angle may indicate instability or a previous injury. In a throwing athlete, it is important to assess UCL instability. This is accomplished by applying a valgus force to the elbow (with forearm supination) at 25° to 30° of flexion while noting laxity and end point (B). The modified milking maneuver is done with the elbow in flexion and UCL stress applied by the examiner grasping the thumb and applying a stress, as pictured, to assess UCL instability (C).

Figures A and B: © 2005 Terry Boyles

Hand/Wrist

The hand and wrist are evaluated for symmetry. Wrists should palmar flex equally to about 80 degrees and dorsiflex to 70 degrees or more. There should be more ulnar deviation than radial deviation. The fingers should be able to close into a full fist, and each fingernail should point at the scaphoid tubercle with the fingers flexed across the palm. Intrinsic muscle function can be checked by having the athlete touch each fingertip with the thumb and spread and close the extended fingers (Figure 5G-10). For individuals reporting persistent pain after a wrist injury, tenderness to palpation in the anatomical snuffbox (Figure 5G-11) suggests possible scaphoid fracture, which can have delayed presentation and warrants further evaluation with radiographs.[18]

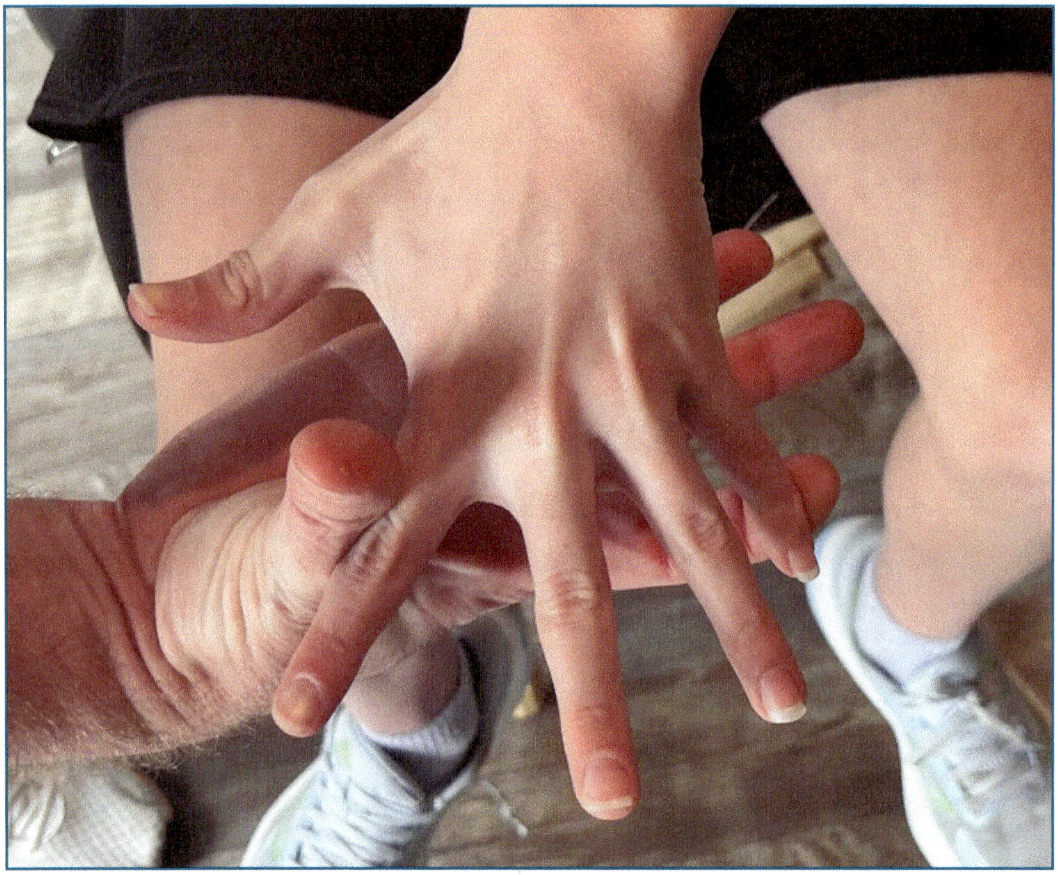

Figure 5G-10. Checking Intrinsic Muscle Function of the Hand
Courtesy of Brian Scott Harvey, DO, FAAP.

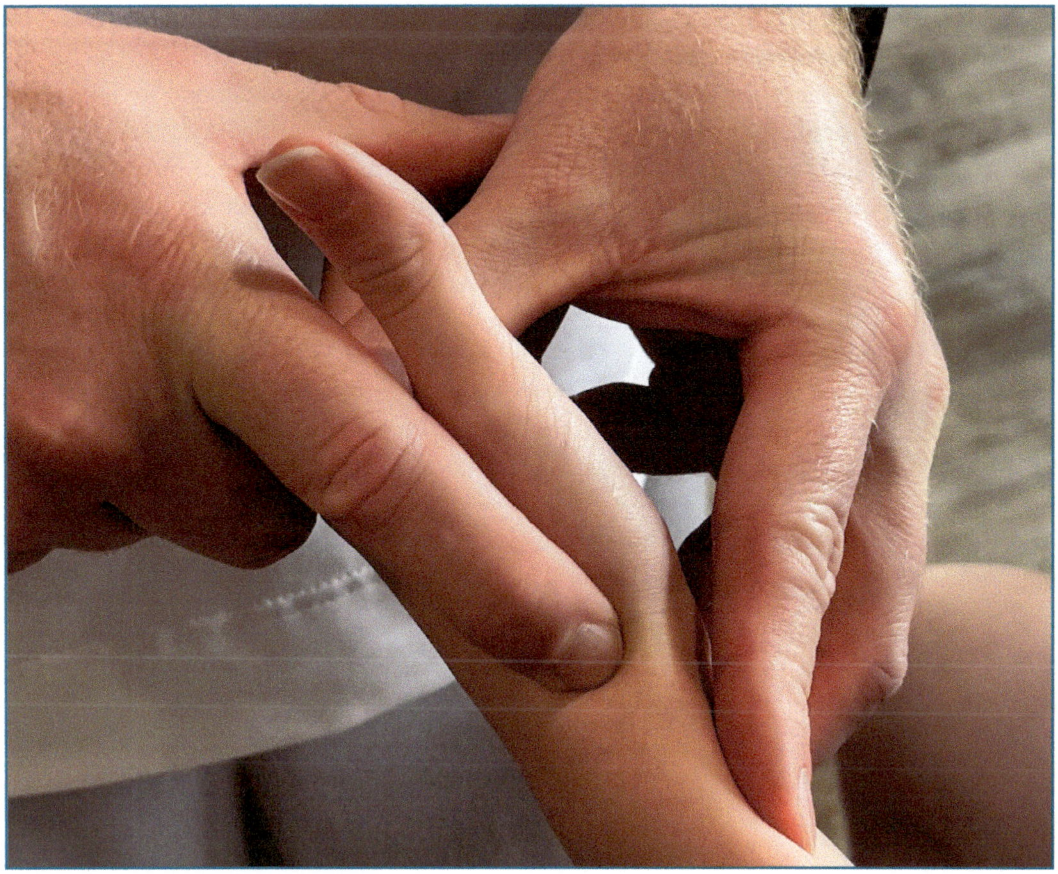

Figure 5G-11. Anatomical Snuff Box
Courtesy of Brian Scott Harvey, DO, FAAP.

Lower Extremity Examination

The lower extremity examination begins with observation of the standing posture. The iliac crest and posterior superior iliac spine heights should be level with the floor when the torso is aligned symmetrically, and the athlete should be able to stand on each flat foot without any translation or tilting of the pelvis.

Hip

Hip range of motion can be assessed with the athlete lying supine or prone. In a supine position, with the hip and the knee fully extended, the hip joint is rotated internally and externally (a "log roll" movement), and any asymmetry is noted. Symmetry of abduction and adduction is also observed. Hip flexion should be beyond 90 degrees, and the knees should come straight toward the chest; any external rotation indicates an intrinsic hip deformity. With the hip and knee flexed to 90 degrees, the hip joint should have 40 degrees of internal rotation and 45 degrees of external rotation (Figure 5G-12). Keeping the hip flexed 90 degrees and passively extending the knee enables the examiner to assess hamstring flexibility. In this position, the *popliteal angle* refers to the angle formed between the long axis of the femur and the anterior tibia. Normal values for popliteal angle can vary depending on the patient's age and sex.[19,20] Significant hamstring tightness (popliteal angle > 50 degrees) can be a risk factor for low back pain or can indicate an underlying neurological or spine issue.

Acetabular labral tears, dysplasia, femoral acetabular impingement (FAI), hip osteochondrosis, and femoral neck stress fractures are recognized as some of the common sources of hip or groin pain and functional limitation. In the skeletally immature individual, loss of hip flexion and internal rotation as well as groin or knee pain can indicate the presence of a slipped capital femoral epiphysis, which warrants emergent orthopedic referral. Passive assessment of the hip in *f*lexion, *ad*duction, and *i*nternal *r*otation (FADIR) is conducted as part of the supine assessment of the hip (Figure 5G-13) and is the most sensitive physical examination for FAI.[21] Loss of internal rotation is also common with anterior superior labral tears and FAI.[22]

The FABER test (Figure 5G-14) involves combining the motion of hip *f*lexion, *ab*duction, and *e*xternal *r*otation. This maneuver tests for pain provocation and range of motion. Posterior hip pain may be indicative of sacroiliac joint involvement, while anterior hip pain or groin pain often indicates intra-articular hip pathology.[23,24]

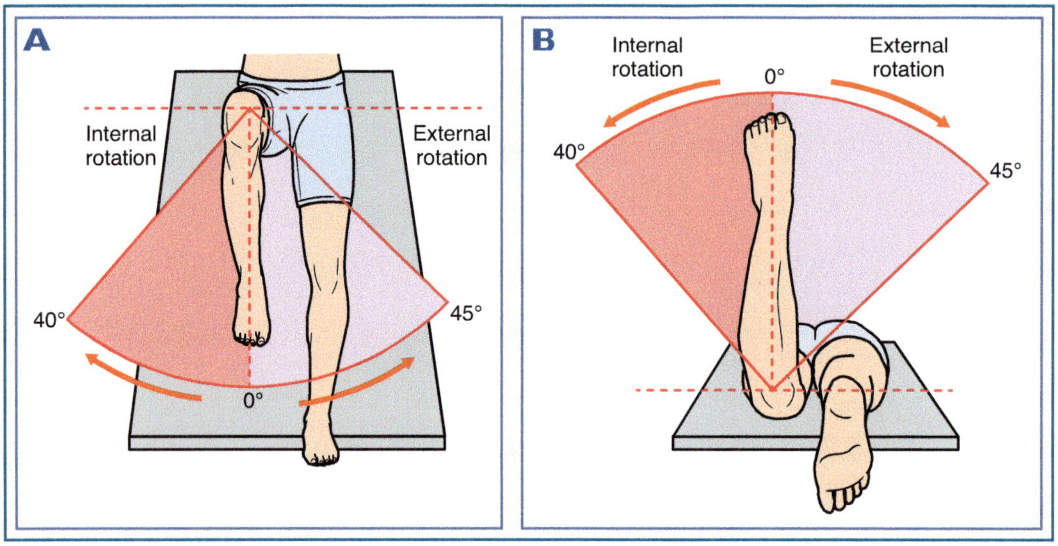

Figure 5G-12. Hip Range of Motion

Hip range of motion can be evaluated either in the supine (A) or prone (B) position. As part of the examination, the hip and knee are flexed to 90° and the hip joint is rotated. A rotation arc of 60° to 85° should be observed. Pain or restriction of motion relative to the opposite side warrants further evaluation.

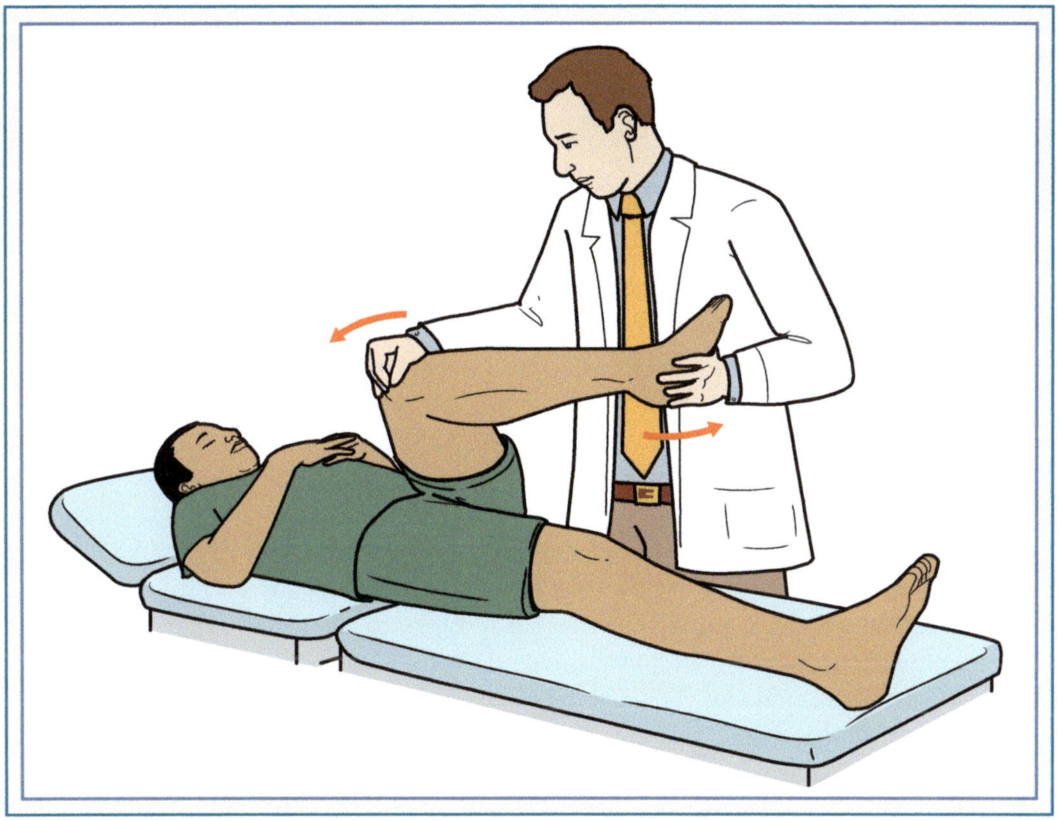

Figure 5G-13. ***F****lexion,* ***Ad****duction, and* ***I****nternal* ***R****otation (FADIR) Test*

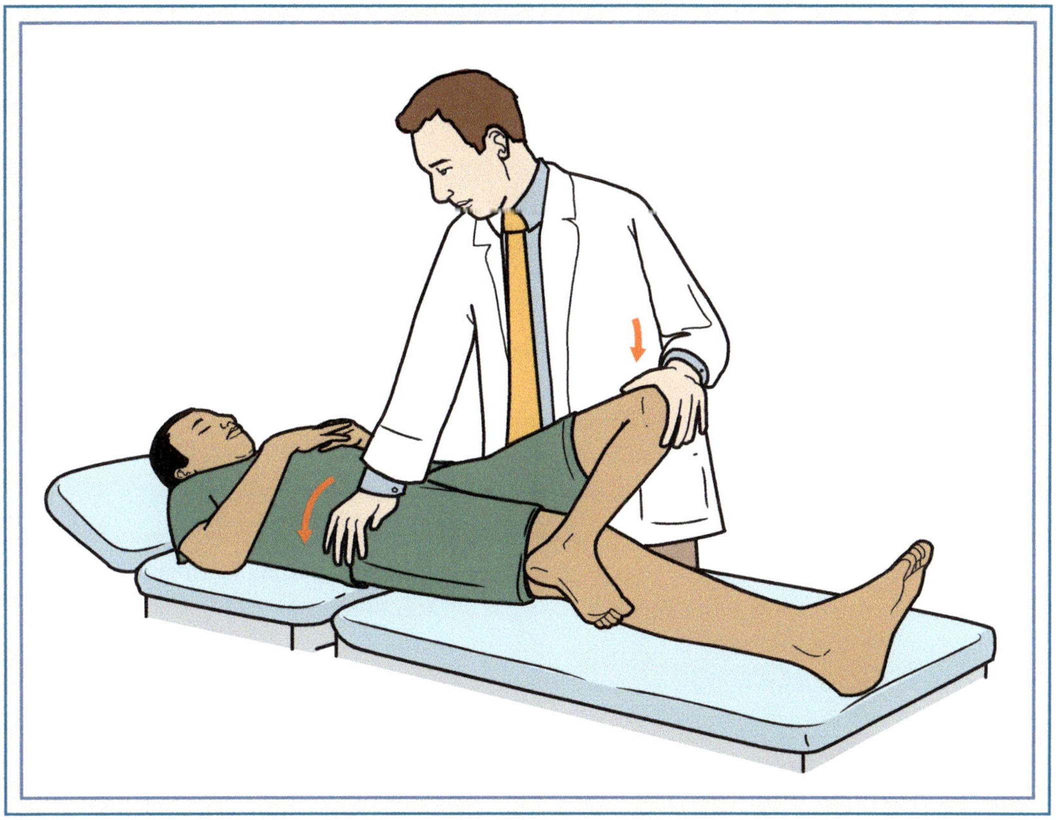

Figure 5G-14. ***F****lexion,* ***Ab****duction, and* ***E****xternal* ***R****otation (FABER) Test*

Knee

With the athlete standing, inspection should reveal a normal thigh-knee valgus angulation of 12 degrees or less in males and 18 degrees or less in females. The knee examination can include observation of the knee and particularly the patella while supine with the knee extended to identify substantial lateral subluxation or while sitting to identify an excessively high position (patella alta), both of which can be risk factors for patellofemoral maltracking and pain.

The remainder of the knee examination is done with the athlete supine. Each patella should be evaluated for hypermobility by translating the patella medially and laterally with the knee fully extended and comparing with the opposite side. A patella apprehension test evaluates for patella instability, and a positive test result is apprehension with lateral translation of the patella and the knee in extension (Figure 5G-15).[25] Joint-line tenderness in conjunction with a positive McMurray or other positive specialized meniscal test result may indicate a meniscal tear. Any amount of knee effusion is important to note and evaluate further. Knee range of motion should be from full extension or hyperextension to approximately 140 degrees of flexion. Knee ligament stability tests include the Lachman test ("gold standard") (Figure 5G-16A) and anterior drawer test (Figure 5G-16B) for ACL deficiency, posterior drawer test for posterior cruciate ligament insufficiency (Figure 5G-16C), and varus and valgus stress tests for collateral ligament laxities (Figures 5G-16D and 5G-16E). It is important to keep in mind that a negative anterior drawer test result does not rule out an ACL tear, and the Lachman test is the better test for ACL integrity.[26]

Palpation of the tibial tubercle is important to assess for Osgood-Schlatter disease (tibial tubercle apophysitis) in the skeletally immature person. It is one of the most frequent causes of knee pain in young children and growing adolescents. Similarly, pain with palpation of the inferior pole of that patella can indicate Sinding-Larsen-Johansson syndrome in a skeletally immature individual.

The lower leg and tibia examination includes the shin edema test (SET) and shin palpation test (SPT) to assess for medial tibial stress syndrome (MTSS). SET is sustained palpation of the distal two-thirds of the medial surface of the tibia bilaterally for at least 5 seconds to evaluate for signs of pitting edema. SPT is palpation of the distal two-thirds of the posteromedial border of the tibiae for focal bony tenderness that may indicate MTSS or bone stress injury (BSI).[27]

The ankles are evaluated with the athlete standing and sitting for normal appearance. In the seated position, active dorsiflexion to 20 degrees and plantar flexion to 40 degrees should be present. Tightness in the Achilles tendon can be identified by limited motion when passively dorsiflexing the individual's ankle with the knee fully extended. The ankle should dorsiflex 15 to 20 degrees past neutral. Stress testing for ligament laxity includes the anterior drawer test for anterior subluxation due to anterior talofibular ligament injury (Figure 5G-17A) and the talar tilt test for injury to the calcaneofibular ligament, causing lateral instability. Decreased motion with the talar tilt test compared to the opposite normal ankle may indicate a tarsal coalition or arthritis of the midfoot (Figure 5G-17B).

At inspection of the foot, pes cavus or rigid flatfoot deformities may be noted. A supple or flexible flatfoot does not affect an individual's athletic performance, but it may be a risk factor for foot pain or upstream problems in the kinetic chain, such as MTSS or patellofemoral joint pain. If the flatfoot is supple, the plantar arch will increase when the individual stands on their toes. Symptomatic abnormalities associated with subtalar, midfoot, and forefoot problems or deformities should be further assessed outside of the PPE.

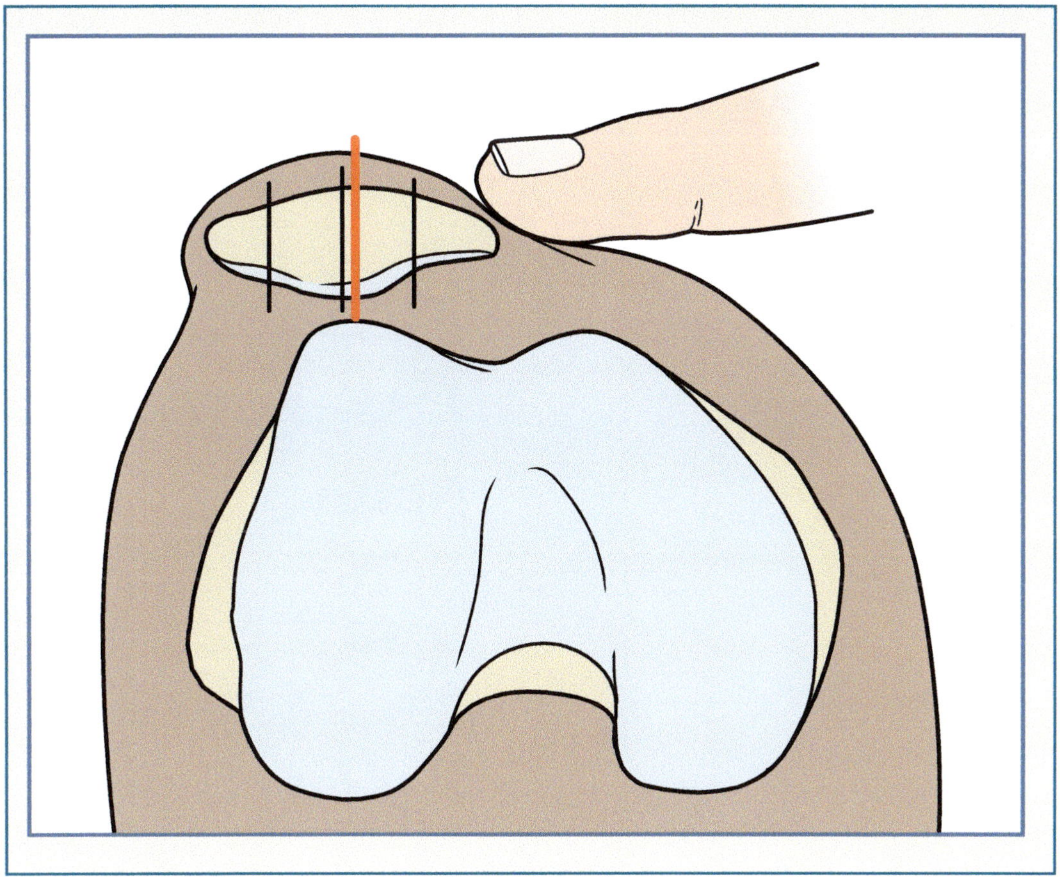

Figure 5G-15. Medial Lateral Patella Translation (Glide Test)

The medial lateral patella translation (glide test) is typically done in full extension. The patella is divided into 4 quadrants; lateral translation or glide > 3 quadrants (more than half of the patella width) represents restraint incompetency or tissue laxity.[25]

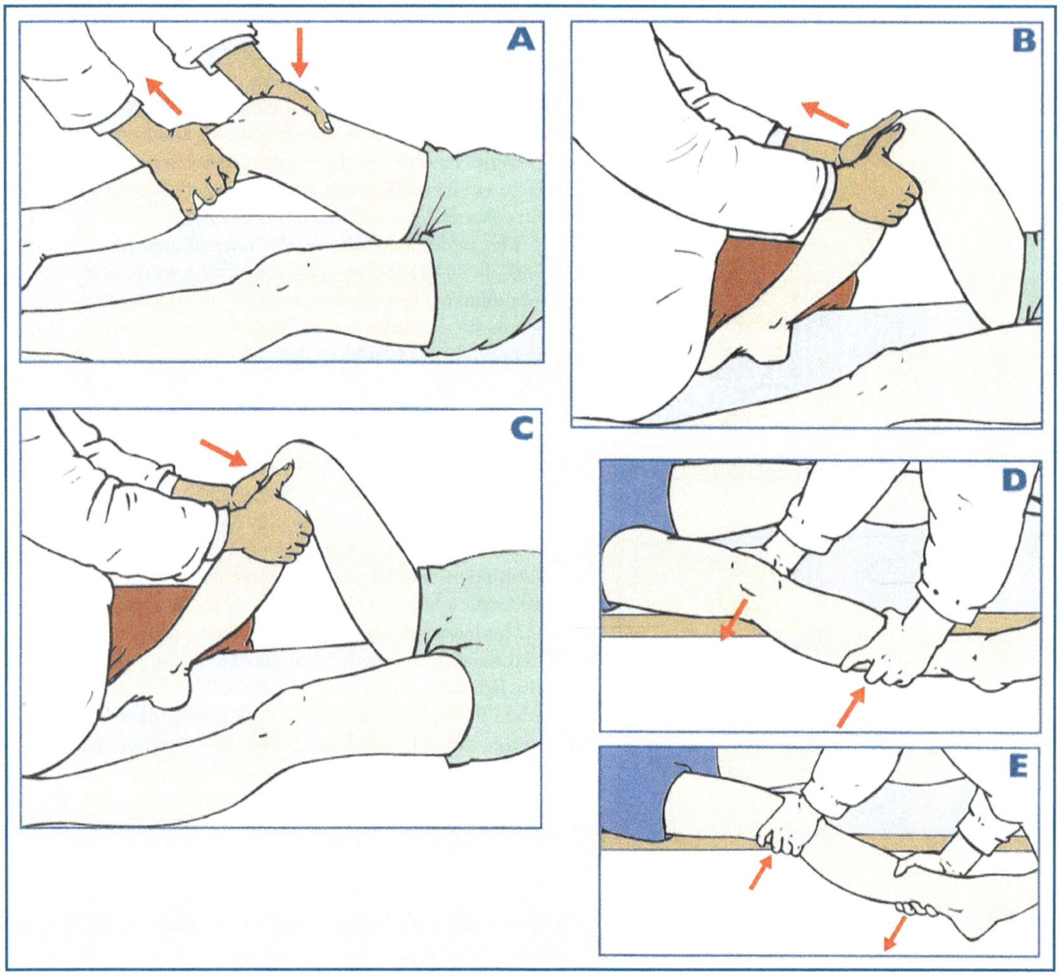

Figure 5G-16. Assessing Ligamentous Instability of the Knee

Abbreviations: ACL, anterior cruciate ligament; PCL, posterior cruciate ligament.

Several tests are used to assess ligamentous instability of the knee. For each test, the degree of excursion and the quality of the end point are noted and compared with the opposite side. The Lachman test (A) is the most sensitive means to assess ACL deficiencies.[26] The patient's knee is flexed approximately 20°, and the muscles are relaxed. The examiner stabilizes the femur with one hand while pulling the tibia anteriorly with the other hand. It is important to note how far the tibial tubercle translates anteriorly and whether there is a soft or firm end point at terminal translation. All findings should be compared with the opposite side. The anterior drawer test (B) is not sensitive (negative test result does not mean an intact ACL), but it does indicate ACL insufficiency when the result is positive. The Lachman test is far superior for determining the integrity of the ACL. The posterior drawer test (C) can reveal PCL insufficiency. With the supine patient's knee bent 90°, the examiner sits on the patient's foot to stabilize it and grasps the proximal tibia. The hamstrings need to be relaxed. The examiner pulls the tibia anteriorly (anterior drawer test, B) and pushes it posteriorly (posterior drawer test, C) from the neutral position. With the anterior drawer test, lack of a firm end point and presence of excessive anterior tibial excursion suggest ACL insufficiency. With the posterior drawer test, the presence of excessive posterior tibial sag suggests PCL insufficiency. With an intact PCL, the tibia is positioned anterior to the femur with the knee in 90° of flexion. During the posterior drawer test, the examiner palpates and quantifies the change in anteromedial femoral-tibial step-off that occurs with and without a posteriorly directed force on the tibia. Varus stress test (D) and valgus stress test (E) gauge instability of the medial and lateral collateral ligaments of the knee. The athlete's knee is extended over the edge of the examination table and flexed to approximately 20°. One of the examiner's hands stabilizes the knee at the joint line, and varus and valgus stresses are applied to the tibia. Once again, comparison with the opposite limb is essential for these tests, given the reference range of variation in joint stability.

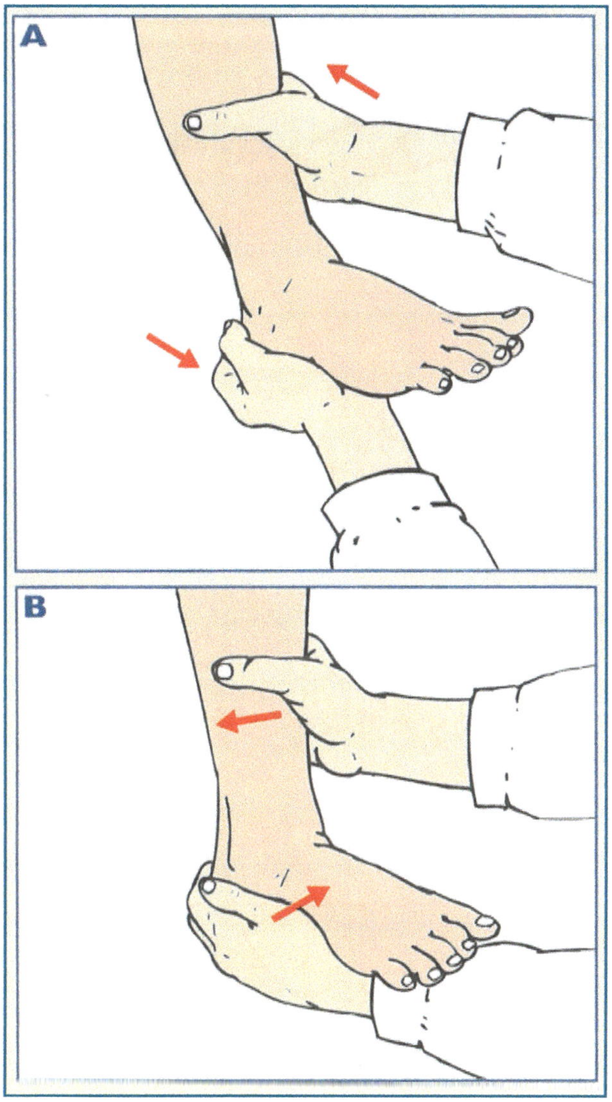

Figure 5G-17. Assessing Instability of the Ankle Ligaments

Two stress tests are used to assess instability of the ankle ligaments. For the anterior drawer test (A), which demonstrates anterior subluxation, the examiner pulls the heel anteriorly while pushing posteriorly on the distal tibia. For the talar tilt test (B), the examiner inverts the ankle by pushing laterally on the medial tibia and medially on the calcaneus. Abnormal motion relative to the opposite ankle indicates a need for further evaluation.

Functional Movement Tests

The data supporting functional movement testing to identify risk factors for injury and improve outcomes are not strong. Testing (eg, the single leg squat) could be considered in players of lateral, pivoting, cutting sports. Poor core strength and inadequate neuromuscular control of the lower extremity are linked to increased risk of patellofemoral pain syndrome and ACL tears.[14,28] A combination of muscle testing to point out individual deficiencies and coaches' education to promote team active warm-ups and neuromuscular training programs may reduce injury risk.[14,28] Athletes in sports requiring lateral, pivoting, and cutting motions could be further assessed with the box drop test and core strength evaluation to identify deficits in neuromuscular control that could be improved upon to decrease the risk of ACL rupture.[29] However, many clinicians may not have the ability to conduct these tests in the office setting, and if concerned can refer the individual for further evaluation with a sports medicine physician, a physical therapist, or an athletic trainer.

Single-Leg Squat Test

A simple screening for potential lower extremity injury risk is the single-leg squat test. Athletes are asked to place their hands onto their hips, stand on 1 limb, and flex the opposing limb to 90 degrees, followed by a single-leg squat to 30 degrees of knee flexion with return to a fully extended knee position. Abnormal responses indicating poor neuromuscular control include arms flailing, Trendelenburg sign, or collapse of the supporting knee into valgus (Figure 5G-18).[30]

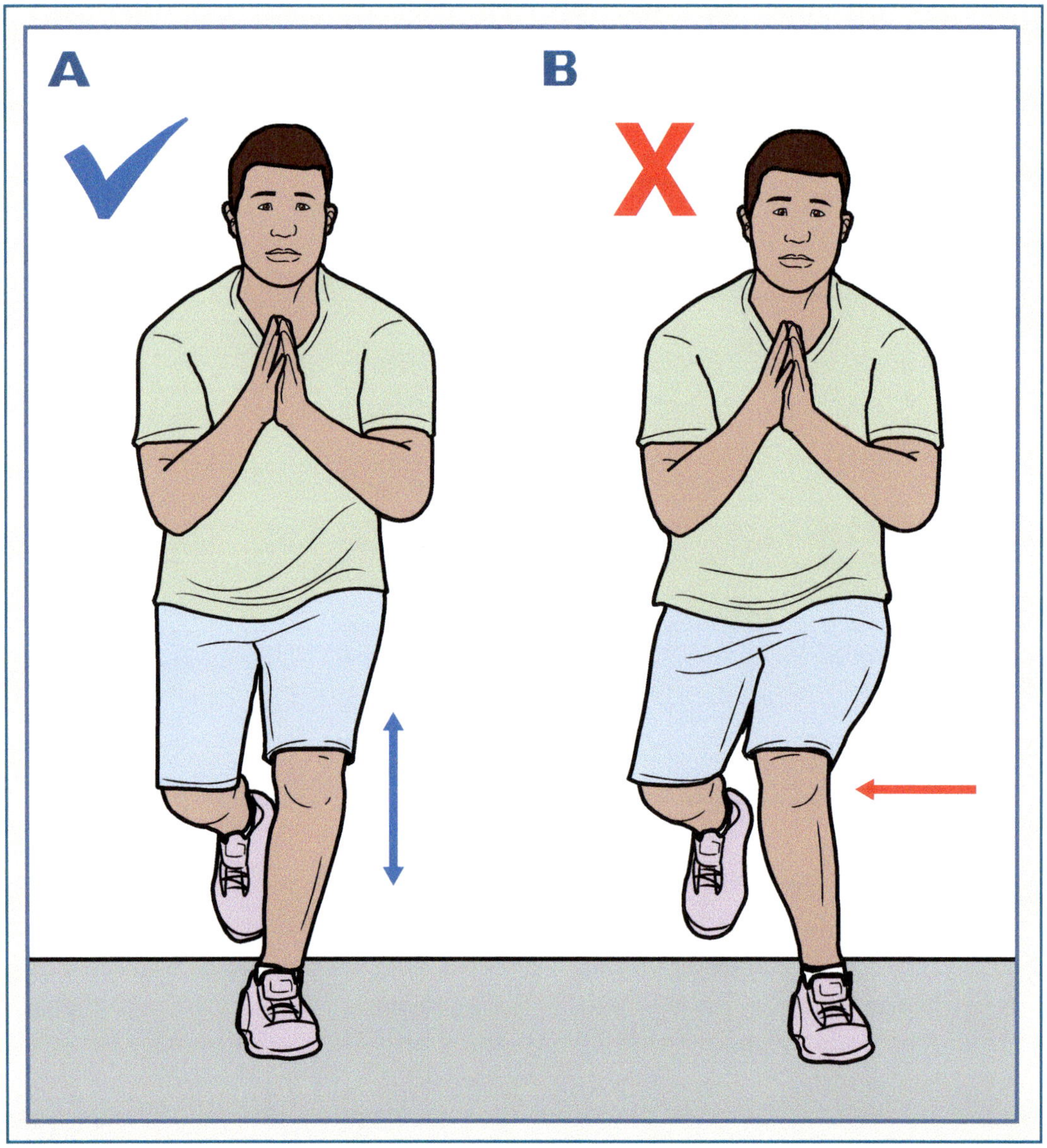

Figure 5G-18. Single-Leg Squat Test

Individuals should place their hands on their hips or in front, as pictured, and stand on 1 limb and flex the opposing limb to 90°. (A) They then should perform 3 single-leg squats to 30° of knee flexion and return to a fully extended knee position. (B) The examiner notes any abnormal responses, which consist of arms flailing, the Trendelenburg sign, or collapse of the supporting knee into valgus.[30]

Box Drop Test

The box drop test addresses dynamic neuromuscular control. The athlete is asked to do a drop vertical jump maneuver from a box height of 31 cm (other heights, such as a low examination table step, are acceptable for the purpose of a PPE). Participants are instructed to drop off the box and immediately perform a maximal vertical jump (Figure 5G-19). In one study, an increase in the knee valgus and abduction angle (knock-knee appearance) at landing the jump was associated with an increased risk for ACL injury, with 73% specificity and 78% sensitivity.[14]

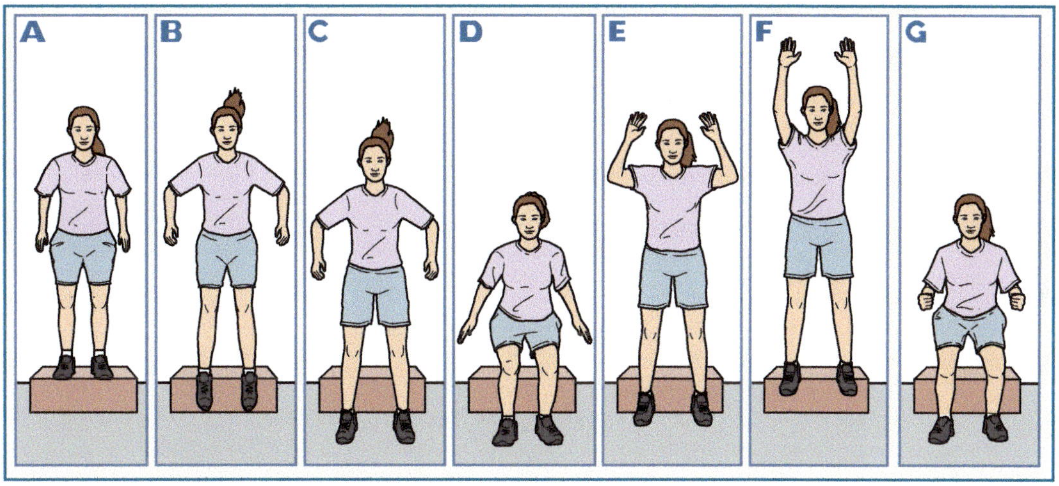

Figure 5G-19. Vertical Jump Maneuver

This series of figures illustrates a normal landing pattern. An abnormal test result would include "kissing knees," flailing arms, or loss of balance. (A) Starting position on 31-cm box. (B) Mid-flight immediately after dropping off the box. (C) Initial contact. (D) Landing phase. (E) Toe off. (F) Maximum vertical jump height. (G) Second landing.[22]

Sport-Specific Examinations

Players of certain sports are at higher risk for injury because of stress placed onto specific joints and muscles. Detailed evaluation of strength, endurance, range of motion, and flexibility may be warranted for these athletes. For example, baseball pitchers can develop adaptive changes in shoulder rotation from repetitive throwing, but also pathological loss of internal rotation (glenohumeral internal rotation deficit) that can increase shoulder and elbow injury risk. If identified, this loss of internal rotation may improve with rehabilitation, decreasing injury risk.

Hockey players are at higher risk for FAI. "Cam"-type impingement affects 79% of ice hockey players.[31,32] The FADIR provocative test for cam-type and "pincer"-type FAI, as noted earlier, would be recommended for evaluating hip pain in these athletes.

Hyperlaxity at joint examination, especially in an individual engaged in overhead arm motions, is also associated with an increased risk of joint injury.[33] For example, an adolescent baseball pitcher, swimmer, or volleyball player with shoulder symptoms and evidence of generalized joint hypermobility may have a connective tissue disorder such as Ehlers-Danlos or Marfan syndrome. Knowledge of the Beighton score (Carter-Wilkinson criteria) can help to objectively make the diagnosis of generalized joint hypermobility spectrum disorder.[34] The Beighton score provides an objective way to risk stratify potentially hypermobile individuals and may aid in determining treatment options in the event of injuries. The Beighton score is determined by the ability to hyperextend the knees and elbows beyond 10 degrees, dorsiflex the metacarpal-phalangeal joints beyond 90 degrees, passively appose the thumb to the forearm, and bend forward and place the palms flat on the ground with the knees in full extension (Table 5G-3). A positive Beighton score is any score greater than or equal to 5/9 points in adults or 6/9 points in children (before puberty).[35] Those with a positive score may require further clinical assessment.

Table 5G-3. Beighton Hypermobility Criteria

Physical Finding	Point Value
Passive dorsiflexion of the metacarpophalangeal joint beyond 90°	1 point for each hand
Passive apposition of the thumb to the flexor aspect of the forearm	1 point for each thumb
Hyperextension of the elbows beyond 10°	1 point for each elbow
Hyperextension of the knees beyond 10°	1 point for each knee
Forward flexion of the trunk with knees fully extended so that the palms of the hands rest flat on the floor	1 point

Adapted with permission from Grahame R, Bird HA, Child A. The revised (Brighton 1998) criteria for the diagnosis of benign joint hypermobility syndrome (BJHS). *J Rheumatol.* 2000;27(7):1777–1779.

MEDICAL ELIGIBILITY FOR PARTICIPATION

The examining provider decides whether an individual is ready to participate in their sport by using information gathered during the history and physical examination. Determining medical eligibility for individuals who have musculoskeletal injuries or disorders requires assessing short- and long-term risks and benefits with respect to the PPE findings. Some problems may exceed the capacity of the PPE venue and require additional evaluation with a repeated visit or consultation with additional providers.

Medical eligibility for participation is based on the degree and type of injury, the ability of the injured individual to compete safely, and the requirements of a given sport. Participation may be possible in activities that do not directly affect the injured site (eg, a wrist sprain might prevent a gymnast from full training but not a runner). Therefore, it is important for the provider to determine which strength and conditioning activities are appropriate during the recovery period so that the individual is able to maintain some level of fitness. Protective padding, taping, or bracing may allow an individual to train and compete safely, as long as the protective device does not increase injury risk for other competitors. The types of protective splinting or bracing permitted in competition vary by sport and the rules of the sport organization or league. If the examiner is not certain of the rules concerning safe participation with protective devices, consultation with a sports medicine specialist is suggested. The final decision on what type of protective padding or bracing is permitted may rest with the on-site officials. In such situations, a change in the original type of protection recommended by the sports medicine staff could be deemed necessary by the official. It is recommended that any alteration required by the on-site official be evaluated by the treating examiner to ensure that it provides the necessary protection for the injury.

Referral or consultation is warranted when the examiner is uncertain of the individual's ability to participate because of the injury or musculoskeletal deficit. The physician(s) who initiated the treatment of an injury that is present at the time of the PPE should be included in the medical eligibility decision whenever possible. Reevaluation for sports participation is required after rehabilitation is completed. Review of every musculoskeletal problem is beyond the scope of this book, but selected problems deserve mention.

Sprains, Strains, Subluxations, Dislocations, and Contusions

Before medical eligibility for sport participation is given for either acute injuries or overuse injuries, the individual needs to be examined and the following conditions ruled out:

- Effusion, swelling, or other signs of inflammation
- Decreased range of motion of the affected joint or joints controlled by the muscle
- Strength less than 85% to 90% of the uninjured side or insufficient for the desired activity
- Ligamentous instability of the affected joint
- Loss or alteration of sport-specific functional ability (ie, inability to complete pain-free functional activity at 80% to 90% effort)

For example, a football defensive back who is rehabilitating a lateral ankle sprain could be assessed with backpedaling and side-to-side movements. If any of the findings are abnormal, further treatment will be needed to allow for return to play. Referral, if necessary, to a provider familiar with the sport-specific requirements and injury assessment is recommended. Ultimately, the decision for medical eligibility is based on the examiner's clinical judgment and may be withheld until the individual is further evaluated and any prescribed treatment or rehabilitation is completed.

Fractures

Medical eligibility for an individual with a fracture should be determined in consultation with the treating physician. The location and type of fracture, the risk of reinjury or complications, and the effect of treatment need to be considered. The possibility of protecting the fracture during participation with a cast or splint should be considered if the risk of worsening the injury is believed to be negligible.

Spinal Deformities

Any history or physical finding of spinal deformity (eg, scoliosis, spondylolysis, or spondylolisthesis, congenital cervical fusion) requires a more thorough evaluation than is generally provided in the PPE.

Follow-up with the individual's primary care physician, sports medicine specialist, or spine specialist is recommended when questions arise. Medical eligibility for individuals with spondylolysis and spondylolisthesis is evaluated individually on the basis of symptoms, physical limitations, and imaging findings. Spondylolysis and spondylolisthesis, along with spinal deformities, may require follow-up imaging to assess progression. Generally, individuals with spinal deformities need not be excluded from play. However, activities may need to be modified according to clinical symptoms and the extent of the abnormality. See Chapter 5B for further information on congenital cervical fusion.

Apophysitis

Clearing individuals with apophysitis of the tibial tubercle (Osgood-Schlatter disease), calcaneus (Sever disease), ileum, or ischium and pain at the infrapatellar insertion of the patellar tendon (Sinding-Larsen-Johansson disease) follows similar criteria to those for overuse injuries and acute strains.

If there are any questions concerning medical eligibility, consultation with a sports medicine specialist is warranted. A systematic approach to history, physical examination, and medical eligibility decisions sets the foundation for a safe sport season for the individual.

REFERENCES

1. Kadel NJ, Teitz CC, Kronmal RA. Stress fractures in ballet dancers. *Am J Sports Med.* 1992;20(4):445–449. PMID: 1357994 doi:10.1177/036354659202000414
2. Brunet ME, Cook SD, Brinker MR, Dickinson JA. A survey of running injuries in 1505 competitive and recreational runners. *J Sports Med Phys Fitness.* 1990;30(3):307–315. PMID: 2266763
3. Korpelainen R, Orava S, Karpakka J, Siira P, Hulkko A. Risk factors for recurrent stress fractures in athletes. *Am J Sports Med.* 2001;29(3):304–310. PMID: 11394600 doi:10.1177/03635465010290030901
4. The team physician and strength and conditioning of athletes for sports: a consensus statement. *Med Sci Sports Exerc.* 2015;47(2):440–445. PMID: 25594944
5. De Souza MJ, Nattiv A, Joy E, et al; Expert Panel. 2014 Female Athlete Triad Coalition Consensus Statement on Treatment and Return to Play of the Female Athlete Triad: 1st International Conference held in San Francisco, California, May 2012 and 2nd International Conference held in Indianapolis, Indiana, May 2013. *Br J Sports Med.* 2014;48(4):289–309. PMID: 24463911 doi:10.1136/bjsports-2013-093218
6. Joy E, De Souza MJ, Nattiv A, et al. 2014 female athlete triad coalition consensus statement on treatment and return to play of the female athlete triad. *Curr Sports Med Rep.* 2014;13(4):219–232. PMID: 25014387 doi:10.1249/JSR.0000000000000077
7. Mountjoy M, Sundgot-Borgen JK, Burke LM, et al. IOC consensus statement on relative energy deficiency in sport (RED-S): 2018 update. *Br J Sports Med.* 2018;52(11):687–697. PMID: 29773536
8. Lundy B, Torstveit MK, Stenqvist TB, et al. Screening for low energy availability in male athletes: attempted validation of LEAM-Q. *Nutrients.* 2022;14(9):1873. PMID: 35565840 doi:10.3390/nu14091873
9. Witkoś J, Błażejewski G, Gierach M. The Low Energy Availability in Females Questionnaire (LEAF-Q) as a useful tool to identify female triathletes at risk for menstrual disorders related to low energy availability. *Nutrients.* 2023;15(3):650. PMID: 36771357 doi:10.3390/nu15030650
10. Melin A, Tornberg AB, Skouby S, et al. The LEAF questionnaire: a screening tool for the identification of female athletes at risk for the female athlete triad. *Br J Sports Med.* 2014;48(7):540–545. PMID: 24563388 doi:10.1136/bjsports-2013-093240
11. Fredericson M, Kussman A, Misra M, et al. The Male Athlete Triad—a consensus statement from the Female and Male Athlete Triad Coalition part II: diagnosis, treatment, and return-to-play. *Clin J Sport Med.* 2021;31(4):349–366. doi:10.1097/JSM.0000000000000948
12. Gomez JE, Landry GL, Bernhardt DT. Critical evaluation of the 2-minute orthopedic screening examination. *Am J Dis Child.* 1993;147(10):1109–1113. PMID: 8213685 doi:10.1001/archpedi.1993.02160340095022
13. Foster HE, Jandial S. pGALS—paediatric Gait Arms Legs and Spine: a simple examination of the musculoskeletal system. *Pediatr Rheumatol Online J.* 2013;11(1):44. PMID: 24219838 doi:10.1186/1546-0096-11-44
14. Hewett TE, Myer GD, Ford KR, et al. Biomechanical measures of neuromuscular control and valgus loading of the knee predict anterior cruciate ligament injury risk in female athletes: a prospective study. *Am J Sports Med.* 2005;33(4):492–501. PMID: 15722287 doi:10.1177/0363546504269591
15. Garrick JG. Preparticipation orthopedic screening evaluation. *Clin J Sport Med.* 2004;14(3):123–126. PMID: 15166899 doi:10.1097/00042752-200405000-00003
16. Burkhart SS, Tehrany AM. Arthroscopic subscapularis tendon repair: technique and preliminary results. *Arthroscopy.* 2002;18(5):454–463. PMID: 11987054 doi:10.1053/jars.2002.30648

17. Speer KP, Hannafin JA, Altchek DW, Warren RF. An evaluation of the shoulder relocation test. *Am J Sports Med.* 1994;22(2):177–183. PMID: 8198184 doi:10.1177/036354659402200205
18. Li NY, Dennison D, Shin A, Pulos NA. Update to management of acute scaphoid fractures. *J Am Acad Orthopaed Surg.* 2023;31(15):e550–e560. doi:10.5435/JAAOS-D-22-01210
19. Katz K, Rosenthal A, Yosipovitch Z. Normal ranges of popliteal angle in children. *J Pediatr Orthop.* 1992;12(2):229–231. PMID: 1552027 doi:10.1097/01241398-199203000-00014
20. Gajdosik R, Lusin G. Hamstring muscle tightness. Reliability of an active-knee-extension test. *Phys Ther.* 1983;63(7):1085–1090. PMID: 6867117 doi:10.1093/ptj/63.7.1085
21. Byrd JW, ed. *Operative Hip Arthroscopy.* 3rd ed. Springer; 2013
22. Martin HD, Shears SA, Palmer IJ. Evaluation of the hip. *Sports Med Arthrosc Rev.* 2010;18(2):63–75. PMID: 20473124 doi:10.1097/JSA.0b013e3181dc578a
23. Martin RL, Enseki KR, Draovitch P, Trapuzzano T, Philippon MJ. Acetabular labral tears of the hip: examination and diagnostic challenges. *J Orthop Sports Phys Ther.* 2006;36(7):503–515. PMID: 16881467 doi:10.2519/jospt.2006.2135
24. Kuhlman GS, Domb BG. Hip impingement: identifying and treating a common cause of hip pain. *Am Fam Physician.* 2009;80(12):1429–1434. PMID: 20000305
25. Arendt EA, Donell ST, Sillanpää PJ, Feller JA. The management of lateral patellar dislocation: state of the art. *J ISAKOS.* 2017;2(4):205–212
26. Kim SJ, Kim HK. Reliability of the anterior drawer test, the pivot shift test, and the Lachman test. *Clin Orthop Relat Res.* 1995(317):237–242. PMID: 7671485
27. Newman P, Adams R, Waddington G. Two simple clinical tests for predicting onset of medial tibial stress syndrome: shin palpation test and shin oedema test. *Br J Sports Med.* 2012;46(12):861–864. PMID: 22966153 doi:10.1136/bjsports-2011-090409
28. Hewett TE, Myer GD, Ford KR, Slauterbeck JR. Preparticipation physical examination using a box drop vertical jump test in young athletes: the effects of puberty and sex. *Clin J Sport Med.* 2006;16(4):298–304. PMID: 16858212 doi:10.1097/00042752-200607000-00003
29. Zazulak BT, Hewett TE, Reeves NP, Goldberg B, Cholewicki J. Deficits in neuromuscular control of the trunk predict knee injury risk: a prospective biomechanical-epidemiologic study. *Am J Sports Med.* 2007;35(7):1123–1130. PMID: 17468378 doi:10.1177/0363546507301585
30. Ugalde V, Brockman C, Bailowitz Z, Pollard CD. Single leg squat test and its relationship to dynamic knee valgus and injury risk screening. *PM R.* 2015;7(3):229–235. PMID: 25111946 doi:10.1016/j.pmrj.2014.08.361
31. Brunner R, Maffiuletti NA, Casartelli NC, et al. Prevalence and functional consequences of femoroacetabular impingement in young male ice hockey players. *Am J Sports Med.* 2016;44(1):46–53. PMID: 26464494 doi:10.1177/0363546515607000
32. Philippon MJ, Ho CP, Briggs KK, Stull J, LaPrade RF. Prevalence of increased alpha angles as a measure of cam-type femoroacetabular impingement in youth ice hockey players. *Am J Sports Med.* 2013;41(6):1357–1362. PMID: 23562808 doi:10.1177/0363546513483448
33. Amir D, Frankl U, Pogrund H. Pulled elbow and hypermobility of joints. *Clin Orthop Relat Res.* 1990(257):94–99
34. Gedalia A, Brewer EJ Jr. Joint hypermobility in pediatric practice—a review. *J Rheumatol.* 1993;20(2):371–374. PMID: 8474078
35. The Ehlers-Danlos Society. Assessing Joint Hypermobility. Accessed August 11, 2026. Available at https://www.ehlers-danlos.com/assessing-joint-hypermobility/

H: Hematology and Oncology Considerations

■ SICKLE CELL DISEASE AND TRAIT

History Form Question

1. *Do you or does someone in your family have sickle cell trait or disease?*

Key Points

- Individuals with sickle cell trait are at risk for sickling during high-intensity physical activity, especially in hot, humid environments before acclimatization, at altitude, early in conditioning, or with dehydration.
- There is no clear evidence that individuals who have sickle cell trait should have additional limitations or modifications in their exercise programs.
- Universal screening is not widely recommended, except for National Collegiate Athletic Association (NCAA) athletes, who are required to show proof of prior testing.

Sickle cell disease involves 2 abnormal genes for hemoglobin, which causes a sickling of the red blood cells that is associated with rhabdomyolysis, splenic infarct or rupture, and stroke. Individual assessment is needed to determine medical eligibility, as some people who are affected with sickle cell disease variants are not too anemic, but they can have splenomegaly and require close monitoring. Overheating, dehydration, and chilling are to be avoided.[1]

Sickle cell disease can become an acute emergency with catastrophic consequences if an individual becomes dehydrated or sustains an internal injury. Such individuals should avoid highly strenuous activities and all contact and collision sports.[1]

Sickle cell disease can become an acute emergency with catastrophic consequences if an individual becomes dehydrated or sustains an internal injury. Such individuals should avoid highly strenuous activities and all contact and collision sports.

Sickle cell trait (SCT) is a descriptive term for an inherited, asymptomatic condition in individuals with 1 copy of the abnormal sickle cell gene. This condition is found in more than 2.5 million people in the United States of African, Mediterranean, Middle Eastern, and Indian heritages; approximately 7% to 10% of African Americans have SCT.[2] SCT does not result in anemia and cannot become sickle cell disease, but SCT is associated with an increased risk of rhabdomyolysis and, in some studies, sudden death.[3] The US Armed Forces reported more than a 20-fold increase in risk of death among recruits with SCT who were engaged in strenuous activity compared with participants in the control group without SCT.[4,5] Other studies have confirmed the significant increased risk of rhabdomyolysis in those with SCT.[5,6] A meta-analysis found an increased risk of rhabdomyolysis in US Army soldiers with SCT, but no increase in sudden cardiac death.[7]

The threat seems greatest when intense exercise occurs in high heat and humidity conditions for which the individual with SCT is not acclimated, or at an altitude greater than 1,500 meters, and may be increased by dehydration or acute illness.[6] Death occurs as a consequence of the complications of sickling, including rhabdomyolysis, profound acidosis, acute renal failure, and multiple-organ system failure.[8] Although sickling events may be confused with exertional heat illness, the risk of heat illness, including heat stroke, for individuals with SCT is similar to that of their peers without SCT.[3,8,9] Individuals with SCT may have episodes of hematuria, which require evaluation.[10] Individuals with SCT may have higher rates of vaso-occlusive phenomena (ie, splenic infarction at high altitudes, complications of traumatic hyphema) and venous thromboembolism. These episodes are rare, and while recognition is important, individuals should not be restricted from any sport in the setting of SCT.

SCT screening prior to athletic participation remains controversial. NCAA Division I, II, and III athletes are required to undergo testing or show proof of previous testing.[11] As of 2006, all 50 states require and provide universal newborn screening for SCT and sickle cell disease. Therefore, any youth or college-aged individual born in the United States in 2006 or later may be able to access their newborn records and obtain SCT status without undergoing repeat screening. However, some states do not retain records permanently, so newborn screening results might not be universally accessible. Other sports conferences and many professional societies recommend voluntary SCT testing and implementation of preventive measures universally for all athletes (those with and without SCT), including gradual introduction of high-intensity conditioning drills, especially at the onset of conditioning training.

Individuals with SCT need to be counseled to stay well hydrated and to immediately report muscle pain or cramping during workouts to the coaching and medical staff. If an individual with SCT has difficulty during training, the activity should be stopped immediately. If rest, supplemental oxygen, and moving to a site with cooler ambient temperature do not immediately improve the condition, the individual should be transported to a hospital emergency department. Use of ice packs may trigger a vaso-occlusive crisis. The American College of Sports Medicine (https://acsm.org/), Civilian Health and Medical Program of the United States, and NCAA (https://www.ncaa.com/) provide useful recommendations for counseling.[11,12] They recommend that individuals with SCT acclimatize gradually and engage in year-round training to maintain physical conditioning and fitness levels, which can reduce oxidative stress and blood viscosity. It is important for athletes, coaches, and medical staff to be educated on how to recognize exercise collapse associated with SCT and to understand the importance of prevention strategies, including maintaining adequate fluid intake and avoiding all-out sprints early in training.[9] Medical eligibility for these athletes should be individualized.

LOW IRON AND ANEMIA

Secondary Questions

- Do you feel fatigued or lightheaded during exercise?
- Does your heart race during exercise?
- Do you have a history of anemia or heavy, frequent menses?
- Do you limit meat in your diet?

Key Points

- Anemia can be associated with heavy or frequent menstrual cycles and nutritional energy deficit.
- Limited evidence supports iron supplementation for low serum ferritin levels without an associated anemia.

The prevalence of iron deficiency anemia in athletes and nonathletes is 3%.[13] An athlete with iron deficiency anemia may present clinically with symptoms of exertional fatigue, tachycardia, dyspnea, and headache. Athletes with iron deficiency anemia may have compromised performance in endurance and nonendurance exercise activities.[14] Symptoms resolve and performance improves after 8 weeks of oral iron supplementation and optimization of dietary energy intake.[14] The activity level and training can be adjusted as symptoms resolve and exercise tolerance improves. However, even after the anemia is corrected, the iron stores often remain low and supplementation may be continued, especially in a symptomatic athlete.[15]

It is a common belief among athletes and coaches, especially those involved in endurance sports and high-altitude activities, that a low ferritin level adversely affects athletic performance. Screening all endurance athletes during the preparticipation evaluation with a complete blood cell count and serum ferritin test is a source of ongoing debate and is not currently recommended as standard of care. Ferritin levels of 12 ng/mL or less correlate with low bone marrow iron stores, although upregulated iron absorption rates have been found even with ferritin values as high as 60 ng/mL.[16] Infection, inflammation, and other disease processes can falsely elevate ferritin levels and confound the assessment of iron status.[17] Endurance athletes have a high prevalence of nonanemic iron deficiency that is based on ferritin cutoff values of 12 to 20 ng/mL. Limited evidence shows that iron supplementation in nonanemic women with iron-depleted ferritin levels less than 16 to 20 ng/mL resulted in improved performance parameters independent of an increase in hemoglobin level.[13] Questions remain regarding the appropriate ferritin level to begin iron supplementation, but most reports advise starting supplementation for a ferritin level of less than 30 to 35 ng/mL, with an aim to continue use of iron supplements empirically for 6 months or until the ferritin level reaches 50 ng/mL.[18] Iron is best obtained through the diet as heme iron found in meat or as nonheme iron from vegetables and grains. Heme iron is better absorbed than nonheme iron, but ascorbic acid and meat proteins can enhance absorption of the latter.[19] Of note, tannins (from tea), calcium, antacids, and phytates (legumes and whole grains) can decrease intestinal absorption of the nonheme iron. Ferrous iron supplements are better absorbed than the ferric iron supplements, with ferrous fumarate, ferrous sulfate, and ferrous gluconate averaging an absorption of 33%, 20%, and 12%, respectively. The amount absorbed is labeled as elemental iron, and supplementation above 45 mg/d of elemental iron increases the risk of gastrointestinal side effects.

BLEEDING DISORDERS

Secondary Questions

- Have you ever been diagnosed with a bleeding disorder?
- Has a doctor restricted your sports participation because of a bleeding disorder?
- Do you have frequent nosebleeds or heavy menstrual bleeding or bruise easily?

Key Point

- Bleeding disorders are rare but complicated when it comes to sport participation.

The most common bleeding disorder is **von Willebrand disease (VWD)**, with a prevalence of 1:1,000.[20]

VWD is an inherited condition with reduced levels of von Willebrand factor or dysfunctional von Willebrand factor. Common features include epistaxis, heavy menstrual bleeding, and easy bruising. Many individuals remain asymptomatic into adulthood. Individuals with known VWD need to be counseled about the risk of participating in contact and collision sports. Sport participation should be a shared decision with the individual, parents or guardians, and medical team.

Hemophilia A and B are hereditary X-linked inherited disorders leading to lifelong bleeding problems, and they generally lead to more severe bleeding episodes than VWD. The spectrum of disease is variable across individuals, and management is complex and evolving.[21]

Exercise and physical activity are recommended for athletes with hemophilia under the supervision of their hematologist. Improvements in strength, flexibility, bone density, and balance contribute to less stress on joints. Additionally, the psychological impact of regular exercise cannot be ignored. Key organizations have produced patient education materials outlining benefits and risks of individual and organized physical activity for those with hemophilia (https://www1.wfh.org/publications/files/pdf-1302.pdf; https://www.bleeding.org/educational-programs/outreach/thrive). Sports like golf, tennis, cycling, and swimming are deemed safe for athletes with hemophilia. Contact and collision sports are generally not recommended, although counseling in partnership with an individual's hematologist is encouraged.

Key organizations have produced patient education materials outlining benefits and risks of individual and organized physical activity for those with hemophilia (https://www1.wfh.org/publications/files/pdf-1302.pdf; https://www.bleeding.org/educational-programs/outreach/thrive).

CANCER AND LONG-TERM EFFECTS OF CHEMOTHERAPEUTIC AGENTS AND RADIATION

Secondary Questions

- Have you ever been diagnosed with any type of cancer?
- Have you ever been treated with chemotherapy?

Key Points

- Chemotherapeutic agents used to treat cancer may have long-term impacts on survivors. Providers need to be aware of possible long-term complications of chemotherapy, including cardiomyopathy, pulmonary toxicity, and peripheral neuropathy.
- Communication with the athlete's managing oncologist needs to be prioritized for those being actively treated or those who have completed chemotherapy.

Cancer survivorship has improved with better health care. Sophisticated treatment regimens allow individuals previously treated for cancer to lead healthy lives. Patients with cancer may feel that physical activity is not encouraged during and after treatment, but physical activity should be encouraged for these patients under the guidance of their oncologist.[22] Cancer survivors are encouraged to participate in physical activity, including but not limited to organized sports. Cancer survivors may present as healthy adolescents wanting to participate in sport, so providers need to be aware of certain chemotherapeutic agents that may impact safe participation.

When released from their oncology team's care, survivors of childhood cancer typically receive a survivorship care plan. This includes date of diagnosis, cancer histology, organs and/or tissues affected, chemotherapeutic agents used, doses of such medications, any radiation therapy and doses used, and history of bone marrow or stem cell transplant. Dosing of chemotherapeutic agents and dosing of radiation therapy guide much of survivorship screening.[23]

For example, doxorubicin[24] with its known cardiac toxicity is the anchor of most pediatric sarcoma treatment and is included in some blood cancer chemotherapy regimens. Dosing of this medication is highly variable and depends on the type of cancer being treated, and cardiotoxicity is dose dependent. Doxorubicin doses are quite low in most blood cancers and much higher in sarcoma, so childhood survivors of sarcoma will likely need specific cardiac screening prior to sport clearance, whereas other cancer survivors will not. Radiation therapy can also have long-term side effects such as osteopenia and osteoporosis that may affect sports participation. For further guidance, consult the individual's managing oncologist/survivorship care plan.

REFERENCES

1. Eichner ER. Sickle cell trait. *J Sport Rehabil.* 2007;16(3):197–203. PMID: 17923725 doi:10.1123/jsr.16.3.197
2. Motulsky AG. Frequency of sickling disorders in U.S. blacks. *N Engl J Med.* 1973;288(1):31–33. PMID: 4681897 doi:10.1056/NEJM197301042880108
3. Kark JA, Ward FT. Exercise and hemoglobin S. *Semin Hematol.* 1994;31(3):181–225. PMID: 7973777
4. Kark JA, Posey DM, Schumacher HR, Ruehle CJ. Sickle-cell trait as a risk factor for sudden death in physical training. *N Engl J Med.* 1987;317(13):781–787. PMID: 3627196 doi:10.1056/NEJM198709243171301

5. Drehner D, Neuhauser KM, Neuhauser TS, Blackwood GV. Death among U.S. Air Force basic trainees, 1956 to 1996. *Mil Med.* 1999;164(12):841–847. PMID: 10628154 doi:10.1093/milmed/164.12.841
6. Kerle KK, Runkle GP. Sickle cell trait and sudden death in athletes. *JAMA.* 1996;276(18):1472. PMID: 8903257 doi:10.1001/jama.1996.03540180028023
7. Nelson DA, Deuster PA, Carter R III, Hill OT, Wolcott VL, Kurina LM. Sickle cell trait, rhabdomyolysis, and mortality among U.S. Army soldiers. *N Engl J Med.* 2016;375(5):435–442. PMID: 27518662 doi:10.1056/NEJMoa1516257
8. Pretzlaff RK. Death of an adolescent athlete with sickle cell trait caused by exertional heat stroke. *Pediatr Crit Care Med.* 2002;3(3):308–310. PMID: 12780975 doi:10.1097/00130478-200207000-00023
9. Kerle KK, Nishimura KD. Exertional collapse and sudden death associated with sickle cell trait. *Am Fam Physician.* 1996;54(1):237–240. PMID: 8677839 doi:10.1093/milmed/161.12.766
10. Kiryluk K, Jadoon A, Gupta M, Radhakrishnan J. Sickle cell trait and gross hematuria. *Kidney Int.* 2007;71(7):706–710. PMID: 17191080 doi:10.1038/sj.ki.5002060
11. National Collegiate Athletic Association (NCAA). Sickle cell trait. Updated February 2023. Accessed April 12, 2025. https://www.ncaa.org/sports/2016/7/27/sickle-cell-trait.aspx
12. O'Connor FG, Bergeron MF, Cantrell J, et al. ACSM and CHAMP summit on sickle cell trait: mitigating risks for warfighters and athletes. *Med Sci Sports Exerc.* 2012;44(11):2045–2056. PMID: 22811029 doi:10.1249/MSS.0b013e31826851c2
13. Fallon KE. Utility of hematological and iron-related screening in elite athletes. *Clin J Sport Med.* 2004;14(3):145–152. PMID: 15166903 doi:10.1097/00042752-200405000-00007
14. Myhre KE, Webber BJ, Cropper TL, et al. Prevalence and impact of anemia on basic trainees in the US Air Force. *Sports Med Open.* 2015;2(1):23–30. PMID: 27239430 doi:10.1186/s40798-016-0047-y
15. Alleyne M, Horne MK, Miller JL. Individualized treatment for iron-deficiency anemia in adults. *Am J Med.* 2008;121(11):943–948. PMID: 18954837 doi:10.1016/j.amjmed.2008.07.012
16. Nielsen P, Nachtigall D. Iron supplementation in athletes. Current recommendations. *Sports Med.* 1998;26(4):207–216. PMID: 9820921 doi:10.2165/00007256-199826040-00001
17. Suedekum NA, Dimeff RJ. Iron and the athlete. *Curr Sports Med Rep.* 2005;4(4):199–202. PMID: 16004828 doi:10.1097/01.CSMR.0000306207.79809.7f
18. Rodenberg RE, Gustafson S. Iron as an ergogenic aid: ironclad evidence? *Curr Sports Med Rep.* 2007;6(4):258–264. PMID: 17618003 doi:10.1097/01.CSMR.0000306481.00283.f6
19. McCormick R, Sim M, Dawson B, Peeling P. Refining treatment strategies for iron deficient athletes. *Sports Med.* 2020;50(12):2111–2123. PMID: 33057935 doi:10.1007/s40279-020-01360-2
20. Nichols WL, Hultin MB, James AH, et al. von Willebrand disease (VWD): evidence-based diagnosis and management guidelines, the National Heart, Lung, and Blood Institute (NHLBI) Expert Panel report (USA). *Haemophilia.* 2008;14(2):171–232. PMID: 18315614 doi:10.1111/j.1365-2516.2007.01643.x
21. Blanchette VS, Key NS, Ljung LR, Manco-Johnson MJ, van den Berg HM, Srivastava A; Subcommittee on Factor VIII, Factor IX and Rare Coagulation Disorders. Definitions in hemophilia: communication from the SSC of the ISTH. *J Thromb Haemost.* 2014;12(11):1935–1939. PMID: 25059285
22. Matuszak JM, O'Connor T. The athlete with cancer. In: O'Connor FG, Davis BA, Hudson KB, et al, eds. *ACSM's Sports Medicine: A Comprehensive Review.* 2nd ed. Wolters Kluwer; 2025
23. Hudson MM, Bhatia S, Casillas J, Landier W; SECTION ON HEMATOLOGY/ONCOLOGY, CHILDREN'S ONCOLOGY GROUP, AMERICAN SOCIETY OF PEDIATRIC HEMATOLOGY/ONCOLOGY. Long-term follow-up care for childhood, adolescent, and young adult cancer survivors. *Pediatrics.* 2021;148(3):e2021053127. PMID: 34462344 doi:10.1542/peds.2021-053127
24. Linders AN, Dias IB, López Fernández T, Tocchetti CG, Bomer N, Van der Meer P. A review of the pathophysiological mechanisms of doxorubicin-induced cardiotoxicity and aging. *NPJ Aging.* 2024;10(1):9. PMID: 38263284 doi:10.1038/s41514-024-00135-7

I: Sports Nutrition and Dietary Supplements

HISTORY FORM QUESTIONS

1. *Medications and supplements: List all current prescriptions, over-the-counter medicines, and supplements (herbal and nutritional).*
2. *Are you happy with your current weight?*
3. *Do you feel pressured to lose/gain weight?*
4. *Do you follow a specific diet plan?*

SECONDARY QUESTIONS

- Have you ever had an eating disorder?
- Have you had a recent weight change?
- Do you worry about gaining weight during the off season or when you can't train because of injury?
- Have you had 3 or more injuries in the past season or did your past season end early because of injury?
- Do you exercise outside of your team's scheduled practices and games to lose weight?
- Have you ever tried weight management medications, diuretics, laxatives, or vomiting to lose weight?
- Are you worried about what you eat?
- Do you have any food allergies or food intolerances?

KEY POINTS

- Low energy availability (LEA) occurs when there is insufficient dietary energy (calorie) intake and/or high exercise energy expenditure.[1]
- Optimized, balanced nutrition plans require individualized assessments of energy requirements, appropriate quantity, quality of food, proper timing of meals/snacks, and maintenance of adequate hydration.
- Individuals with restrictive eating behaviors are considered at higher risk for disordered eating (DE) and may need nutrition education or interventions (eg, gluten allergy or sensitivity, lactose intolerant, vegan or vegetarian, calorie restrictive for weight-based and esthetic sports).[2–5]
- Dietary supplements, except for creatine (see Chapter 5C), do not enhance sport performance in youth athletes and are not recommended unless they have a predetermined clinical need for them identified by a health care provider (HCP) or a dietitian.
- DE, if unrecognized and untreated, can lead to the development of a true eating disorder (ED) and result in potentially irreversible health consequences.

OVERVIEW

The preparticipation evaluation (PPE) is an opportunity to discuss nutrition and healthy eating habits and provide education for individuals participating in sports and physical activity. It should aid in identifying at-risk individuals who have disordered eating habits, who have concerns about their weight or body image, or who are inappropriately using dietary supplements. A well-balanced diet can provide sufficient nutrients and meet energy needs to support normal growth and development and help optimize physical and mental performance. Individual training programs and sport-specific demands pose additional risks for nutritional deficiencies in competitive athletes.

Adequate nutrition is a difficult goal to achieve. Most youths in the United States do not meet national nutrition recommendations for a wide variety of reasons. As a result, DE is a universal problem of almost epidemic proportions in the young and adolescent populations.[6–8] Disordered eating is an ill-defined, descriptive phrase referring to food- and diet-related behaviors that have negative effects on an individual's physical, mental, and emotional health, and it falls along a spectrum of severity ending in EDs.[8] DE encompasses both overeating and undereating behaviors as well as various food avoidance patterns (eg, skipping meals).[2–5] Orthorexia (ie, an obsession with eating healthy food) is increasingly seen in the preadolescent age groups and can cause nutritional deficits through both intentional and unintentional restrictive and avoidance behaviors. In athletes, fueling with good nutrition is a prerequisite for sports performance, but many lack the knowledge to prioritize incorporating healthy eating habits into their training regimens and recovery strategies.

Before puberty, energy requirements are similar for both sexes. Dietary energy intake in the form of food and liquid calories creates energy availability (EA) that supports both basic physiological functions and exercise energy expenditure. Energy needs in adolescents are more variable and fluctuate with physical maturity, individual metabolism, genetic influences, gender, age, hormones, growth spurts, and, particularly, level of activity. Adolescence is a critical period when long-term dietary habits, eating behaviors, body image, and relationships with food and exercise are being cultivated and reinforced.[9] Common maladaptive behaviors include intentional or unintentional calorie restriction; binging; purging; use of laxatives, diuretics, and weight loss medications; avoidance of food groups; food aversion; and a variety of negative psychological associations with diet (eg, guilty feelings from eating, fear of being overweight, compulsive exercise to offset calorie intake, constant preoccupation with or worries about food intake or weight, obsession with weight loss/gain, body image misperceptions).[1] DE behaviors (eg, restrictive eating, binging, purging) and EDs (eg, anorexia nervosa and bulimia nervosa) are more common in athletes than nonathletes and are highest in weight class, endurance, and esthetic sports where leanness is emphasized and desired.[10–12] Youth athletes should pay particular attention to energy balance, portion size, meal timing, and hydration to maximize energy levels, optimize performance, aid in recovery, and reduce injury risk.

MEDICAL HISTORY

Obtaining an accurate, detailed, and current diet history is a crucial, yet challenging, component of the PPE when screening for nutrition-related concerns.[13] Individuals often have poor dietary recall, withhold key details, or report inaccurate information out of fear of restricted athletic participation, loss of self-control, and uncovering underlying personal stressors. Dietary energy intake should represent an average 24-hour dietary intake or even a weekly average. Caloric intake calculations are challenging. Consider referral to a registered dietitian to assist with further nutritional intake/expenditure calculations and formulation of dietary guidance in at-risk individuals. It is also important to identify external pressures that "force" athletes to alter their weight (see Chapter 9). A weight loss recommendation from a coach is a known risk factor for developing maladaptive weight loss behaviors.[14]

A review of recorded vital signs (eg, low blood pressure, bradycardia < 50 beats per minute), anthropometrics for baseline measurements (eg, body mass index [BMI] < 5th percentile for age), or any recent changes (eg, recent increase in height, weight ≥ 10% loss/month, drop in ≥ 1 weight percentile line on growth chart) can identify at-risk individuals who require additional evaluation. BMI is commonly used to determine appropriate weight for height and screen for weight-related health concerns.[15] In children and teens, "BMI for age" is both sex specific and age specific and is plotted on sex-specific growth charts for ages 2 to 20 years (see Table 5C-1 in Chapter 5C for the BMI categories). BMI is notoriously inaccurate for athletes because it does not account for body composition (eg, ratio of muscle to fat), so it can overestimate adiposity (body fat) in athletes with significant muscle mass.[16]

Identification of any recent significant injuries or illnesses in which poor nutrition was a causal contributing factor is also a red flag for potential DE/EDs (eg, bone stress injuries, iron deficiency, chronic fatigue).[17] Screening for DE/EDs is challenging as there are a wide range of physiological, behavioral, and psychological characteristics that contribute to these conditions. Supplement use is common among individuals with known or intentional nutritional deficits. Since nutritional supplement intake is common among young individuals, there is a significant need for HCPs to both inquire about and counsel on appropriate use or avoidance.[18]

ENERGY EXCESS AND ENERGY DEFICITS

While the athlete population is often at risk for underfueling to replace energy used during sports participation, many more (athletes and nonathletes) overconsume low-nutrient-dense foods that are high in calories, saturated fat, and sugar while underconsuming the recommended daily intake of lean protein, fruits, and vegetables. Energy (caloric) excess is the primary cause of overweight and obesity in youth. It is estimated that 33% of children aged 6 to 11 years and 50% of children aged 12 to 19 years will have overweight or obesity by 2030.[19,20] Almost 20% of today's youth are considered obese.[19,20]

Obesity in children and adolescents is associated with health-related problems in every organ system, such as hypertension, hyperlipidemia, asthma, obstructive sleep apnea, insulin resistance, renal disease, slipped capital femoral epiphysis, and various mental health issues (see Chapter 5C). Similarly, energy (caloric) deficits and LEA may be associated with many health problems in every organ system, such as EDs, hormonal dysregulation, menstrual irregularities, erectile dysfunction, low libido, impaired bone health, bone stress injuries, growth restriction, and delayed puberty. Furthermore, a general increase in illnesses, injury risks, fatigue, overtraining syndrome, cognitive deficits, poor academic performance, and/or decreased physical performance may result (see Chapter 6).[17] Proper nutritional intake is vital for normal physiological maturation. Inadequate nutritional intake can impact future adult dietary behaviors, psychological relationships with body image, and the development of some chronic diseases related to unhealthy eating practices. Maintaining adequate levels of hydration daily also influences general health and wellness, improves digestion of food, facilitates delivery of nutrients and oxygen to the body, enhances cognitive and physical function, regulates body temperature, and helps optimize physical performance.

DISORDERED EATING AND EATING DISORDER SCREENING

Normal, Overweight, Underweight

Given that DE/EDs are widely prevalent in the preadolescent, adolescent, and emerging adult populations, consideration has been given to the benefit of screening.[6,7,21,22] The US Preventive Services Task Force (USPSTF) published a scoping review[23] that evaluated ED screening in **normal or overweight adolescents and adults** and concluded that the **evidence is insufficient** to assess the balance of benefits and harms of screening for EDs in that population. The USPSTF recommended that HCPs **screen children over the age of 6 years for obesity** and refer them to intensive, comprehensive, behavioral health interventional programs with a goal of improving weight statuses. The USPSTF identified psychological, social, environmental, and biological risk factors that contribute to the development of DE/ED, but evidence for ED screening in the underweight or known DE/ED population was not considered in the scoping review. Athletes, females, and younger adults (aged 18–29 years) are considered at highest risk, with the highest reported prevalence.[12] Girls as young as 5 to 7 years participating in appearance-oriented sports report weight concerns more often than girls in nonesthetic sports or those who are not physically active.[24] Race, ethnicity, gender, and sexual orientation affect the prevalence of EDs in each respective population. Anorexia nervosa is higher in non-Latino whites, and bulimia nervosa is higher in Asians, African Americans, and Latinos.[25] Transgender adolescents have a higher prevalence of self-reported ED diagnoses than cisgender heterosexual females.[26] Comorbid psychiatric disorders also are associated with an increased incidence of diagnosed EDs.[23] HCPs need to be aware that in adolescent and collegiate athletes with DE and/or LEA, there is a strong association with increased anxiety, and they need to take proactive steps to screen for and initiate early intervention when appropriate (see Chapter 6).[27,28]

DE and EDs associated with LEA are more prevalent in athletes but are also influenced by age, gender, and the sport of choice.[22] In athletes, LEA is often responsible for hormonal effects of hypothalamic suppression such as the development of low libido and/or oligomenorrhea or amenorrhea in females and low sex drive, erectile dysfunction, decreased spermatogenesis, and smaller testicular/phallus size in males. LEA can have adverse effects on bone health such as osteopenia or osteoporosis.[29,30] Causes of LEA are multifactorial, but the most common are intentional dietary restriction, excessive exercise, rapid weight loss, and maintaining a body weight that is too low for height and age. Not all individuals with LEA are underweight, but some may have LEA as a result of abnormal dietary behaviors (eg, binging and purging) often associated with an intense desire to lose weight or be thinner. The history of a past or current ED is a consistent risk factor for future DE/EDs.[31] Modifying diet, exercise, body weight, and/or body composition is necessary to increase energy availability, restore regular menstruation, improve libido and sexual function, and optimize bone mineral density (BMD).[32–34] Early recognition and intervention for young individuals with DE habits is essential to prevent escalation to EDs and/or chronic health conditions.[32]

Relative Energy Deficiency Syndrome (RED-S)/Female and Male Athlete Triad

RED-S is a multisystem physiological response due to a negative imbalance in energy availability. It affects up to 50% of adolescent athletes.[27,35] The definition of RED-S was updated in 2023 as a multifactorial "syndrome of impaired physiological and/or psychological functioning experienced by female and male athletes that is caused by exposure to problematic (prolonged and/or severe) LEA."[35] LEA occurs on a spectrum from adaptable to problematic. Adaptable LEA refers to short-term LEA, resulting in benign effects such as body composition changes that can either have no effect on or slightly improve performance. Conversely, problematic LEA occurs when long-term exposure (eg, exercise energy expenditure or insufficient dietary energy intake) causes a maladaptive response that impairs health, well-being, and/or performance.[35] RED-S symptomology was first described as the Female Athlete Triad ("the Triad") and includes specifically LEA (with or without DE), menstrual dysfunction, and low BMD.[36] More recently, the Male Athlete Triad was described as a similar syndrome of 3 interrelated conditions commonly seen in adolescent and young adult males who are in a state of underfueling. Similar to female athletes, participation in endurance and weight-class sports or those that emphasize lean physiques put male athletes at highest risk. Both triads include the interrelatedness of (1) energy deficiency/LEA with or without DE/EDs, (2) functional hypothalamic hypogonadism, and (3) osteoporosis or low BMD with or without bone stress injury, all occurring on a spectrum of varying severity.[37,38] Adding to the complexity of diagnosing RED-S are the overlapping characteristics with overtraining syndrome and the original Triad. Both involve stresses or suppression of the hypothalamic-pituitary-adrenal axis that results in the multiorgan system effects and the vast array of signs and symptoms. RED-S/Triad screening using evidence-based risk assessment protocols is recommended beginning in middle school or high school and continuing through college in at-risk individuals, regardless of gender, to promote early identification and optimize bone health and general wellness.[38,39] Indications for bone density screening are discussed in Chapter 5G. Deficits in whole-body bone mineral content and BMD at the lumbar spine, total hip, and femoral neck in both sexes are significantly, and similarly, associated with the degree of malnutrition present.[40] The need for bone density screening may be greater when a bone stress injury is present and DE/ED screening is positive (see Tables 5G-1 and 5G-2).[41,42]

SCREENING TOOLS FOR DE/ED/RED-S/TRIAD

The importance of performing some type of screening is recognized because of the widespread prevalence of DE/EDs in the youth and young adult population, and screening supports the PPE goal to identify conditions that may be life threatening or disabling, or those that may predispose to injury or illness related to participation in physical activity (see Chapter 1). Examiners are advised to screen for signs of RED-S/Triad/DE/EDs during PPEs and whenever an individual presents with one component of the Triad (eg, bone stress injury, menstrual dysfunction, or DE).[43] The National Athletic Trainers' Association, American College of Sports Medicine, and International Olympic Committee have released statements supporting regular screening for DE in athletes; however, they did not identify a current, universal screening tool, validated in both male and female athletes, to easily screen for DE, and not specifically EDs. There is a lack of consensus among leading experts on ideal screening tools. In adult athletes, the Triad Cumulative Risk Assessment Tool (Triad CRA), the RED-S questionnaires (eg, Low Energy Availability in Male Athletes [LEAM-Q] and Low Energy Availability in Female Athletes [LEAF-Q]), and Relative Energy Deficiency in Sport Clinical Assessment Tool [RED-S CAT]) have been validated and may be useful for individuals aged 18 and older.[27,36,44–47]

Since there is no single screening tool that has been validated in adolescent athletes to incorporate into a PPE, this has led to multiple combinations, revisions, and variations of questions extracted from available tools attempting to identify individuals at risk for ED/DE. There are 6 ED athlete-specific screening tools, but they were validated in collegiate athletes only or designed to be used only in females, and/or they do not screen for DE.[48,49] There is emerging evidence in male athletes that can help guide screening practices. A scoping review by Hoogenboom et al[22] in 2025 analyzed the clinical use of specific tools for screening young male and female athletes for ED/DE risk. The Eating Disorder Examination (EDE 17.0D) is the current "gold standard" for diagnosing ED, but not DE alone.[50] The EDE is a psychometrically validated, semistructured, in-person interview about 1 hour in length, with 62 items grouped into 4 subscales. It was not designed specifically for athletes. The Eating Attitudes Test (EAT-26) has the longest history of use.[51] It is a 26-item self-report screen that is designed with a 6-point Likert scale ranging from 1 (never) to 6 (always) for each item. It is a validated psychometric measure to identify risk for EDs in the general population and is also validated in athletes. A score of 20 or higher indicates risk for ED. Expert opinions from sports psychiatrists have suggested that a score of 12 can indicate someone "at risk" for DE. In 2021, Kennedy et al[49] validated the Disordered Eating Screening for Athletes (DESA-6), which is a yes/no 6-question screening tool for detecting DE and not ED. It has only been validated for athletes 18 years and older. In the process of creating and validating the DESA-6, the researchers identified 6 key elements that were most effective (frequency and severity of injuries, fear of weight gain, happiness with weight, intensity of dissatisfaction with current weight, presence of dieting, and external pressure to lose weight). A positive score is 3 or more "yes" answers. The DESA-6 pilot study in 18- to 19-year-old adolescent athletes found that the prevalence of DE was 12.84% (n = 148) in males (sensitivity 100%; specificity 85.0%) and 34.38% (n = 16) in females (sensitivity 90.9%; specificity 86.5%). With a combined prevalence of 30.86%, the results of the DESA-6 were similar to those in previous research that screened for ED/DE using validated ED scales in various mixed populations of elite adolescent and young adult or collegiate athletes. The applicability to 13- to 17-year-olds or to the nonathletic adolescent population has yet to be studied. The Eating Disorder Screening Tool for Primary Care (ESP) is a 5-item questionnaire that is widely used as an ED screen but was not originally designed for use in athletes. In the ESP, the best individual questions for ruling out an ED screened for satisfaction with eating patterns and if weight affects the way one feels about oneself. The best individual questions for ruling in an ED are worrying about eating, lack of control, feeling full or sick, eating in secret, and a personal history of a prior ED.[52] Lastly, a RED-S screening tool (RST) has been developed for use in a younger age population, takes activity levels into account, is applicable to both genders, and can be used in females who have not yet menstruated. However, further research is needed to fully validate the RST for widespread screening; further, it contains 25 questions with several subsections, so it is not easily administered during the typical PPE.[53]

In the ESP, the best individual questions for ruling out an ED screened for satisfaction with eating patterns and if weight affects the way one feels about oneself. The best individual questions for ruling in an ED are worrying about eating, lack of control, feeling full or sick, eating in secret, and a personal history of a prior ED.

In addition to less-than-ideal screening methods or tests, other barriers to screening include limited time and lack of resources.[43] Lastly, in the adolescent athlete population, the HCP's specialty influences screening practices, with orthopedic surgeons being less likely to screen for DE conditions such as RED-S or Triad. Red flags in the general health history that indicate a need to screen for RED-S/Triad include identification of an ED (88%), menstrual dysfunction (76%), and bone stress injury (74%).[43]

The current PPE dietary habits and nutrition screening questions are primarily based on data that have a high probability of accurate risk stratification to identify a need for further detailed DE/ED screening. This is a daunting task to accomplish with 3 primary screening questions on the PPE History Form. Answering "yes" to question 2 (Are you happy with your current weight?) is an encouraging sign that the presence of DE/ED is less likely. However, a positive screening response to any of the primary or secondary questions (eg, pressured to gain or lose weight, unhappy with current weight, restrictive eating behaviors to change body weight or shape, body image issues, negative feelings of guilt or fear regarding food, or nonprescribed supplement use) merits further investigation for the presence of DE/EDs. HCPs may find DE/ED screening questionnaires helpful adjuncts in their assessments.

CLEARANCE FOR SPORTS PARTICIPATION

Dietary screening tools are not intended to definitively diagnose DE/EDs. Attempts at screening are simply initial steps to identify individuals at risk who would benefit from a more thorough investigation. The decision to withhold sports participation in high-risk or symptomatic individuals with LEA during the PPE is to prevent escalation of the condition(s). It is important to include a plan for close follow-up, ideally in the medical home or with the team physician. A multidisciplinary team (eg, physician, dietitian, psychologist, behavioral therapist, and/or exercise physiologist) approach to management of DE/RED-S/Triad/EDs is beneficial in achieving a successful postintervention outcome.[36] Improving energy availability through optimal nutrition is the mainstay of treatment. Factors identified during the PPE that influence clearance decisions include very low BMI, recent rapid or severe weight loss, significant malnutrition, or any signs of acute or chronic physical injury or illness (eg, physiological or mental) where future physical activity or sports participation could result in an adverse health outcome for the individual being screened.[48] Depending on the individual situation, medical eligibility may be denied until the athlete has undergone more extensive medical, psychiatric, or nutritional assessment and has made progress toward recovery. Using clearance and return-to-play guidelines such as those from the Female and Male Athlete Triad Coalition Consensus Statements is recommended to optimize treatment and prevent problems.[27,37,38,53]

Using clearance and return-to-play guidelines such as those from the Female and Male Athlete Triad Coalition Consensus Statements is recommended to optimize treatment and prevent problems. See https://doi.org/10.1136/bjsports-2018-099193 and https://doi.org/10.1097/JSM.0000000000000948

Engaging athletes to undergo treatment for DE/EDs is challenging as they are often reluctant to cooperate. The treatment goals for athletes with LEA are to optimize overall nutritional status, normalize eating behavior(s), attain and maintain a healthy weight, manage physical complications, modify unhealthy thought processes that maintain the disorder, treat underlying emotional issues contributing to the disorder, and prevent future relapse. Conditional participation can be successful at keeping the individual engaged and accountable during treatment if their caloric intake is sufficient to support the permitted amount of energy expenditure related to physical activity; however, imposing any restrictions on participation can harm the physician–patient relationship. Disengaging an athlete from team participation and training does not prevent unsupervised physical activity; therefore, the more actively involved the athlete stays with their team and their HCP, the more likely a positive outcome can be achieved. Often, an individual in treatment for an ED/DE (and parents or guardian if a minor) may be asked to sign a contract stipulating the requirements to resume or continue participating in their sport.[36] Examples include adherence to treatment, regular visits with the health care team, and modification of training. If the contract is broken, or weight and eating behaviors do not improve, the athlete could be restricted from athletic participation on the basis of the language in the contract.

Once the athlete is medically eligible for full participation, they may be less compliant with treatment recommendations. It is important for athletes, parents or guardians, and coaches to understand that inadequate caloric intake, DE behaviors, and subsequent hormonal dysfunction that result in adverse health consequences and injury will compromise the individual's ability to train and compete, regardless of clearance status.[36]

DIETARY SUPPLEMENTS

History Form Question

1. *Medications and supplements: List all current prescriptions, over-the-counter medicines, and supplements (herbal and nutritional).*

Secondary Questions

- Do you take any herbals, minerals, or vitamins?
- Do you use anything to help with your exercise or workouts?
- Do you take any protein or muscle-building supplements?

Supplements: Nutritional and Dietary

Youth athletes should not consume dietary supplements unless they have a predetermined clinical need for them identified by an HCP or a dietitian. They are not an appropriate substitute for a good diet. The PPE is an opportunity to provide education on nutrition guidelines and help young individuals avoid the common pitfalls associated with inadequate nutrition, poor hydration, and supplement use/abuse. Therefore, HCPs performing PPEs need to be familiar with the risks and benefits of the supplements that are commonly used in the physically active youth, adolescent, and young adult populations. Teaching young individuals and their parents to read food labels is one strategy to help them compare products and make healthier food and beverage choices. In light of the widespread popularity of nutritional supplements, more research is needed to better understand the effects on the young, maturing body; however, ethical concerns make such an undertaking extremely challenging. Most of the current research is conducted in adults only.

Many individuals are hesitant to reveal their use of supplements or ergogenic aids, so an open and inviting questioning style may help elicit an accurate history. It may take time to investigate the components and potential risks/benefits of unfamiliar substances. Asking individuals about their motivation for taking supplements may allow insight into body image issues, competitive pressures, and the potential likelihood for future supplement or ergogenic aid use. Individuals should be informed about the risks of supplements that are not regulated by the US Food and Drug Administration (FDA) or have not undergone testing certification, as up to 58% of supplements contain components not listed on product labels, and these undisclosed components may have health risks and/or may be on the banned substance list for elite or collegiate athletes.[54] The safest sources of vitamins and minerals come from a healthy, balanced diet. However, if supplements are used, more reliable products with a greater likelihood of containing the ingredients on the label and being free of harmful contaminants often have third-party certifications from independent testing organizations that have verified the ingredients. It is also wise to read labels carefully and check for FDA warnings.

Very few dietary supplements have been proven to possess clinically relevant effectiveness, and others are dangerous and illegal. The vulnerable youth population has been effectively targeted by the supplement industry, and this is a major cause of concern.

Unfortunately, many young individuals resort to using nutritional supplements as a means of preventing or treating micronutrient and macronutrient deficiencies, and for health promotion, injury prevention, manipulation of physique, pain management, recovery, mood enhancement, or improvement of athletic performance (eg, power, speed, agility, and endurance). Athletes desiring to improve performance often intentionally use supplements as ergogenic aids.[55,56] An ergogenic aid is any mechanical device, training technique, pharmacologic agent, or nutritional substance that either enhances training adaptations or improves exercise capacity and performance.[57] A nutritional ergogenic aid is a naturally occurring food substance that is packaged in artificially high doses, exceeding what could be consumed in a typical diet (eg, caffeine in energy drinks versus caffeine in chocolate). Athletes who are motivated to advance in their sport to elite levels are often particularly vulnerable to external pressures and marketing strategies that imply certain supplements can enhance performance (eg, protein/amino acid supplements, sports drinks, electrolytes).[58] The rise in youth supplement use is attributed in part to promotional strategies with adult sport role models, easy accessibility in stores, and various other marketing strategies (eg, colorful packaging, candy-like flavorings). Understanding the motivation for supplement use allows the HCP to address health issues or provide education (eg, fatigue and poor sleep, anxiety, and excess caffeine consumption).

An ergogenic aid is any mechanical device, training technique, pharmacologic agent, or nutritional substance that either enhances training adaptations or improves exercise capacity and performance.

Vitamin and Mineral Micronutrients: Iron, Calcium, and Vitamin D

The most frequently used vitamin and mineral supplements are vitamin C and D, multivitamins, calcium, and iron. There is a role for prescribed supplementation in youths who are nutritionally deficient in certain micronutrients if improvements in the diet alone are not sufficient or until long-term lifestyle changes are successfully implemented (eg, increased dietary iron, calcium, or vitamin D). However, large doses of vitamins and minerals can lead to toxicity and adverse interactions with other nutrients.[55] The lack of regulation means that the safety and composition of vitamin and mineral supplementation is not guaranteed. Some products may even contain substances banned in National Collegiate Athletic Association (NCAA) or Olympic sports, and use can result in negative consequences for athletes undergoing drug tests.

The 3 most important vitamins and minerals for adolescents, and particularly athletes, are calcium, vitamin D, and iron.[59] Iron is discussed in Chapter 5H. Deficiencies in micronutrients can occur independently of overall adequate or insufficient macronutrient (eg, carbohydrate, protein, fat) intake. Identified micronutrient deficiencies are also red flags to perform more thorough screening of an individual's overall nutritional status, which often leads to further, sometimes extensive, diagnostic testing.[60]

Calcium

The recommended dietary allowance (RDA) is the dietary intake that meets the requirements of almost all (97.5%) of the population. The RDA for calcium in adolescents is 1,300 mg/d with an upper limit of 3,000 mg/d. (See Table 51-1.) The upper limit represents the highest average total daily intake that minimizes the risks of age-related adverse health effects for most individuals in that age group. Only 10% of adolescent girls achieve the recommended dietary intake of calcium.[39] Adequate calcium intake is encouraged through good dietary habits. Routine calcium supplementation is not recommended for healthy children and adolescents unless they have dairy intolerance or another medical condition that does not allow for adequate calcium intake through food. Calcium is necessary for healthy bone development, muscle function, and normal enzyme activity. Calcium demand increases during periods of rapid growth and during recovery from bone stress injuries. Virtually all calcium is stored in bone. Milk intake during adolescence is associated with higher bone mineral content and reduced fracture risk in adulthood.[61] Typical dietary sources of calcium are dairy products (eg, milk, cheese, yogurt), green leafy vegetables, salmon, sardines, tomatoes, beans, tofu, orange juice, and calcium-fortified grains (eg, cereals). Natural calcium-containing food sources have better bioavailability than fortified foods or supplements; therefore, encouraging the development of healthy dietary behaviors and eating a well-balanced diet are preferred.

Typical dietary sources of calcium are dairy products (eg, milk, cheese, yogurt), green leafy vegetables, salmon, sardines, tomatoes, beans, tofu, orange juice, and calcium-fortified grains (eg, cereals).

Table 51-1. Calcium and Vitamin D Dietary Reference Intakes

Age, y	Calcium		Vitamin D	
	RDA (mg/d) (Intake That Meets Needs of ≥ 97.5% of Population)	UL (mg/d)[a]	RDA (IU/d) (Intake That Meets Needs of ≥ 97.5% of Population)	UL (IU/d)[a]
9–13	1,300	3,000	600	4,000
14–18	1,300	3,000	600	4,000
19–50	1,000	2,500	600	4,000

Abbreviation: RDA, recommended daily allowance.

[a] Upper limit (UL) indicates a level above which there is a risk of adverse events. The UL is not intended as a target intake (no consistent evidence of greater benefit at intake levels above the RDA).

Reproduced from Golden NH, Abrams SA; American Academy of Pediatrics Committee on Nutrition. Optimizing bone health in children and adolescents. *Pediatrics.* 2014;134(4):e1229–e1243.

Vitamin D

Vitamin D (calciferol) is a fat-soluble hormone necessary for calcium absorption, regulation, and utilization. Without it, only 10% to 15% of dietary calcium is absorbed. Vitamin D encompasses endogenous conversion of vitamin D_2, dietary animal-derived cholecalciferol (vitamin D_3), and plant-derived ergocalciferol (vitamin D_2). The RDA for vitamin D is 600 IU/day for children, adolescents, and adults, with a maximum of 4,000 IU/day.[62] See Table 5I-1. The AAP endorses these daily allowances. Universal or routine screening for vitamin D deficiency is not recommended because there is not enough evidence of a sufficient cost-benefit ratio in reducing fracture risk.[39] Conversely, vitamin D is increasingly recognized for its critical role in bone health and the management of osteoporosis, as well as potential benefits on cardiometabolic risk factors, immune system function, and cancer prevention.[63] Testing for vitamin D deficiency in children and adolescents at risk for bone fragility is supported on an individual case-by-case basis (see Chapter 5G). Darker-skinned individuals, those with inadequate sunlight exposure, those living in northern climates, and those with obesity are at higher risk for deficiency. Cross-sectional studies in adolescents found vitamin D deficiency in 17% to 47% of adolescents, with an additional increased risk in Black and Hispanic teenagers.[61] Serum concentration of 25-hydroxyvitamin D (25[OH]D) is the best indicator of vitamin D status. The National Academy of Medicine concluded that people are vitamin D deficient with serum 25(OH)D concentrations of less than 12 ng/mL and are at potential risk with levels ranging from 12 ng/mL to 20 ng/mL.[62]

Universal or routine screening for vitamin D deficiency is not recommended because there is not enough evidence of a sufficient cost-benefit ratio in reducing fracture risk.

Electrolyte Supplements

Electrolyte supplements (other than sports drinks) are gaining in popularity due in part to marketing ploys stating that electrolytes can improve energy and concentration. These supplements are readily available, usually in liquid or powder form, and are being increasingly used on a daily basis, or even several times a day, as routine beverage supplements and not in association with exercise. There are notable health risks associated with excessive use of electrolyte supplements (eg, sodium and potassium overload), as an imbalance of electrolytes can overwhelm the body's ability to regulate, leading to fluid overload, congestive heart failure, acute kidney injury, seizures, brain edema, clotting disorders, cramping, gastrointestinal upset, breathing difficulties, and other adverse effects.[64]

Creatine

Creatine is naturally synthesized in the body by combining the amino acids of glycine, arginine, and methionine and is produced in physiological amounts by the liver, kidneys, and pancreas. Creatine is also found in protein-rich foods such as meat and fish. In 2001, 1,103 school-aged competitive sport athletes ranging from 10 to 18 years old were surveyed; 10.6% reported using creatine in middle school, and use steadily rose until 12th grade when 44% reported using creatine.[65] Creatine as an ergogenic aid came into popularity because creatine facilitates the production of adenosine triphosphate from adenosine diphosphate, thus increasing the amount of free energy available for muscle contraction. This can increase strength, lean body mass, and anaerobic performance when combined with a structured training program, even in adolescents and across both genders.[62,65] In adults, short-term and long-duration creatine use has been extensively studied and has been found to pose minimal risk for adverse events or significant negative impact on general health. While studies in children and adolescents are more limited, they also have shown improvements in athletic performance and low risk for adverse events.[62] However, given that creatine supplements are unregulated, there is no guarantee that these products are free of substances on the World Anti-Doping Agency or NCAA banned substances lists. Therefore, it would be safer for individuals who are subject to drug testing to increase creatine in their diets by eating larger amounts of protein, rather than by taking creatine supplements.

Caffeine

Caffeine is a central nervous system stimulant that has a drug-like effect on the body. It is the world's most widely used psychoactive substance at any age. It has no nutritional value and is not a necessary part of a healthy diet. The AAP recommends no caffeine intake for individuals younger than 12 years and 100 mg per day for those between ages 12 and 18 years; adults are advised to limit caffeine intake to 200 to 400 mg daily. Ingestion of small amounts of caffeine naturally occurring in foods such as chocolate is considered low risk. Most energy drinks contain 80 to 300 mg of caffeine per serving. Serving sizes can range from 2 to 24 oz, which can add to consumer confusion. It is estimated that nearly two-thirds of all adolescents in the United States consume energy drinks. Caffeine is also available in a variety of other forms (eg, pills, powders, bars, and gum). Side effects include palpitations, tachycardia, hypertension, jitteriness, acute myocardial infarctions, sudden cardiac arrest, gastrointestinal disturbances (eg, pain, diarrhea, nausea, vomiting), acute kidney injury, rhabdomyolysis, headaches, seizures, strokes, sleep disturbances, insomnia, mood disorders, anxiety, addiction, and even death related to overdoses or cross-reactions with other stimulant substances in the body (eg, attention-deficit/hyperactivity disorder or migraine medications, recreational drugs).[66,67]

The AAP recommends no caffeine intake for individuals younger than 12 years and 100 mg per day for those between ages 12 and 18 years; adults are advised to limit caffeine intake to 200 to 400 mg daily. Ingestion of small amounts of caffeine naturally occurring in foods such as chocolate is considered low risk. Most energy drinks contain 80 to 300 mg of caffeine per serving. Serving sizes can range from 2 to 24 oz, which can add to consumer confusion.

The AAP recommends against the use of energy drinks as ergogenic aids and discourages their use as routine beverages in the diet because of the high caffeine and sugar content. For the overweight and obese population, energy drinks provide unnecessary calories with low nutritional value.[66] Additionally, there is high acidity in these drinks that can be associated with tooth decay and poor dentition, even in sugar-free beverages.

Hydration

The body is composed of approximately 50% water. Daily hydration is required to maintain fluid balance, replenish ongoing losses (eg, breathing, sweating, urination), aid in digestion of food, aid in thermoregulation, and optimize health and performance. General guidelines state that 0.5 to 1.0 oz of fluid per pound of body weight is sufficient to maintain fluid balance for nonexertional activities of daily living.[68] Proper hydration in physically active individuals usually requires additional fluid intake before, during, and after physical activity to help replace sweat losses during exercise and regulate body temperature. Fluid deficiency at the beginning of training sessions is common, with 1 study finding that 20% to 44% of high-performance adolescent athletes were underhydrated prepractice.[69] Both dehydration and overhydration can have negative effects on athletic performance and general health. Failure to maintain adequate fluid intake can lead to dehydration. Water losses of 2% or more of total body weight can have detrimental effects on performance.[8] Individual sweat rates, ambient temperature, and humidity of the environment all affect an individual's ability to maintain adequate hydration status. Individuals with heavy sweat rates who have insufficient compensatory habits (eg, impaired thirst, inability to ingest adequate amounts of fluid) are at highest risk for dehydration compared to individuals with lighter sweat rates or a better ability to ingest fluids during exercise.[8] Some common signs and symptoms of dehydration include thirst, headaches, dizziness, impaired concentration, muscle cramps, weakness, tachycardia, and elevated body temperature, particularly if the environment is hot and/or humid. Unrecognized or unaddressed dehydration can result in serious or life-threatening conditions such as heat stroke, seizures, and shock (see Chapter 5C). Simple methods to monitor for signs of dehydration include noticing thirst, dark yellow urine color, decreased body weight, or the development of additional signs and symptoms of dehydration.

The AAP identifies plain water, plain pasteurized milk, and limited amounts of watered down 100% fruit and vegetable juice as healthy beverage choices.[70] The routine ingestion of carbohydrate-containing sports drink throughout the day, with meals, during short bouts of physical activity, or during light-intensity exercise is unnecessary and can lead to excess calorie intake, overweight, and obesity conditions. For physical activity of an hour or less in a moderate environment without extreme exertion, ad lib water-only intake, drinking to thirst, is appropriate.[66] In general, adolescents should drink 8 to 20 oz of fluids 1 hour before exercise, followed by an average of 5 oz every 15 minutes during exercise and then 20 oz of fluids per pound of weight lost during the postexercise recovery period. The amount of exercise, intensity, environment, and individual sweat rates all influence the actual amount of fluid needed to maintain hydration, and recommendations should be individualized for ongoing sports participation whenever possible. Every individual participating in physical activity must have access to fluids at all times.

In general, adolescents should drink 8 to 20 oz of fluids 1 hour before exercise, followed by an average of 5 oz every 15 minutes during exercise and then 20 oz of fluids per pound of weight lost during the postexercise recovery period.

Sports drinks are carbohydrate-electrolyte–containing beverages that have a role in replenishing losses sustained during prolonged or intense exercise, usually lasting more than 1 hour. There are risks associated with failure to replenish carbohydrate and electrolyte losses, as electrolyte imbalances (eg, sodium and potassium) can adversely affect performance and exercise tolerance and can impair health.[66]

Energy Sources: Macronutrients

Macronutrients, including carbohydrates, protein, and fat, are the source of energy in all individuals.[71] Basic energy requirements for young individuals vary based on age, sex, and physical activity level.[72] (See Table 51-2.) Additional daily caloric needs vary in relation to physical maturity, growth spurts, age, basal metabolic rate, quantity of physical activity, and degree of strenuousness. Additional caloric intake is needed primarily during growth spurts and for replenishment of energy expenditure during physical activity.

Carbohydrates

One gram of carbohydrate provides 4 kcal of energy. Approximately 45% to 65% of total caloric intake should be in the form of carbohydrates in the pediatric population. The basic building block for energy is glucose. Excess glucose is stored in muscles and the liver as glycogen and can be mobilized as an energy source promptly during exercise.

Table 51-2. Summary Table of EER Equations by Age, Sex, and Physical Activity and Energy Cost of Growth: Children and Adolescents (2023)

Age Group	Sex	PAL Category	EER Equation (kcal/d)
3–13.99 years	M	Inactive	EER = −447.51 + (3.68 × age) + (13.01 × height) + (13.15 × weight) + 20/15/25[a]
		Low active	EER = 19.12 + (3.68 × age) + (8.62 × height) + (20.28 × weight) + 20/15/25
		Active	EER = −388.19 + (3.68 × age) + (12.66 × height) + (20.46 × weight) + 20/15/25
		Very active	EER = −671.75 + (3.68 × age) + (15.38 × height) + (23.25 × weight) + 20/15/25
	F	Inactive	EER = 55.59 − (22.25 × age) + (8.43 × height) + (17.07 × weight) + 15/30[b]
		Low active	EER = −297.54 − (22.25 × age) + (12.77 × height) + (14.73 × weight) + 15/30
		Active	EER = −189.55 − (22.25 × age) + (11.74 × height) + (18.34 × weight) + 15/30
		Very active	EER = −709.59 − (22.25 × age) + (18.22 × height) + (14.25 × weight) + 15/30

(continued)

Table 5I-2. Summary Table of EER Equations by Age, Sex, and Physical Activity and Energy Cost of Growth: Children and Adolescents (2023) (*continued*)

14–18.99 years	M	Inactive	EER = −447.51 + (3.68 × age) + (13.01 × height) + (13.15 × weight) + 20
		Low active	EER = 19.12 + (3.68 × age) + (8.62 × height) + (20.28 × weight) + 20
		Active	EER = −388.19 + (3.68 × age) + (12.66 × height) + (20.46 × weight) + 20
		Very active	EER = −671.75 + (3.68 × age) + (15.38 × height) + (23.25 × weight) + 20
	F	Inactive	EER = 55.59 − (22.25 × age) + (8.43 × height) + (17.07 × weight) + 20
		Low active	EER = −297.54 − (22.25 × age) + (12.77 × height) + (14.73 × weight) + 20
		Active	EER = −189.55 − (22.25 × age) + (11.74 × height) + (18.34 × weight) + 20
		Very active	EER = −709.59 − (22.25 × age) + (18.22 × height) + (14.25 × weight) + 20

Abbreviations: EER, estimated energy requirement; kcal/d, kilocalories per day; PAL, physical activity level.

Age is in years, weight is in kilograms, and height is in centimeters.

[a]Energy cost of growth for boys: 3 y: 20 kcal/d; 4 to 8 y: 15 kcal/d; 9 to 13 y: 25 kcal/d.

[b]Energy cost of growth for girls: 3 y: 15 kcal/d; 4 to 8 y: 15 kcal/d; 9 to 13 y: 30 kcal/d.

Reproduced from National Academies of Sciences, Engineering, and Medicine; Health and Medicine Division; Food and Nutrition Board; Committee on the Dietary Reference Intakes for Energy. *Dietary Reference Intakes for Energy.* National Academies Press; 2023.

Protein

Protein also provides 4 kcal of energy per gram. The primary function of protein is as a building block for muscle, nails, skin, and hair. Protein can act as a secondary source of energy through gluconeogenesis in the liver when the carbohydrate supply is exhausted through exercise or a period of starvation. Approximately 10% to 30% of total caloric intake should be in the form of protein in the pediatric and young adult population. High-quality protein comes from specific animal (eg, beef, poultry, fish, eggs, milk) and plant-based (eg, beans, nuts, and seeds) sources. More information about protein content of various foods can be found at https://www.healthychildren.org/English/ages-stages/teen/nutrition/Pages/Protein-for-the-Teen-Athlete.aspx.

Fat

Fat provides the greatest amount of energy per gram at 9 kcal. Fat provides essential fatty acids, helps to absorb fat-soluble vitamins (A, D, E, K), and protects the body's vital organs. Approximately 25% to 35% of total caloric intake should be in the form of fat in the pediatric population, primarily in the form of unsaturated fat. More information about healthy fat choices can be found at https://www.healthychildren.org/English/ages-stages/gradeschool/nutrition/Pages/Making-Healthy-Food-Choices.aspx.

REFERENCES

1. Landolfi E. Exercise addiction. *Sports Med.* 2013;43(2):111–119. PMID: 23329605 doi: 10.1007/s40279-012-0013-x
2. Gonzalez VM, Vitousek KM. Feared food in dieting and non-dieting young women: a preliminary validation of the Food Phobia Survey. *Appetite.* 2004;43(2):155–173. PMID: 15458802 doi: 10.1016/j.appet.2004.03.006
3. Aloufy A, Latzer Y. Diet or health—the linkage between vegetarianism and anorexia nervosa. Article in Hebrew. *Harefuah.* 2006;145(7):526–531, 549. PMID: 16900745
4. Klopp SA, Heiss CJ, Smith HS. Self-reported vegetarianism may be a marker for college women at risk for disordered eating. *J Am Diet Assoc.* 2003;103(6):745–747. PMID: 12778048
5. Cialdella-Kam L, Kulpins D, Manore MM. Vegetarian, gluten-free, and energy restricted diets in female athletes. *Sports (Basel).* 2016;4(4):50. PMID: 29910298 doi: 10.3390/sports4040050
6. Bonci CM, Bonci LJ, Granger LR, et al. National Athletic Trainers' Association position statement: preventing, detecting, and managing disordered eating in athletes. *J Athl Train.* 2008;43(1):80–108. PMID: 18335017 doi: 10.4085/1062-6050-43.1.80
7. Grunbaum JA, Kann L, Kinchen SA, et al. Youth risk behavior surveillance—United States, 2001. *MMWR Surveill Summ.* 2002;51(4):1–62. PMID: 12102329 doi: 10.1111/j.1746-1561.2002.tb07917.x
8. Hecht C, Bank N, Cook B, Mistovich RJ. Nutritional recommendations for the young athlete. *J Pediatr Soc North Am.* 2024;5(1):599. PMID: 40433081 doi: 10.55275/JPOSNA-2023-599
9. Desbrow B. Youth athlete development and nutrition. *Sports Med.* 2021;51(suppl 1):3–12. PMID: 34515968 doi: 10.1007/s40279-021-01534-6
10. Nattiv A, Loucks AB, Manore MM, Sanborn CF, Sundgot-Borgen J, Warren MP; American College of Sports Medicine. American College of Sports Medicine position stand. The female athlete triad. *Med Sci Sports Exerc.* 2007;39(10):1867–1882. PMID: 17909417
11. Dane A, Bhatia K. The social media diet: a scoping review to investigate the association between social media, body image and eating disorders amongst young people. *PLOS Glob Public Health.* 2023;3(3):e0001091. PMID: 36962983 doi: 10.1371/journal.pgph.0001091
12. Sundgot-Borgen J, Torstveit MK. Prevalence of eating disorders in elite athletes is higher than in the general population. *Clin J Sport Med.* 2004;14(1):25–32. PMID: 14712163 doi: 10.1097/00042752-200401000-00005PubMedGoogle
13. Tanner SM. Preparticipation examination targeted for the female athlete. *Clin Sports Med.* 1994;13(2):337–353. PMID: 8013037
14. Sundgot-Borgen J. Risk and trigger factors for the development of eating disorders in female elite athletes. *Med Sci Sports Exerc.* 1994;26(4):414–419. PMID: 8201895 doi: 10.1249/00005768-199404000-00003
15. Dewi RC, Rimawati N, Purbodjati P. Body mass index, physical activity, and physical fitness of adolescence. *J Public Health Res.* 2021;10(2):2230. PMID: 33855415 doi: 10.4081/jphr.2021.2230
16. Campa F, Toselli S, Mazzilli M, Gobbo LA, Coratella G. Assessment of body composition in athletes: a narrative review of available methods with special reference to quantitative and qualitative bioimpedance analysis. *Nutrients.* 2021;13(5):1620. PMID: 34065984 doi: 10.3390/nu13051620
17. Harmon KG. Lower extremity stress fractures. *Clin J Sport Med.* 2003;13(6):358–364. PMID: 14627867 doi: 10.1097/00042752-200311000-00004
18. Tiwari K. Supplement (mis)use in adolescents. *Curr Opin Pediatr.* 2020;32(4):471–475. PMID: 32520823 doi: 10.1097/MOP.0000000000000912
19. Hampl SE, Hassink SG, Skinner AC, et al. Clinical practice guideline for the evaluation and treatment of children and adolescents with obesity. *Pediatrics.* 2023;151(2):e2022060640. PMID: 36622115 doi: 10.1542/peds.2022-060640

20. Hooper L, Framson C, Donaldson A, et al. The American Academy of Pediatrics guideline for obesity: an adolescent health perspective. *J Adolesc Health.* 2024;75(4):535–537. PMID: 39115469 doi: 10.1016/j.jadohealth.2024.07.006
21. Feltner C, Peat C, Reddy S, et al. Screening for eating disorders in adolescents and adults: an evidence review for the U.S. Preventive Services Task Force. Evidence synthesis No. 212. Agency for Healthcare Research and Quality; 2022. AHRQ publication 21-05284-EF-1. www.ncbi.nlm.nih.gov/books/NBK578988/
22. Hoogenboom BJ, Capulong Z, Teeter M. Examination of the clinical utility of eating disorder and disordered eating screening tools in young athletes: a scoping review. *Int J Sports Phys Ther.* 2025;20(1):1–14. PMID: 39758700 doi: 10.26603/001c.126965
23. US Preventive Services Task Force. Screening for eating disorders in adolescents and adults: US Preventive Services Task Force recommendation statement. *JAMA.* 2022;327(11):1061–1067. PMID: 35289876 doi: 10.1001/jama.2022.1806
24. Davison KK, Earnest MB, Birch LL. Participation in aesthetic sports and girls' weight concerns at ages 5 and 7 years. *Int J Eat Disord.* 2002;31(3):312–317. PMID: 11920993 doi: 10.1002/eat.10043
25. Marques L, Alegria M, Becker AE, et al. Comparative prevalence, correlates of impairment, and service utilization for eating disorders across US ethnic groups: implications for reducing ethnic disparities in health care access for eating disorders. *Int J Eat Disord.* 2011;44(5):412–420. PMID: 20665700 doi: 10.1002/eat.20787PubMedGoogle
26. Diemer EW, Grant JD, Munn-Chernoff MA, Patterson DA, Duncan AE. Gender identity, sexual orientation, and eating-related pathology in a national sample of college students. *J Adolesc Health.* 2015;57(2):144–149. PMID: 25937471 doi: 10.1016/j.jadohealth.2015.03.003
27. Mountjoy M, Sundgot-Borgen JK, Burke LM, et al. IOC consensus statement on relative energy deficiency in sport (RED-S): 2018 update. *Br J Sports Med.* 2018;52(11):687–697. PMID: 29773536
28. Scheid JL, Basile S, West SL. Low energy availability risk is associated with anxiety in female collegiate athletes. *Sports (Basel).* 2024;12(10):269. PMID: 39453235 doi: 10.3390/sports12100269
29. De Souza MJ, Williams NI. Physiological aspects and clinical sequelae of energy deficiency and hypoestrogenism in exercising women. *Hum Reprod Update.* 2004;10(5):433–448. PMID: 15231760 doi: 10.1093/humupd/dmh033
30. Loucks AB, Verdun M, Heath EM. Low energy availability, not stress of exercise, alters LH pulsatility in exercising women. *J Appl Physiol.* 1998;84(1):37–46. PMID: 9451615 doi: 10.1152/jappl.1998.84.1.37
31. Windauer U, Lennerts W, Talbot P, Touyz SW, Beumont PJ. How well are 'cured' anorexia nervosa patients? An investigation of 16 weight-recovered anorexic patients. *Br J Psychiatry.* 1993;163(2):195–200. PMID: 8075911 doi: 10.1192/bjp.163.2.195
32. Dominguez J, Goodman L, Sen Gupta S, et al. Treatment of anorexia nervosa is associated with increases in bone mineral density, and recovery is a biphasic process involving both nutrition and return of menses. *Am J Clin Nutr.* 2007;86(1):92–99. PMID: 17616767 doi: 10.1093/ajcn/86.1.92
33. Warren MP, Brooks-Gunn J, Fox RP, Holderness CC, Hyle EP, Hamilton WG. Osteopenia in exercise-associated amenorrhea using ballet dancers as a model: a longitudinal study. *J Clin Endocrinol Metab.* 2002;87(7):3162–3168. PMID: 12107218 doi: 10.1210/jcem.87.7.8637
34. Zanker CL, Cooke CB, Truscott JG, Oldroyd B, Jacobs HS. Annual changes of bone density over 12 years in an amenorrheic athlete. *Med Sci Sports Exerc.* 2004;36(1):137–142. PMID: 14707779 doi: 10.1249/01.MSS.0000106186.68674.2C
35. Mountjoy M, Ackerman KE, Bailey DM, et al. 2023 International Olympic Committee's (IOC) consensus statement on Relative Energy Deficiency in Sport (REDs). *Br J Sports Med.* 2023;57(17):1073–1097. PMID: 37752011. Published correction appears in *Br J Sports Med.* 2024;58(3):e4. doi: 10.1136/bjsports-2023-106994corr1
36. De Souza MJ, Nattiv A, Joy E, et al; Expert Panel. 2014 Female Athlete Triad Coalition consensus statement on treatment and return to play of the female athlete triad: 1st international conference held in San Francisco, California, May 2012 and 2nd international conference held in Indianapolis, Indiana, May 2013. *Br J Sports Med.* 2014;48(4):289–309. PMID: 24463911 doi: 10.1136/bjsports-2013-093218
37. Nattiv A, De Souza MJ, Koltun KJ, et al. The Male Athlete Triad—a consensus statement from the Female and Male Athlete Triad Coalition Part 1: definition and scientific basis. *Clin J Sport Med.* 2021;31(4):335–348. PMID: 34091537 doi: 10.1097/JSM.0000000000000946
38. Fredericson M, Kussman A, Misra M, et al. The Male Athlete Triad—a consensus statement from the Female and Male Athlete Triad Coalition Part II: diagnosis, treatment, and return-to-play. *Clin J Sport Med.* 2021;31(4):349–366. PMID: 34091538 doi: 10.1097/JSM.0000000000000948

39. Golden NH, Abrams SA; American Academy of Pediatrics Committee on Nutrition. Optimizing bone health in children and adolescents. *Pediatrics.* 2014;134(4):e1229–e1243. PMID: 25266429 doi: 10.1542/peds.2014-2173
40. Nagata JM, Golden NH, Peebles R, et al. Assessment of sex differences in bone deficits among adolescents with anorexia nervosa. *Int J Eat Disord.* 2017;50(4):352–358. PMID: 27611361 doi: 10.1002/eat.22626
41. Weiss Kelly AK, Hecht S, et al; American Academy of Pediatrics Council on Sports Medicine and Fitness. The female athlete triad. *Pediatrics.* 2016;138(2):e20160922. PMID: 27432852
42. American Academy of Family Physicians, American Academy of Orthopaedic Surgeons, American College of Sports Medicine, American Medical Society for Sports Medicine, American Orthopaedic Society for Sports Medicine, American Osteopathic Academy of Sports Medicine. Female athlete issues for the team physician: a consensus statement—2017 update. *Med Sci Sports Exerc.* 2018;50(5):1113–1122. PMID: 29652732 doi: 10.1249/MSS.0000000000001603
43. Sweeney E, Brna M, Howell D, Armento A, Gilmer G, Franklin C. Screening for Relative Energy Deficiency in Sport and Female Athlete Triad: a survey of pediatric sports medicine professionals. *J Women Sports Med.* 2024;4(1):30–38. doi: 10.53646/vxe7wx77
44. Joy E, De Souza MJ, Nattiv A, et al. 2014 female athlete triad coalition consensus statement on treatment and return to play of the female athlete triad. *Curr Sports Med Rep.* 2014;13(4):219–232. PMID: 25014387 doi: 10.1249/JSR.0000000000000077
45. Melin A, Tornberg AB, Skouby S, et al. The LEAF questionnaire: a screening tool for the identification of female athletes at risk for the female athlete triad. *Br J Sports Med.* 2014;48(7):540–545. PMID: 24563388 doi: 10.1136/bjsports-2013-093240
46. Lundy B, Torstveit MK, Stenqvist TB, et al. Screening for low energy availability in male athletes: attempted validation of LEAM-Q. *Nutrients.* 2022;14(9):1873. PMID: 35565840 doi: 10.3390/nu14091873
47. Witkos J, Błażejewski G, Gierach M. The Low Energy Availability in Females Questionnaire (LEAF-Q) as a useful tool to identify female triathletes at risk for menstrual disorders related to low energy availability. *Nutrients.* 2023;15(3):650. PMID: 36771357 doi: 10.3390/nu15030650
48. Sim A, Burns SF. Review: questionnaires as measures for low energy availability (LEA) and relative energy deficiency in sport (RED-S) in athletes. *J Eat Disord.* 2021;9(1):41. PMID: 33789771 doi: 10.1186/s40337-021-00396-7
49. Kennedy SF, Kovan J, Werner E, Mancine R, Gusfa D, Kleiman H. Initial validation of a screening tool for disordered eating in adolescent athletes. *J Eat Disord.* 2021;9(1):21. PMID: 33588900 doi: 10.1186/s40337-020-00364-7
50. Cooper Z, Fairburn C. The Eating Disorder Examination: a semi-structured interview for the assessment of the specific psychopathology of eating disorders. *Int J Eat Disord.* 1987;6(1):1–8. doi: 10.1002/1098-108X(198701)6:1<1:AID-EAT2260060102>3.0.CO;2-9
51. Garner DM, Olmsted MP, Bohr Y, Garfinkel PE. The eating attitudes test: psychometric features and clinical correlates. *Psychol Med.* 1982;12(4):871–878. PMID: 6961471 doi: 10.1017/S0033291700049163
52. Cotton MA, Ball C, Robinson P. Four simple questions can help screen for eating disorders. *J Gen Intern Med.* 2003;18(1):53–56. PMID: 12534764 doi: 10.1046/j.1525-1497.2003.20374.x
53. Foley Davelaar CM, Ostrom M, Schulz J, Trane K, Wolkin A, Granger J. Validation of an age-appropriate screening tool for female athlete triad and relative energy deficiency in sport in young athletes. *Cureus.* 2020;12(6):e8579. PMID: 32670715 doi: 10.7759/cureus.8579
54. McDowall JA. Supplement use by young athletes. *J Sports Sci Med.* 2007;6(3):337–342. PMID: 24149420
55. Barretto JR, Gouveia MADC, Alves C. Use of dietary supplements by children and adolescents. *J Pediatr (Rio J).* 2024;100(suppl 1):S31–S39. PMID: 38529679 doi: 10.1016/j.jped.2023.09.008
56. Stierman B, Mishra S, Gahche JJ, Potischman N, Hales CM. Dietary supplement use in children and adolescents aged ≤19 years—United States, 2017-2018. *MMWR Morb Mortal Wkly Rep.* 2020;69(43):1557–1562. PMID: 33119556 doi: 10.15585/mmwr.mm6943a1
57. Dietary reference intakes for calcium and vitamin D. *Pediatrics.* 2012;130(5):e1424. doi: 10.1542/peds.2012-2590
58. Vitamin D. Fact sheet for health professionals. National Institutes of Health, Office of Dietary Supplements. Updated June 27, 2025. Accessed December 21, 2025. https://ods.od.nih.gov/factsheets/VitaminD-HealthProfessional
59. Tenforde AS, Sayres LC, Sainani KL, Fredericson M. Evaluating the relationship of calcium and vitamin D in the prevention of stress fracture injuries in the young athlete: a review of the literature. *PM R.* 2010;2(10):945–949. PMID: 20970764 doi: 10.1016/j.pmrj.2010.05.006

60. Martínez-Sanz JM, Sospedra I, Ortiz CM, Baladía E, Gil-Izquierdo A, Ortiz-Moncada R. Intended or unintended doping? A review of the presence of doping substances in dietary supplements used in sports. *Nutrients.* 2017;9(10):1093. PMID: 28976928 doi: 10.3390/nu9101093
61. Maughan RJ, Burke LM, Dvorak J, et al. IOC consensus statement: dietary supplements and the high-performance athlete. *Int J Sport Nutr Exerc Metab.* 2018;28(2):104–125. PMID: 29589768 doi: 10.1123/ijsnem.2018-0020
62. Jagim AR, Stecker RA, Harty PS, Erickson JL, Kerksick CM. Safety of creatine supplementation in active adolescents and youth: a brief review. *Front Nutr.* 2018;5:115. PMID: 30547033 doi: 10.3389/fnut.2018.00115
63. Bell A, Dorsch KD, McCreary DR, Hovey R. A look at nutritional supplement use in adolescents. *J Adolesc Health.* 2004;34(6):508–516. PMID: 15145408 doi: 10.1016/j.jadohealth.2003.07.024
64. Maughan R, Shirreffs S. Exercise in the heat: challenges and opportunities. *J Sports Sci.* 2004;22(10):917–927. PMID: 15768725 doi: 10.1080/02640410400005909
65. Metzl JD, Small E, Levine SR, Gershel JC. Creatine use among young athletes. *Pediatrics.* 2001;108(2):421–425. PMID: 11483809 doi: 10.1542/peds.108.2.421
66. Schneider MB, Benjamin HJ; American Academy of Pediatrics Committee on Nutrition and the Council on Sports Medicine and Fitness. Sports drinks and energy drinks for children and adolescents: are they appropriate? *Pediatrics.* 2011;127(6):1182–1189. PMID: 21624882 doi: 10.1542/peds.2011-0965
67. Bartelt K, Higgs E, Kazaglis L, Deckert J. Caffeine-related ED visits, although uncommon, doubled for middle school and high school aged children since 2017. Epic Research. November 5, 2024. Accessed March 2, 2025. https://epicresearch.org/articles/caffeine-related-ed-visits-although-uncommon-doubled-for-middle-school-and-high-school-aged-children-since-2017
68. Popkin BM, D'Anci KE, Rosenberg IH. Water, hydration, and health. *Nutr Rev.* 2010;68(8):439–458. PMID: 20646222 doi: 10.1111/j.1753-4887.2010.00304.x
69. Suppiah HT, Ng EL, Wee J, et al. Hydration status and fluid replacement strategies of high-performance adolescent athletes: an application of machine learning to distinguish hydration characteristics. *Nutrients.* 2021;13(11):4073. PMID: 34836328 doi: 10.3390/nu13114073
70. Healthy Eating Research. Accessed June 2025. https://healthyeatingresearch.org/
71. American Academy of Pediatrics. Adolescent nutrition. In: Greer FR, Abrams SA, eds. *Pediatric Nutrition.* 9th ed. American Academy of Pediatrics; 2025:259–276. https://doi.org/10.1542/9781610027700-ch8
72. National Academies of Sciences, Engineering, and Medicine; Health and Medicine Division; Food and Nutrition Board; Committee on the Dietary Reference Intakes for Energy. *Dietary Reference Intakes for Energy.* National Academies Press; 2023

J: Gynecologic Considerations

HISTORY FORM QUESTIONS

1. *How old were you when you had your first menstrual period?*
2. *When was your most recent menstrual period?*
3. *How many periods have you had in the past 12 months?*

SECONDARY QUESTIONS

- Are you presently taking any hormones or hormone-blocking medications (pill or patch) or do you have an internal or implantable hormone device (estrogen-containing device, progesterone-containing device, or birth control pills)?
- Do you frequently miss school or practices because of menstrual cramps or heavy menstrual bleeding?

KEY POINTS

- Menstrual cramping—or dysmenorrhea—and heavy menstrual bleeding are common problems among adolescents, and either can affect school attendance and sports performance. The preparticipation evaluation (PPE) is an ideal opportunity to provide relevant information on treatment options.
- Low energy availability, disordered eating, and eating disorders are associated with menstrual dysfunction.
- Low energy availability, disordered eating, and eating disorders may be associated with amenorrhea and oligomenorrhea, persistent or recurrent injury, or bone stress injuries (stress reaction and stress fracture).
- Use of hormonal contraception may mask menstrual dysfunction associated with low energy availability.
- Anemia is often associated with heavy or frequent menstrual cycles.

INTRODUCTION

Menstrual history is important because menstrual cycle abnormalities may be a sign of low energy availability, intentional or unintentional suppression of the hypothalamic-pituitary-adrenal axis, pregnancy, or other gynecologic or medical conditions. A detailed menstrual history is important if answers to any of the History Form questions indicate a possible menstrual problem. Amenorrhea, both primary and secondary, needs to be evaluated with additional history. Primary amenorrhea is defined as the absence of menarche by age 15 years.[1] In addition, individuals who lack physical changes associated with the onset of puberty by age 13 years or have a delay in the progression of pubertal development, including menarche within 5 years of initial breast development, need *further* endocrine and gynecologic evaluations.[1] Secondary amenorrhea refers to missing at least 3 consecutive menstrual periods in a previously menstruating female. Pregnancy is a common cause that is often overlooked in physically active individuals and athletes and should be considered as part of the initial evaluation. Oligomenorrhea is defined as having intervals between menstrual cycles that are between 35 days and 90 days once regular menses have been established.

Menstrual dysfunction is 2 to 3 times more common in athletes than in nonathletes, and 10% to 15% of female athletes have amenorrhea or oligomenorrhea.[2] Amenorrhea occurs more frequently in individuals participating in sports emphasizing leanness, such as running, gymnastics, cheerleading, dance, and figure skating.[3] Athletes with amenorrhea or oligomenorrhea need to undergo a thorough evaluation for causes of menstrual disturbance (eg, pregnancy, polycystic ovary syndrome, thyroid disease) before attributing amenorrhea or oligomenorrhea to low energy availability. Consequences of low energy availability–associated amenorrhea or oligomenorrhea include inadequate bone mineralization, bone stress injuries, changes in lipid profiles, and disturbances of vascular dilation. Amenorrheic and oligomenorrheic individuals also need to have their nutritional status assessed, as menstrual dysfunction is often related to low energy availability.

Menstrual dysfunction is 2 to 3 times more common in athletes than in nonathletes, and 10% to 15% of female athletes have amenorrhea or oligomenorrhea.

Low energy availability is often responsible for the development of oligomenorrhea or amenorrhea, and osteopenia or osteoporosis.[4,5] Low energy availability may occur as a result of intentional dietary restriction (as is seen in athletes who practice disordered eating or have eating disorders), unintentional underfueling, excessive exercise, or maintaining a body weight that is too low for height and age. Modifying diet, exercise, body weight, and/or body composition is necessary to increase energy availability, restore regular menstruation, and optimize bone mineral density (BMD).[6–8] See Chapter 5I for more information about screening for eating disorders and disordered eating and determining medical eligibility for these individuals.

Further diagnostic testing can be requested following the PPE. Laboratory testing may detect electrolyte disturbances and metabolic disruption that result from eating disorders. Self-induced vomiting, diuretic use, and laxative use can result in hypokalemia. Excessive water intake may cause hyponatremia. Elevated liver enzyme and low triiodothyronine (free) levels may be observed in athletes who have malnutrition caused by dietary caloric restriction. Functional hypothalamic amenorrhea is a diagnosis of exclusion but can result in laboratory findings of low or normal levels of luteinizing hormone, follicle-stimulating hormone, and serum estradiol in individuals who are not taking any forms of exogenous hormones.[9] Additional testing includes measuring prolactin level and thyroid-stimulating hormone level to screen for other causes of amenorrhea or oligomenorrhea.

Hypermenorrhea, menorrhagia, and polymenorrhea alone or together may lead to iron deficiency from excessive blood loss, resulting in anemia, fatigue, and poor athletic performance. Hypermenorrhea is excessive menstruation flow and duration at regular cycle intervals. Polymenorrhea is menstrual cycles occurring at greater than normal frequency. If any of these conditions is present, an evaluation is recommended for possible anemia and to determine the underlying cause. This evaluation includes asking about any previous gynecologic assessments; examining for physical signs of anemia such as pale conjunctiva, pale mucous membranes, rapid pulse, or high-output flow murmur, or signs of pregnancy; and advising the individual to follow up for further evaluation.

Oral contraceptives, and other forms of hormonal birth control (eg, injectable medroxyprogesterone acetate, progestin-containing intrauterine devices [IUDs], implantable progesterone), may be overlooked by athletes when answering the medication question on the medical History Form. Hormone-based medications may be prescribed for contraception and/or used for managing irregular menstrual cycles, menorrhagia, or dysmenorrhea, as well as for nonmenstrual-related conditions such as acne. However, the use of hormonal contraception can mask the loss of menstruation as a sign of low energy availability. It is important to educate athletes that the bleeding occurring while on the week of placebo oral contraceptive pills is only withdrawal bleeding and is not the same as a naturally occurring menstrual period. Individuals taking oral contraceptives may continue to have a "monthly" blood flow caused by hormone manipulation despite having low energy availability. Individuals using progesterone-only medications such as injectable medroxyprogesterone acetate injections, etonogestrel implant rods, or progesterone-containing IUDs often experience cessation of menstrual periods. In highly active females, it can be difficult to discern whether the loss of menstruation is caused by hormonal medications or low energy availability.

Some forms of hormone replacement therapy can have a positive impact on bone health. Transdermal forms of estrogen have been shown to improve BMD in adolescents with anorexia nervosa (especially when combined with improvements in dietary energy intake).[10] Combined oral contraceptive pills (containing both estrogen and progesterone) have a mixed effect on BMD.[10] Oral estrogen undergoes first-pass metabolism in the liver, resulting in a downregulation of insulin-like growth factor 1, especially in the setting of low energy availability. The consequence of this is a negative impact on BMD.[10] Alternatively, in energy-replete females, use of combined oral contraceptive pills is *not* associated with a decrease in BMD. It is also important to note that progestin-only birth control methods are associated with lower BMD in both teenagers and adults.[11] Following cessation of progestin-only contraception, BMD typically increases back to baseline; however, for weight-bearing athletes, even temporary decreases in BMD may increase the likelihood of bone stress injuries.

PHYSICAL EXAMINATION

Breast, Pelvic, and Genitourinary Examinations

Breast, pelvic, and genitourinary examinations are not routinely part of a PPE. If a pelvic or breast examination is necessary to evaluate symptoms from the individual's medical history or findings on the general physical examination, it is best to schedule it for a separate time. Prior to any gynecologic examination taking place, obtain informed consent from the individual as well as from a parent or legal guardian for any patient younger than 18 years. A chaperone is recommended.[12]

DETERMINING MEDICAL ELIGIBILITY

Gynecologic Disorders and Pregnancy

Because ovarian injury is highly unlikely during any form of athletic participation, there are no restrictions for individuals with only 1 ovary. Anyone with an identified menstrual disorder needs an evaluation by a physician and needs to be screened for common causes such as polycystic ovarian syndrome and hypothalamic suppression. Athletes with oligomenorrhea or amenorrhea usually may be allowed to participate while undergoing further evaluation, but it is important to explain to them that menstrual irregularities and low BMD increase fracture risk,[3] and they should report any symptoms that develop or worsen during training.

Pregnancy is the most common cause of amenorrhea. If pregnancy is confirmed, medical eligibility should be determined by the clinician who is following the pregnancy. For athletes with an identified team physician who is ultimately responsible for clearance to participate, the team physician should be involved in the eligibility determination. Most athletes with normal pregnancies can safely continue to participate, with progressive modifications as the pregnancy develops.[13]

REFERENCES

1. Klein DA, Poth MA. Amenorrhea: an approach to diagnosis and management. *Am Fam Physician.* 2013;87(11):781–788. PMID: 23939500
2. Female athlete issues for the team physician: a consensus statement—2017 update. *Med Sci Sports Exerc.* 2018;50(5):1113–1122. PMID: 29652732 doi:10.1249/MSS.0000000000001603
3. Nattiv A, Loucks AB, Manore MM, Sanborn CF; American College of Sports Medicine. American College of Sports Medicine position stand. The female athlete triad. *Med Sci Sports Exerc.* 2007;39(10):1867–1882. PMID: 17909417
4. Loucks AB, Verdun M, Heath EM. Low energy availability, not stress of exercise, alters LH pulsatility in exercising women. *J Appl Physiol.* 1998;84(1):37–46. PMID: 9451615 doi:10.1152/jappl.1998.84.1.37
5. De Souza MJ, Williams NI. Physiological aspects and clinical sequelae of energy deficiency and hypoestrogenism in exercising women. *Hum Reprod Update.* 2004;10(5):433–448. PMID: 15231760 doi:10.1093/humupd/dmh033
6. Dominguez J, Goodman L, Sen Gupta S, et al. Treatment of anorexia nervosa is associated with increases in bone mineral density, and recovery is a biphasic process involving both nutrition and return of menses. *Am J Clin Nutr.* 2007;86(1):92–99. PMID: 17616767 doi:10.1093/ajcn/86.1.92
7. Warren MP, Brooks-Gunn J, Fox RP, Holderness CC, Hyle EP, Hamilton WG. Osteopenia in exercise-associated amenorrhea using ballet dancers as a model: a longitudinal study. *J Clin Endocrinol Metab.*

2002;87(7):3162–3168. PMID: 12107218 doi:10.1210/jcem.87.7.8637

8. Zanker CL, Cooke CB, Truscott JG, Oldroyd B, Jacobs HS. Annual changes of bone density over 12 years in an amenorrheic athlete. *Med Sci Sports Exerc.* 2004;36(1):137–142. PMID: 14707779 doi:10.1249/01.MSS.0000106186.68674.2C
9. Meczekalski B, Katulski K, Czyzyk A, Podfigurna-Stopa A, Maciejewska-Jeske M. Functional hypothalamic amenorrhea and its influence on women's health. *J Endocrinol Invest.* 2014;37(11):1049–1056. PMID: 25201001 doi:10.1007/s40618-014-0169-3
10. Misra M, Katzman D, Miller KK, et al. Physiologic estrogen replacement increases bone density in adolescent girls with anorexia nervosa. *J Bone Miner Res.* 2011;26(10):2430–2438. PMID: 21698665 doi:10.1002/jbmr.447
11. World Health Organization. WHO statement on hormonal contraception and bone health. September 2, 2005. Accessed March 18, 2026. https://www.who.int/publications/i/item/WER8035-302-304
12. Berhane A, Hackell JM, Wallace S; Committee on Practice and Ambulatory Medicine; Committee on Adolescence. Use of chaperones for the pediatric and adolescent encounter: policy statement. *Pediatrics.* 2025;155(6):e2025071810. PMID: 40383537 doi:10.1542/peds.2025-071810
13. Hogshead-Makar N, Sorensen EA. *Pregnant and Parenting Student-Athletes: Resources and Model Policies.* National Collegiate Athletic Association; 2008. Accessed December 22, 2025. https://www.uncp.edu/_files/NCAA%20Pregnant%20and%20Parenting%20Students%20Resources%20and%20Model%20Policies.pdf

CHAPTER 6

Mental Health

HISTORY FORM QUESTION

1. *List past and current medical conditions (including mental health disorders such as attention-deficit/hyperactivity disorder [ADHD], anxiety, and depression).*

Patient Health Questionnaire Version 4 (PHQ-4)[1–3]

Over the last 2 weeks, how often have you been bothered by any of the following problems?

1. Feeling nervous, anxious, or on edge. Responses: Not at all (0), Several days (1), More than half the days (2), Nearly every day (3).
2. Not being able to stop or control worrying. Responses: Not at all (0), Several days (1), More than half the days (2), Nearly every day (3).
3. Little interest or pleasure in doing things. Responses: Not at all (0), Several days (1), More than half the days (2), Nearly every day (3).
4. Feeling down, depressed, or hopeless. Responses: Not at all (0), Several days (1), More than half the days (2), Nearly every day (3).

The total score is determined by adding together the scores for each of the 4 items. Psychological distress is rated as normal (0–2), mild (3–5), moderate (6–8), and severe (9–12).

A sum of ≥ 3 is considered positive on either subscale (questions 1 and 2 for anxiety or questions 3 and 4 for depression) for screening purposes.

Suicide Screen (PHQ-9: question No. 9 addressing suicide)[4]

1. Over the past 2 weeks, have you had thoughts that you would be better off dead, or thoughts of hurting yourself in some way? Responses: Not at all (0), Several days (1), More than half the days (2), Nearly every day (3).

Any response other than 0 requires further investigation.

SECONDARY QUESTIONS

- Screening for alcohol use disorder

For adults 21 years and older, use the NIAAA Single Alcohol Screening Question (SASQ)[5,6]:

— How many times in the past year have you had 'X' or more drinks in a day? X = 4 for women, X = 5 for men. *A response of > 1 time in past year is positive.*

For individuals < 21 years of age, CRAFFT (Box 6-1) is a 6-question tool endorsed by the American Academy of Pediatrics (AAP) assessing alcohol and drug use in adolescents, with the questions pertaining to the focus words: *C*ar, *R*elax, *A*lone, *F*orget, *F*amily/Friends, and *T*rouble (https://crafft.org).

Box 6-1. CRAFFT

- **C** Have you ever ridden in a CAR driven by someone (including yourself) who was "high" or had been using alcohol or drugs?
- **R** Do you ever use alcohol or drugs to RELAX, feel better about yourself, or fit in?
- **A** Do you ever use alcohol or drugs while you are by yourself, or ALONE?
- **F** Do you ever FORGET things you did while using alcohol or drugs?
- **F** Do your FAMILY or FRIENDS ever tell you that you should cut down on your drinking or drug use?
- **T** Have you ever gotten into TROUBLE while you were using alcohol or drugs?

NOTICE TO CLINIC STAFF AND MEDICAL RECORDS:

The information on this page is protected by special federal confidentiality rules (42 CFR Part 2), which prohibit disclosure of this information unless authorized by specific written consent.

crafft@childrens.harvard.edu

www.crafft.org

For more information and versions in other languages, see www.crafft.org.

Two or more YES answers suggest a serious problem, and appropriate referrals should be made.

- Screening for abuse and sexual violence (see Chapter 9)
  - —Has anyone ever touched you in a way or pressured you to engage in any physical or sexual acts that made you uncomfortable?
  - —Have you ever felt bullied, harassed, threatened, neglected, or placed into situations in sport in which your health may have been at risk?

Mental Health Conditions Covered in This Chapter

- Depression
- Suicide
- Overtraining syndrome
- Anxiety disorders
- Attention-deficit/hyperactivity disorder
- Obsessive-compulsive disorder
- Posttraumatic stress disorder
- Substance use and addiction
- Bipolar and psychotic disorders
- Sleep
- Connections between mental health and abuse

KEY POINTS

- Mental health is increasingly recognized as a major health issue in the adolescent and young adult years.
- Screening for mental health disorders and addressing mental health issues is an important component of the preparticipation evaluation (PPE).
- US Preventive Services Task Force (USPSTF) recommends screening 12- to 18-year-olds for depression.
- USPSTF recommends screening all individuals 18 years and older for unhealthy drug use, including cannabis, in primary care settings, but there is insufficient evidence to screen adolescents. However, the AAP recommends screening adolescents with the CRAFFT tool.
- USPSTF recommends screening 8- to 18-year-olds for anxiety.
- USPSTF states that there is insufficient evidence on harms and benefits to screen for suicide and eating disorders in children and adolescents. The AAP recommends screening for suicide.
- Several screening and diagnostic tools to help providers identify mental health disorders have been validated in many groups including children. However, most are not currently validated specifically for athletes other than those who are elite athletes.
- To effectively screen for mental health issues, it is recommended that providers have resources available and/or an established emergency action plan for any acute or subacute mental health crisis.

To effectively screen for mental health issues, it is recommended that providers have resources available and/or an established emergency action plan for any acute or subacute mental health crisis.

Note, the PHQ-4 is a simple, easily administered screening tool for depression and anxiety. It is not exhaustive or validated in all age groups. The question on suicide was added to the 6th edition of *PPE: Preparticipation Evaluation* because it is the most urgent mental health issue to screen for in order to prevent the most catastrophic outcomes from depression and anxiety. Many mental health disorders exist in young people and athletic populations. Additional screening tools for these disorders are presented in this chapter (See Table 6-1).

A secondary question, using either the SASQ (Single Alcohol Screening Question) or CRAFFT to screen for alcohol use disorder, may be helpful in the young adult and adolescent populations, respectively. SASQ is a single question endorsed by the National Institute on Alcohol Abuse and Alcoholism.[5,6] CRAFFT is a 6-question tool endorsed by the AAP. Questions assessing for abuse are also included in the mental health assessment given the high rates of coexistence. There is significant overlap between mental health and substance use disorders, commonly alcohol, tetrahydrocannabinol (THC), and vaping. However, much of it may be beyond the scope of the PPE. The USPSTF recommends screening all adults 18 years and older for unhealthy drug use, including cannabis, in primary care settings, but there is insufficient evidence to screen adolescents. Screening for substance use disorders—including THC, vaping, and other less commonly used substances in teens—using validated self-report questionnaires such as the CRAFFT may be reasonable in the appropriate clinical context during the PPE. See Chapter 9 on Preventing and Addressing Abuse and Sexual Violence.

Table 6-1. Summary of Mental Health Conditions and Some Recommendations on Screening

Condition	Screening Tools	Comments
General athlete strain (which can lead to mental health disorders)	• APSQ (Athlete Psychological Strain Questionnaire)	• Designed for elite athletes • Looks for psychological strain • Intended to lead to other, more specific testing • Endorsed by IOC
Mental health disorders overall	• SMHAT-1 (Sport Mental Health Assessment Tool-1–clinical screening) • SMHRT-1 (Sport Mental Health Recognition Tool-1-nonclinician, used to recognize mental health problems)	• Recommended for use by NCAA and IOC
Depression	• PHQ-2 (Patient Health Questionnaire), PHQ-9, PHQ-A • CES-D (Centers for Epidemiological Studies Depression Scale)	• (PHQ-A for adolescents) • All validated for youth • Available in multiple languages
Suicide	• ASQ (Ask Suicide Questions) • C-SSRS (Columbia-Suicide Severity Rating Scale)	• ASQ is a tool validated for youth to identify elevated risk of suicide, AAP recommended[7] • C-SSRS helps identify risk and severity of suicide, AAP recommended[7]
Overtraining syndrome (OTS)	• REST-Q (Recovery Stress Questionnaire for Athletes) • POMS (Profile of Mood State)	• There is no validated tool for OTS • REST-Q measures frequency of current stress[8] • POMS provides insights into a person's mood state[9]
Anxiety	• GAD-7 (Generalized Anxiety Disorder-7 item) • SCARED (Screen for Child Anxiety Related Disorders) • SPIN-17b (Social Phobia Inventory)	• GAD-7 is validated for general anxiety in primary care[10] • SCARED is validated for youth to screen for anxiety symptoms[10] • SPIN-17b is good for screening for social phobias[11]
Obsessive compulsive disorder	• CY-BOCS (Children's Yale-Brown Obsessive Compulsive Scale) • CBCL-OCS (Child Behavior Checklist-OCD subscale)	• AAP noted CY-BOCS to be more effective in specialized mental health offices rather than in primary care[12] • CBCL-OCS shows promise as an introductory screening tool leading to further workup[12]

Table 6-1. Summary of Mental Health Conditions and Some Recommendations on Screening (*continued*)

Condition	Screening Tools	Comments
Performance anxiety	—	• No screening tests for athletes
Posttraumatic stress disorder (PTSD)	• PC-PTSD (Primary Care-PTSD Screen) • CAPS-CA5 (Clinician Administered PTSD Scale-Child/Adolescent)	• PC-PTSD is a 4-question screen for adults[13] • CAPS-CA5, considered "gold standard," but is clinician administered[14]
Addictions, substance use and misuse	• SASQ (Single Alcohol Screening Question) • SBIRT (Screening, Brief Intervention, and Referral to Treatment) (includes the CRAFFT tool)	• Single question recommended by National Institute on Alcohol Abuse and Alcoholism for alcohol use disorder[5,6] • SBIRT recommended by AAP for routine visits to screen for substance use[15]
Attention-deficit/hyperactivity disorder (ADHD)	• ADHD Rating Scale-5 • Vanderbilt rating scale (VADRS)	• ADHD Rating Scale-5 used by clinicians is a parent questionnaire[16] • VADRS parent and teacher forms for screening[17]
Bipolar, psychotic	• MDQ (Mood Disorder Questionnaire)	• Clinical use, brief survey
Interpersonal violence	• PVS (Partner Violence Screen) • WAST (Woman Abuse Screening Tool)	• Both tests USPSTF recommended for screening[18] • PVS: 3 questions • WAST: starts with 2 questions; if score above a value, 6 more questions
Sleep	• ASSQ (Athlete Sleep Screening Questionnaire • ASBQ (Athlete Sleep Behavior Questionnaire) • STOP-Bang	• ASSQ and ASBQ recommended by NCAA and IOC • ASSQ is a clinical tool to assess sleep and daytime dysfunction[19,20] • ASBQ is designed to detect the impact of sleep quality, helps guide sleep hygiene recommendations[21] • STOP-Bang for sleep apnea

Abbreviations: AAP, American Academy of Pediatrics; IOC, International Olympic Committee; NCAA, National Collegiate Athletic Association; USPSTF, US Preventive Services Task Force.

INTRODUCTION

The intent of this chapter is to increase awareness of mental health conditions encountered in those who participate in sport by briefly describing the most important mental health conditions encountered. Key resources are provided for more in-depth screening as needed.

Awareness of mental health issues in elite athletes, recreational athletes, and active children and adolescents has increased in recent years. Since publication of the last edition of this book, 3 position statements have been published on mental health concerns in athletes by the International Olympic Committee (IOC), American Medical Society for Sports Medicine (AMSSM), and Canadian Centre for Mental Health and Sport.[22–24] The National Collegiate Athletic Association (NCAA) also published the *Mental Health Best Practices*.[25] Studies report that rates of mental health issues are similar for athletes and their nonathletic colleagues in these age groups.

The goals of this chapter are to (1) call attention to mental health issues, (2) encourage providers to look for ways to identify mental health issues, and (3) facilitate connecting individuals to helpful resources. To achieve these goals, the most common mental health issues are summarized.

The team physician, as well as the primary care provider, may be best able to advocate for the wellness of the individual and direct appropriate care. Although recent attention on mental health issues has helped to alleviate the historical stigma, it nonetheless persists in certain contexts and may cause athletes to avoid seeking help. Perceived barriers to pursuing mental health services include stigma about mental health, negative past experiences with seeking treatment, a sense of toughness, and the athlete's busy schedule.[26] Poor mental health literacy has also been a reported barrier. This can include a lack of prevention strategies and awareness of symptoms and warning signs, not knowing how to seek help, lack of available resources, and lower socioeconomic means.[27]

Differences exist in mental health prevalence and presenting symptoms across sport, gender, age, and level of competition. Further, mental health disorders may be exacerbated by a time-loss injury or surgery and transitioning out of sport.

Medications for mental health conditions may have a positive and/or negative effect on performance. Health care providers need to be familiar with these medications, their safety profile, as well as approved use by the World Anti-Doping Agency (WADA).

To effectively screen, it is important to have available resources for management of mental health disorders. These include a network of (preferably sports-experienced) mental health clinicians (counselors, psychologists, and psychiatrists) for consultation and referral, and a mental health emergency crisis plan that is in place and rehearsed on a regular basis (see NCAA for more information: https://ncaaorg.s3.amazonaws.com/ssi/mental/SSI_MentalHealthBestPractices.pdf). Finally, encourage open discussion about mental health issues in athletics to encourage a healthier environment for these active individuals.

To implement an effective screen for any mental health condition, several factors are important. First, choose an instrument validated and appropriate for the population to be screened, and take into account the amount of time needed to conduct the screening. It is also important to determine ahead of time what cutoff score will be considered "positive." Additional considerations include the following: How will the person screened be informed of their positive result? What is in place for follow-up testing and evaluation? What are the referral options? Do you have a plan for follow-up if one chooses not to engage at the time of screening? Will the individual need reevaluation? Are they able to attend follow-up sessions? Do they have the means and time allocated? Finally, when screening for a mental health condition, it is important to demonstrate empathy, be engaged with those screened, not rush the screen, and emphasize expectations of confidentiality.

This chapter should be used as a starting point in improving awareness of and screening for mental health disorders in physically active individuals. At a minimum, the PHQ-4 screening tool can be used to briefly and quickly assess anxiety and depression, along with the last question on the PHQ-9 validated instrument, which is used to screen for suicide. Asking about and discussing suicide is beneficial because it introduces a topic that is uncomfortable, typically taboo, and yet if addressed in a forthcoming manner as part of the PPE, it paves the way for potential future conversations and indicates that it is indeed a safe topic to broach. Conversations can improve opportunities to prevent future successful attempts. Similarly, providers are encouraged to address alcohol consumption and alcohol use disorder for potential early intervention. The additional questions on alcohol use disorder in the CRAFFT have a much greater upside than downside. There is ongoing active discussion of the negative effects of alcohol use in adults, including cancer risks, even at the "recommended" levels of use.[28]

More detailed information on screening for mental health disorders is available from these sources: AAP Bright Futures (https://www.aap.org/en/practice-management/bright-futures), *NCAA Mental Health Best Practices* (https://ncaaorg.s3.amazonaws.com/ssi/mental/SSI_MentalHealthBestPractices.pdf), and IOC mental health screening tools (https://pubmed.ncbi.nlm.nih.gov/32948518/).

The IOC has been working to develop tools for mental health screening for elite athletes. The SMHAT-1 (Sport Mental Health Assessment Tool 1–for clinicians) and SMHRT-1 (Sport Mental Health Recognition Tool 1–for nonclinicians) are great starting points. They advocate using a brief screening tool, which uses the Athlete Psychological Strain Questionnaire (APSQ) to identify stressors in an individual; if the results are positive, providers should follow up with 6 disorder-specific screening tools (for generalized anxiety, depression, sleep, alcohol use disorders, substance use disorder, and eating disorder). The next step is a clinical assessment by a sports medicine physician or licensed registered mental health professional.[29,30] The APSQ is a 10-question screen for athlete mental strain of self-regulation, performance, and external coping that uses a 5-point Likert scale. Any score above 17 warrants further evaluation.[29,31–33] While this is a good starting point for an organized approach to mental health screening, the tool was developed for elite athletes older than 16 years. Further, it continues to be tested for validity.[30] Some authors recommend using the ASPQ and all 6 disorder-specific screening tools to improve predictive ability.[30] Another good resource is the NCAA publication *Mental Health Best Practices: Understanding and Supporting Student-Athlete Mental Health*.[25] In addition, position statements from the American Medical Society for Sports Medicine[23] and the IOC[22] were published since the 5th edition of this book.

MOOD DISORDERS (DEPRESSION)

Depression is one of the most frequently encountered mental health conditions in youth activities. Rates of depression over a 5-year period for college athletes and nonathletes were similar at 23.7%,[34] with females at higher risk.[35] The reported prevalence among elite athletes aged 18 to 26 years ranges from 4% to 68%.[36] Data from 2019 showed a nearly doubling rate of 15% of youth aged 0 to 17 years having at least 1 major depressive disorder episode over a 5-year period.[37] Some argue that depression among elite athletes has been historically underreported because of the associated stigma. Athletics entails some unique risks with respect to becoming depressed: time demands on the athlete, performance expectations (intrinsic and extrinsic), identity of being an athlete, and time loss due to injury or surgery. Further, these risk factors may be amplified for the athlete by social media forces and, for college athletes, by name, image, and likeness deals.[23] Other risk factors for depression include positive family history of depression, relationship issues, lack of social or team support, failure to achieve or to remain competitive, concussion, and retirement from sport. At the collegiate level, those participating in individual sports may be at higher risk than those in team sports.[38]

In addition to experiencing common diagnostic symptoms of depressed mood and anhedonia, individuals may experience other symptoms of depression. These include anger, guilt, low self-esteem, concentration or attention problems, feeling of helplessness, irritability, and sleep disturbance. Other symptoms associated with depression include risk-taking behavior, substance misuse or use, prolonged or incomplete recovery from injuries, staleness, or decreased performance.

In addition to experiencing common diagnostic symptoms of depressed mood and anhedonia, individuals may experience other symptoms of depression. These include anger, guilt, low self-esteem, concentration or attention problems, feeling of helplessness, irritability, and sleep disturbance. Other symptoms associated with depression include risk-taking behavior, substance misuse or use, prolonged or incomplete recovery from injuries, staleness, or decreased performance.

Key to recognizing and diminishing associated stigma and treating and managing depression are having a greater sense of awareness, having an open discussion about mental health, and frequently screening for disorders. There are several reliable screening tools for depression with variable characteristics, including the intended age group, language, and time to complete. The USPSTF recommends the PHQ-9 as a good clinical-based test. Other screens are the CES-D (Centers for Epidemiological Studies Depression Scale)[39] and the IOC's SMHAT-1/SMHRT-1 (endorsed by the NCAA), in which the PHQ-9 is embedded.[29] The PHQ-9 is widely available in many languages and is appropriate for individuals 12 years and older, and there is a modified version (PHQ-A) for adolescents (https://www.phqscreeners.com/). The PHQ-9 can be used to help determine the severity of major depression. The sensitivity ranges from 88% to 95% and specificity from 85% to 88%, depending on what cutoff value is used. The PHQ-2 is a short version of the PHQ-9, using 2 questions (No. 3 and No. 4 of the PHQ-4). A score greater than 3 warrants administering the PHQ-9. The sensitivity and specificity of the PHQ-2 ranges from 83% to 88% and 78% to 92%, respectively.[1,2] The CES-D is currently available in multiple languages and consists of 20 questions, and there is a CES-D-10 with 10 questions. The sensitivity and specificity of the CES-D ranges from 71% to 84% and 57% to 60%, respectively, depending on the cutoff value used.

SUICIDE

Suicide may be associated with depression, substance use disorder, risk-taking behavior, bullying, certain anxiety disorders (eg, panic), and posttraumatic stress disorder (PTSD). Anabolic and androgenic steroid use has been associated with increased risk of suicide and aggressive behavior such as assault and murder.[40] Sports participation may have a protective effect against suicide.[41]

Suicide is the second leading cause of death for 10- to 34-year-olds, and is more common in males than in females. Firearms are the most common method for males in this age group, whereas for females in this age group the most common method is suffocation.[42] A 20-year study by the NCAA (2002–2022) reported that 11.6% of student-athlete deaths were from suicide and pointed out that the incidence doubled in the second decade from 7.6% to 15.3%, with rates higher in males than in females. Of note, cross-country athletes had the highest rate of suicide per sport.[43] Suicide, which is associated with major depression, may often occur in response to life events such as time-loss injury, performance expectations (intrinsic and extrinsic), harassment, hazing and bullying, as well as abuse (psychological, physical, and sexual).

In recent years, much attention has been drawn to the identification of risk, prevention, and intervention to prevent suicide. Drum and Denmark[44] identified ways to address this on college campuses by first having a robust clinical intervention to identify and intervene for those at risk and, second, promoting a campus-wide environment to improve coping skills and resilience.[44] The Substance Abuse and Mental Health Services Administration (SAMHSA) Suicide Prevention Resource Center[45] has posited 4 key ways to help prevent suicide: (1) promote social networks and connectedness in schools and on campuses, (2) improve access to mental health services, (3) identify and assist those who may be at risk, and (4) be prepared to respond when a suicide occurs.[45] In the United States, there is a 24/7 suicide crisis lifeline: call 988 (https://afsp.org/).

Drum and Denmark identified ways to address suicide prevention on college campuses by first having a robust clinical intervention to identify and intervene for those at risk and, second, promoting a campus-wide environment to improve coping skills and resilience.

Four key ways to help prevent suicide: (1) promote social networks and connectedness in schools and on campuses, (2) improve access to mental health services, (3) identify and assist those who may be at risk, and (4) be prepared to respond when a suicide occurs. In the United States, there is a 24/7 suicide crisis lifeline: call 988 (https://afsp.org/).

The AAP recommends 2 screening tools for suicide; the ASQ (Ask Suicide Screening Question) is a brief 5-question screening tool (https://www.nimh.nih.gov/research/research-conducted-at-nimh/asq-toolkit-materials). This can be followed by the C-SSRS (Columbia-Suicide Severity Rating Scale) to help identify risk and severity of risk for suicide (https://cssrs.columbia.edu/the-columbia-scale-c-ssrs/about-the-scale/). This tool is validated, progressing to 6 questions based on the initial 2 screening questions. A very important point is to "ask" and "talk about" suicide.

A very important point is to "ask" and "talk about" suicide.

OVERTRAINING SYNDROME

Overtraining syndrome (OTS) is a well-known condition within athletics that results from an accumulation of multifactorial physical and mental stressors leading to a state of underperformance. It results from the imbalance created from excess exertion and inadequate recovery.[46–48] OTS has been characterized as a chronic fatigue that impairs both sporting and nonsporting aspects of life, including a decline in performance and a rise in illness and injury; OTS also negatively affects several body systems.[46,48] OTS represents the far end of a continuum that begins with acute and mild fatigue, unexplained reduced performance, sleep problems, and/or mood changes over the course of a few days identified as functional overreaching (FOR) or over the course of weeks as nonfunctional overreaching (NFOR). If uncorrected, these stressors continue to amass for months to years, resulting in OTS and heterogenous decrements in physiological, immunological, and neuroendocrine function and, secondarily, in psychological function. Incidence may be as high as 65% in elite-level sports; however, recreational youth athletes are also at risk because of unique stressors including academic and schedule considerations[49] (See Box 6-2). Risk factors include endurance and esthetic sports, sports favoring a power-to-weight ratio advantage (eg, cycling, running, and swimming), year-round or multiple sports participation, elite-level sport, poor sleep habits, and high-stress environments.[47,48] These risk factors—alone or in conjunction—tip the balance of health unfavorably toward inadequate recovery. This underrecovery can be further identified as excessive energy expenditure or unintentional/intentional underfueling.[47,50] No validated diagnostic tool exists for OTS; it is a diagnosis of exclusion. Tools such as the Recovery-Stress Questionnaire for Athletes (RESTQ) and Profile of Mood State (POMS) may assist in assessing athlete well-being.[51,52] The time required for restoration to baseline function differentiates the less concerning FOR/NFOR from the much more serious OTS, as individuals with the former typically take less time to return to baseline health.

Burnout is a similar condition often used synonymously with OTS but differs in that it is characterized more as a decrease in enjoyment or motivation, leading to emotional and psychological fatigue. It can result in withdrawal from sport if not addressed.[46]

Recent literature points out commonalities between OTS and relative energy deficiency in sport (RED-S) (see Chapter 51). Similar to OTS, RED-S is the syndrome of impaired physiological and psychological pathways attributed specifically to chronic, problematic low-energy availability, with emerging data underscoring the amplified role that low carbohydrate availability may confer to this pathological pathway. RED-S, too, is a multifactorial process diagnosed via exclusion. Because of similarities in the processes, underfueling needs to be considered with any case in which OTS is being considered, as the more appropriate diagnosis may be RED-S.[47,50] Similarly, there exists a large overlap between OTS and depression. Varying definitions, inconsistent terminology, and related dysregulation pathways further confuse matters. Depression is a less limited, more overarching concept affecting all aspects of life. OTS, on the other hand, is classically applied to the specific realm of sport, with some consequences extending beyond sport. The 2 conditions are often tightly interwoven; thus, it is important to address potential depression when considering a diagnosis of OTS.[52] (See Box 6-3.)

Box 6-2. Signs and Symptoms of Overtraining Syndrome

- Academic decline
- Anorexia
- Bradycardia/tachycardia
- Chronic pain
- Difficulty concentrating/easily distracted
- Fatigue
- Hypertension
- Sleepiness/insomnia/unrestful sleep
- Mental fog
- Mood changes
  - Anhedonia
  - Agitation
  - Anxiety
  - Depression
  - Irritability
- Muscle soreness
- Restlessness
- Sports performance decline
- Weight loss

Box 6-3. Differential Diagnosis of Overtraining Syndrome

- Nutritional deficiencies
  - relative energy deficiency in sport (RED-S)
  - Eating disorders/disordered eating
  - Unbalanced diet
  - Vitamin deficiency
    - Vitamins E, D
    - Iron deficiency/anemia
    - Magnesium
    - Potassium
- Sleep disorders
  - Insomnia
  - Obstructive sleep apnea
  - Restless leg syndrome
- Psychological disorders
  - Anxiety
  - Depression
- Medical conditions
  - Cardiac
  - Postconcussive syndrome
  - Diabetes
  - Environmental
    - Allergies
    - Heat
    - Poor air quality
  - Infection
  - Medication side effects
  - Postviral syndromes
  - Pregnancy
  - Substance abuse/misuse
  - Thyroid

ANXIETY AND ANXIETY DISORDERS

Anxiety has been cited as the most common mental health diagnosis among the general population, and similar rates exist among athletes.[53] According to the *Diagnostic and Statistical Manual of Mental Disorders, 5th edition, Text Revision (DSM-5-TR)*,[54] generalized anxiety disorder is defined by the presence of excessive fear or worry sustained most days of the week for at least 6 months that persists beyond developmentally appropriate stages and disrupts function of work, play, social interactions, and interpersonal relations. Avoidant behaviors, unpleasant feelings, stress, and tension commonly accompany anxiety. Somatic complaints include increased heart rate, sweating, gastrointestinal distress including dry mouth and stomach pain, as well as disrupted sleep.

Anxiety may impact performance in sport as it affects attention, executive functioning, muscle tension, and processing of stimulation.[55] Anxiety is also consistently and negatively associated with injury in sport, as well as with the resultant recovery and return to sport.[56] Athletes may experience symptoms of anxiety during training and performance, but attention is warranted when symptoms routinely interfere with participation or competition. Providers need to be aware of the symptoms and risk factors of anxiety disorders among athletes to diagnose, treat, and refer individuals appropriately.

Clinicians should also consider the sources of the athlete's psychological, social, and physiological demands in relation to the symptoms of anxiety. Specific factors inherent to sports may impact athletes or worsen anxiety symptoms and disorders differently from the general population. The unique biopsychosocial constructs within sport culture and stressors such as pressure to perform, public scrutiny, securing career or team position, and injury are unique to the athlete.[55] Compared to those who participate in team sports, individual sport participants may have increased relative risk for anxiety.[53] Sports in which judges score athletes to determine success and matriculation to the next level of competition (eg, gymnastics, figure skating, dance, diving) are correlated with anxiety.[57] Participants who focus on perfection and personal goal attainment over fun, and individuals who internalize failure, as well as those who begin sport specialization at a younger age, may also show increased rates of anxiety.[58] Individuals who lack support systems and exhibit poor coping skills may experience loneliness and focus on failure when goals are not achieved.[58] Alternatively, individuals who participate in sports that are high risk for injury (aerial sports, motor sports, sliding sports) are least associated with anxiety disorders.[53]

Athletes may seek attention to manage anxiety when symptoms inhibit their ability to perform. Alternatively, individuals may not recognize that symptoms are secondary to anxiety until they thoroughly discuss them with their health care provider. Female athletes and older athletes more commonly report worry regarding poor performance, whereas male athletes more often report difficulties with concentration.[59]

Female athletes and older athletes more commonly report worry regarding poor performance, whereas male athletes more often report difficulties with concentration.

It is common for athletes to feel anxiety. Sometimes this is a manifestation of a specific anxiety disorder. Diagnostic symptoms, patterns of symptom onset, and duration and severity help to differentiate anxiety subtypes. Anxiety disorders can be classified as generalized anxiety disorder (GAD), panic disorder, social anxiety disorder (SAD), competitive performance anxiety, or specific phobias.[54]

Generalized anxiety disorder is the most common mental health disorder among athletes. Female gender, younger age, and less athletic experience have been associated with GAD among athletes.[55] Men are more likely to be diagnosed solely with GAD, while women may experience multiple additional anxiety disorders concurrently (eg, obsessive-compulsive disorder, social phobia, panic disorder).[53] Symptoms of depression, eating disorders, and substance use and dependence[60] also coexist with GAD among the general population as well as among athletes. Individuals with GAD experience consistent and persistent worry that interferes with daily function most days of the week.

Panic disorder is defined by unexpected and recurrent episodes of intense fear accompanied by pronounced symptoms of heart racing and shortness of breath.[61] Exercise may introduce panic episodes even though it also relieves symptoms of anxiety for most individuals. Like the general population, approximately 4.5% of athletes report symptoms associated with panic disorder. Importantly, panic disorder is considered a risk factor for suicide.

Social anxiety disorder focuses on fear of being judged by others in social or public environments. Specific to athletes, individuals fear negative evaluation of sports performance, public appearance, and social interactions. Social phobia affects 14.7% of athletes, comparable to the general population rate of 13%.[61] Individuals may avoid public interaction, public appearances, and social settings.

Separation anxiety disorder is excessive and developmentally inappropriate anxiety/fear about being separated from home or a major attachment figure lasting for at least 4 weeks in children and at least 6 months in adults. The feelings of fear and worry experienced interfere with daily activities and responsibilities. Individuals with separation anxiety disorder may be distracted during practice or when traveling away from their loved one. They may repeatedly contact the significant person during training or check their communication devices to connect with the individual. Somatic complaints may also escalate before and during times of separation. For individuals experiencing separation anxiety disorder, it is important to assess when behaviors and attention to connect with loved ones prohibit the ability to perform, focus, and interact when apart from them.

Specific phobias are marked by fear about a specific object or situation that typically develops prior to age 11 years but can persist into adulthood. Common examples include fear of airplane travel or fear of mascots in sporting venues. Avoidance behaviors and somatic complaints are typical.

Competitive performance anxiety (CPA) is categorized as a subtype of SAD in *DSM-5-TR*. It involves fear near competition that the individual will not be able to perform successfully. CPA is common to athletes and more common among females, younger participants, and those with lower athletic skill, as well as among individual sport participants.[62,63] Somatic presentation of fight-flight-freeze response includes dry mouth, flushed or pale skin, increased heart rate, sweaty hands, and gastrointestinal symptoms.[62] Athletic deterioration lasting weeks or months has been termed a *slump*.[64] A *choke* refers to behavioral and physical signs that debilitate one to the point of inability to participate. *The yips* refers to involuntary, fine motor movements that prevent accurate sport task performance. The term *twisties* is used for gymnasts who lose the sense of control midair, preventing the ability to twist and tumble.

Diagnosis and Treatment

No athlete-specific screening tools for anxiety disorders have been validated. The IOC recommends the SMHAT-1, which includes the GAD-7, as a screening tool that should be introduced preseason, midseason, and at the end of the season.[29] The PHQ-4 serves as a quick screening tool for generalized anxiety. Individuals who report escalation of symptoms need to be closely monitored and referred to a mental health provider as part of standard protocol. Medical and substance-related conditions that may contribute to anxiety also need to be evaluated and appropriately treated. Psychotherapy, specifically cognitive-behavioral therapy, serves as primary treatment to reduce anxiety, introduce gradual exposure, and prevent undesirable responses by targeting and addressing the negative thoughts and behaviors. Mindfulness-based programs (yoga, meditation, tai chi, qi gong) have also been shown to be efficacious.[65,66] Exercise is an adjunctive nonpharmacologic treatment. Recommendations vary based on presentation and severity of symptoms.

Selective serotonin reuptake inhibitors (SSRIs) commonly serve as initial medication treatment for anxiety disorders.[67] SSRIs prevent the reuptake of serotonin into presynaptic neurons and secondarily increase its neurotransmission. Escitalopram, sertraline, and fluoxetine are first-line options.[67] Treatment with these agents is typically maintained for a minimum of 4 weeks. The dose may then be adjusted, or a different SSRI may be trialed. Tricyclic antidepressants and buspirone, a partial serotonin receptor agonist, are less commonly considered. Intermittent use of anxiolytics is not recommended for those who occasionally report symptoms of anxiety with sport; however, beta-blockers (eg, propranolol) may be used to treat performance anxiety and acute anxiety with associated symptoms such as tremors.[68,69] Beta-blockers are prohibited by the NCAA and WADA in sports that rely on stability of the extremities (eg, archery, racing, billiards, darts, golf, shooting, and fishing). Therefore, their use needs to be individualized. Caution should be exercised when using dietary or natural supplements because of the lack of regulation of contents. Poorly defined ingredients cause undesirable side effects, and prohibited additives may disqualify elite athletes from competition. Athletes consuming cannabidiol (CBD) should be made aware that CBD products may also contain THC, which is prohibited by many sports governing bodies.[70]

Beta-blockers are prohibited by the NCAA and WADA in sports that rely on stability of the extremities (eg, archery, racing, billiards, darts, golf, shooting, and fishing). Therefore, their use needs to be individualized.

Athletes may worry that treatment of anxiety will negatively impact sport performance by decreasing motivation, dedication, and focus. Undesirable side effects of medications include change in sleep quality and body weight, cardiac symptoms, heat intolerance, impaired concentration, blurred vision, dizziness, and agitation.[67] Research has not demonstrated that treatment of anxiety with medication leads to detrimental outcomes in training; however, the athlete may avoid medications because of potential undesirable side effects.

A multidisciplinary team including a mental health professional offers a comprehensive support network to prevent, intervene in, and manage anxiety disorders. Key strategies of psychological management including self-regulation, intrinsic motivation, self-confidence, effective coping skills, and positive mindset are fundamental to assist the athlete in sustaining success in life and in sport.[55] Athletes are particularly well-positioned for psychotherapeutic interventions as they are accustomed to discipline and following direction.[67]

When symptoms of anxiety are identified on the initial screen with PHQ-4 and anxiety-related disorders are suspected, further evaluation with additional screening tools and prompt intervention are needed. Individuals who exhibit or report increased feelings of anxiety warrant close follow-up. Effective treatment options include psychotherapy, mindfulness techniques, medications, and referral to a mental health provider. Organized, comprehensive, and timely treatment supports successful participation in sport, promotes psychological wellness, and prevents further symptom exacerbation.

Individuals who exhibit or report increased feelings of anxiety warrant close follow-up. Effective treatment options include psychotherapy, mindfulness techniques, medications, and referral to a mental health provider. Organized, comprehensive, and timely treatment supports successful participation in sport, promotes psychological wellness, and prevents further symptom exacerbation.

OBSESSIVE-COMPULSIVE DISORDER

Obsessive-compulsive disorder (OCD) involves recurrent unwanted thoughts, ideas, or sensations that compel the repeated performance of specific behaviors. OCD has been identified at higher rates among collegiate athletes (5.2%) in comparison to the general population (2.3%).[71] In children and adolescents, the prevalence of OCD is 1% to 3%.[72] OCD symptoms may occur at an increased prevalence among athletes without meeting the criteria for OCD diagnosis, as perfectionism and compliance with strict routines as well as superstitions and rituals are inherent to the culture of sports.[22] OCD requires intervention when the obsessions prevent the individual from successfully functioning or when attention cannot remain focused because of intrusive thoughts.

POSTTRAUMATIC STRESS DISORDER

Posttraumatic stress disorder involves intrusive thoughts and feelings and associated behavioral changes following a traumatic event. PTSD is more likely experienced by females, youth athletes, and those who have experienced an injury. Individuals with PTSD may experience inconsistent sport performance, excessive somatic complaints, or avoidance behaviors.

SUBSTANCE USE AND ADDICTION

Screening for addiction during the PPE is essential for ensuring the holistic health and well-being of student-athletes. Athletes often face unique pressures, such as intense competition, academic responsibilities, and the need to maintain peak physical performance. These factors can increase the risk of substance use, subsequent addiction, or exacerbating or exposing existing mental health conditions such as anxiety, depression, or substance-induced psychotic disorders. By incorporating substance use and addiction screening into PPEs, physicians and other health care providers can identify athletes who may be at risk and intervene early, potentially preventing the escalation of substance use disorder (SUD) or other conditions that may impact an athlete's mental health and athletic performance.

Early detection of SUD in student-athletes can lead to timely referrals for treatment and support, which are critical for recovery.[73] SUD is notably prevalent among high school and college athletes. According to the 2024 NCAA Student-Athlete Health and Wellness Study, a significant proportion of student-athletes reported using substances such as alcohol (72%), marijuana (26%), vape/e-cigarette (22%), tobacco (spit, cigar, cigarette, 31%), and narcotic pain medication (8%).[74] While there have been declines in certain areas, such as binge drinking and use of narcotic pain medication, the study reports that the overall prevalence remains a concern.

According to the 2024 NCAA Student-Athlete Health and Wellness Study, a significant proportion of student-athletes report using substances such as alcohol (72%), marijuana (26%), vape/e-cigarette (22%), tobacco (spit, cigar, cigarette, 31%), and narcotic pain medication (8%).

During the PPE, screening for SUD is recommended based on the individual population risk. However, given the wide use of alcohol, the NIAAA Single Alcohol Screening Question (SASQ) (https://www.niaaa.nih.gov/health-professionals-communities/core-resource-on-alcohol/screen-and-assess-use-quick-effective-methods#pub-toc7), a quick validated screening tool, can help identify individuals 21 years and older at increased risk of SUD and, when indicated, refer them to appropriate resources.[5] For individuals younger than 21 years, CRAFFT is a validated screening tool for SUD (https://crafft.org).

According to the AAP, incorporating SUD screening into PPEs and screening for addiction can help identify adolescents and young adults who may be at risk for substance use disorder, thereby facilitating timely referrals for treatment and support. Furthermore, screening for SUD during PPEs can contribute to creating a culture of awareness and prevention within athletic programs. By addressing the issue openly, coaches, athletic trainers, and physicians can educate athletes about the dangers of substance use and the importance of seeking help when needed. This proactive approach can reduce the stigma associated with SUD, encouraging more athletes to come forward if they are struggling.

ATTENTION-DEFICIT/HYPERACTIVITY DISORDER

Attention-deficit/hyperactivity disorder (ADHD) is a common neurodevelopmental disorder that affects more than 10% of children and adolescents.[75] It is characterized by symptoms of inattention, hyperactivity, and impulsivity that are present in multiple settings (eg, home, school, sports). Athletes are diagnosed with ADHD at rates comparable to those in the general population, although there may be a sport-specific overrepresentation, including in contact sports.[76] Athletes with ADHD may be drawn to sports as a method of self-treatment, as even small amounts of physical activity can improve executive function and self-regulation. However, athletes with ADHD, especially those who are untreated or undertreated, may experience challenges with focus, task completion, adherence to coaching instructions, and impulse control. These have the potential to increase the risk of injury.[76] The PPE provides an opportunity to assess ADHD symptoms, current treatment, and considerations for athletic participation.

Diagnosis and Screening in Athletes

The diagnosis of ADHD is made clinically, in accordance with *DSM-5-TR* criteria. Screening tools (eg, ADHD Rating Scale-5, Vanderbilt [https://nichq.org/wp-content/uploads/2024/09/NICHQ-Vanderbilt-Assessment-Scales.pdf]) may aid in the evaluation. ADHD diagnosis and treatment disparities exist across gender, socioeconomic, and racial groups. Girls may be underdiagnosed, or diagnosed later, because of differing symptom presentation. Children from marginalized communities are less likely to receive proper diagnosis and treatment. Socioeconomic factors influence treatment adherence, with those in lower-income families having poorer adherence.[77] For individuals who report a past or current diagnosis of ADHD on their PPE History Form, it is important for the provider to ask about medication use and academic accommodations, with attention to equitable evaluation and management strategies for all athletes. Some conditions can present with overlapping symptoms and can be distinguished through screening tools (see Table 6-2).

Table 6-2. Common Mimics for ADHD and Validated Screening Tools

Condition	Key Symptoms Overlapping With ADHD	Validated Screening Tools
Autism spectrum disorder	Social communication challenges, focus difficulties	Autism Diagnostic Observation Schedule (ADOS), Social Responsiveness Scale (SRS)
Bipolar disorder	Impulsivity, mood instability, distractibility	Mood Disorder Questionnaire (MDQ)
Generalized anxiety disorder (GAD)	Inattention, restlessness, difficulty concentrating	GAD-7, Hamilton Anxiety Scale
Learning disabilities	Poor academic performance, difficulty processing information	Woodcock-Johnson Tests of Cognitive Abilities, Wechsler Intelligence Scale for Children (WISC)
Major depressive disorder	Low motivation, poor concentration, fatigue	PHQ-9 (Patient Health Questionnaire-9), Beck Depression Inventory
Oppositional defiant disorder	Defiance, impulsivity, emotional dysregulation	Vanderbilt ADHD Diagnostic Rating Scale, SNAP-IV
Posttraumatic stress disorder (PTSD)	Hypervigilance, irritability, difficulty concentrating	PCL-5 (PTSD Checklist), CAPS-5 (Clinician-Administered PTSD Scale)

Table 6-2. Common Mimics for ADHD and Validated Screening Tools (*continued*)

Condition	Key Symptoms Overlapping With ADHD	Validated Screening Tools
Sensory processing disorder	Overresponsiveness or underresponsiveness to sensory stimuli	Sensory Processing Measure (SPM), Sensory Profile
Sleep disorders (eg, sleep apnea)	Daytime sleepiness, poor focus, hyperactivity	Epworth Sleepiness Scale, polysomnography
Substance use disorder	Impulsivity, inattentiveness, mood instability	Single Alcohol Screening Question (SASQ), CRAFFT

Abbreviations: ADHD, attention-deficit/hyperactivity disorder; SNAP-IV, Swanson, Nolan and Pelham Teacher and Parent Rating Scale.

Treatment Considerations

ADHD management in athletes may include a combination of behavioral and pharmacologic intervention. Stimulant medications (eg, methylphenidate, amphetamines) are effective but require monitoring because of their potential for abuse/misuse and because their use in elite competitive sports is highly regulated (see Table 6-3).

Table 6-3. Common Medications Used to Treat ADHD and Regulatory Considerations

Medication	Classification	NCAA and WADA Status	Considerations
Methylphenidate	Stimulant	Banned (TUE required)	Requires documentation for TUE; potential cardiovascular effects
Dextroamphetamine	Stimulant	Banned (TUE required)	Requires documentation for TUE; risk of increased blood pressure
Amphetamine	Stimulant	Banned (TUE required)	Requires documentation for TUE; potential for misuse
Lisdexamfetamine	Stimulant	Banned (TUE required)	Requires documentation for TUE; appetite suppression common
Atomoxetine	Nonstimulant	Permitted	No TUE required; alternative for those avoiding stimulants
Guanfacine	Nonstimulant	Permitted	No TUE required; may cause drowsiness or fatigue
Clonidine	Nonstimulant	Permitted	No TUE required; used primarily for symptom management

Abbreviations: ADHD, attention-deficit/hyperactivity disorder; NCAA, National Collegiate Athletic Association; TUE, Therapeutic Use Exemption; WADA, World Anti-Doping Agency.

- Stimulant medications and doping regulations: Stimulants are prohibited by WADA and NCAA unless a Therapeutic Use Exemption (TUE) is granted. Athletes should be informed of documentation requirements and alternative treatment options.
- Nonstimulant medications: Atomoxetine, guanfacine, and clonidine provide alternatives for those unable to tolerate stimulants or for those seeking treatment options that reduce concerns about stimulant use, side effects, or anti-doping regulations. Providers can also consider bupropion.
- Nutritional and behavioral strategies: Cognitive-behavioral therapy, sleep hygiene, structured routines, mindfulness techniques, and dietary adjustments (eg, omega-3 fatty acids) may help with symptom management.
- Potential for abuse: Stimulants are subject to abuse or misuse because of their perceived ergogenic effects, such as euphoria, enhanced focus, and faster reaction time. However, actual performance benefits remain largely unproven, and misuse raises concerns about dependency and adverse effects. Some athletes, especially those in weight-controlled sports, may use stimulants for appetite suppression properties.[77] While there is potential for abuse or misuse, the fear of potential abuse of stimulants is not justification for withholding pharmacologic management of ADHD in patients in whom it is indicated.

Stimulants are prohibited by WADA and NCAA unless a Therapeutic Use Exemption is granted. Athletes should be informed of documentation requirements and alternative treatment options.

Safety Consideration

Stimulants have been shown to cause a mild increase in blood pressure and heart rate; however, current evidence does not demonstrate an increase in sudden cardiac death risk among otherwise healthy individuals.[77] For individuals without underlying cardiac conditions, a pretreatment electrocardiogram is not required.

Stimulant medications may raise core temperature and affect its regulation; however, the risk of exertional hyperthermia is largely theoretical and speculative and is extrapolated from data on ephedra or other stimulants. No association between elevated core temperature and prescription stimulants used at therapeutic doses has been established.[77]

ADHD, Concussion, and Neurocognitive Testing

Athletes with ADHD, especially when untreated, may exhibit baseline neurocognitive testing scores that are outside of the normal range, especially in those domains related to attention, memory, and reaction time.[77] These ADHD-related deficits may complicate postconcussion evaluation. Athletes with ADHD may need individualized concussion management plans. While a diagnosis of ADHD does not appear to worsen outcomes, some data suggest prolonged recovery time and increased symptom burden among some affected athletes.[77] It is recommended that ADHD medications not be discontinued while recovering from a concussion.

BIPOLAR AND PSYCHOTIC DISORDERS

Bipolar and psychotic disorders are relatively uncommon among adolescent and college athletes (84.97 per 100,000 population in 2019).[78] Bipolar and psychotic disorders can significantly impact quality of life and athletic performance. During the PPE, it may be beneficial to screen for these mental health conditions, as they can predispose athletes to injury or illness. The typical age of onset for bipolar and psychotic disorders coincides with peak performance years in athletes, making early detection and management essential.[79] However, diagnosing these disorders in athletes can be challenging because of the modifying role of exercise and potential substance use. Medications used to treat these disorders may also have side effects that are problematic for athletes. Therefore, tailored approaches and referral for specialty care are recommended to address the specific needs of this population.

DISORDERED EATING AND EATING DISORDERS

Disordered eating (DE) patterns are widespread across sports and can range from mild to more serious manifestations, including meeting diagnostic criteria for an eating disorder (ED) such as anorexia nervosa, bulimia nervosa, binge eating disorder, and others. Orthorexia (compulsively healthy eating associated with mental preoccupation) and RED-S (syndrome of physiological and psychological outcomes from chronic energy unavailability) are not identified in the *DSM-5-TR* as diagnoses but are common in sporting environments.[54] Athletes have higher rates of EDs than the general population, with higher rates in females than in males and rates increasing longitudinally over an athletic career.[80–82] DE and EDs are often associated with other mental health conditions such as anxiety, depression, bipolar disorder, substance use, PTSD, and suicide.[80] Mental health disorders can lead to the development of RED-S or vice versa, in which mental health disorders prove to be a manifestation of RED-S.[50] See Chapter 5I for more information.

SLEEP

Sleep has become a very important area for study in an active population. A summary of the consensus statement by the American Academy of Sleep Medicine and Sleep Research Society noted the importance of sleep on overall health and mortality (see Table 6-4).[83]

Table 6-4. The Effect of Adequate and Inadequate Sleep on Health

Effect of Sleep on Human Health	Effect of Inadequate Sleep on Mortality
• Brain function • Neurobehavioral function • Cognitive function • Performance • Safety-related performance • Memory • Clearance of brain metabolites • Appetite regulation • Immune function • Hormone function • Cardiovascular system	• Cardiovascular disease and hypertension • Cerebrovascular disease • Diabetes • Obesity • Cancers • Depression and suicide

Derived from Watson NF, Badr MS, Belenky G, et al; Consensus Conference Panel. Joint consensus statement of the American Academy of Sleep Medicine and Sleep Research Society on the recommended amount of sleep for a healthy adult: methodology and discussion. *J Clin Sleep Med.* 2015;11(8):931–952.

Individuals experiencing problems with initiating sleep were 5.1 times more likely to think about suicide, 9.1 times more likely to plan suicide, and 7.5 times more likely to have attempted suicide in the past 12 months than those without a sleep problem.[84]

Sleep is important for the body to process information and recover mentally and physically. Healthy sleep requires an adequate duration, good quality, appropriate timing and regularity, and the absence of sleep disturbances or disorders.

Athletes have been shown to have different sleep habits compared with nonathletes.[21] Postulated causes include varying demands on their schedule with training and competition, an increase in muscle tension, fatigue, pain, elevated core body temperature from training, an increase in psychological distress (competition-related), travel, and disruption due to light and noise.[21] Sixty-five percent of college athletes reported suboptimal sleep health,[83] and 49% of Olympic athletes were classified as poor sleepers.[85] In addition to improving performance, sufficient sleep is important to prevent overtraining and injuries while improving recovery and maximizing training gains.[22]

Sleep function is a dance between a person's sleep drive and circadian rhythm. Sleep drive is the internal process whereby pressure to sleep builds, and this drive increases the longer one is awake. Circadian rhythm (Figure 6-1) is the internal biological clock that keeps one awake. It is modulated by the effect of light on the production of melatonin and countered by cortisol production. Chronotype refers to the effects of the circadian rhythm and genetic and environmental factors that define the natural tendency to be a morning or evening person. Those with an evening chronotype tend to have more sleep issues. Circadian rhythm changes with age. For example, adolescents' body clocks are more evening chronotypes favoring later bedtimes, longer sleep, and later morning awakenings.

Stages of sleep are of 2 main types defined by eye movements and electrical brain patterns. Rapid-eye-movement (REM) sleep increases as the night goes on and is noted by a paralyzed motor system. Non–rapid-eye-movement (NREM) sleep has 3 stages: N1, N2, and N3, with N1 reflecting a lighter sleep pattern and N3 reflecting a deep sleep

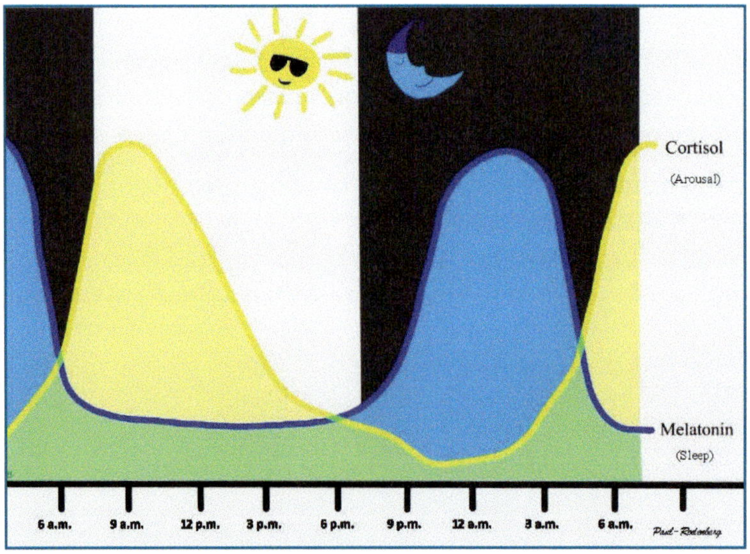

Figure 6-1. Sleep-Wake Cycle
Reproduced with permission from Paul S, Benjamin H. *Sleep Essentials.* Healthy Learning; 2020.

pattern (deep slow wave sleep). In a normal night's sleep, one cycles through the stages and brief awakenings can occur during the transitions between stages. Memory consolidation requires both REM and NREM sleep. As we age, we spend less time in REM sleep.

Jet lag can adversely affect sleep. Traveling across time zones adversely affects the circadian rhythm because of environmental cues of natural daylight and darkness. In addition, air travel compounds this effect because of discomfort, ambient air pressure, and dehydration. The overall effect can be daytime sleepiness and fatigue as well as difficulty concentrating and gastrointestinal problems such as diarrhea or constipation. Traveling east is more difficult because one is "losing" time, whereas traveling west may be easier because one is "gaining" time and flying in the direction of the sun.

The conflict between the circadian rhythm and sleep drive due to a social sleep schedule is referred to as "social jet lag." Examples include sleeping late on weekends, late night social activities, training, studies, and use of blue light from electronic devices. Social jet lag can have the same effect as true jet lag from flying 2 to 3 hours across time zones.[83]

Components of Healthy Sleep

One component of good sleep is quality, which is reflected in an optimal environment: dark, quiet, cool, and comfortable. Further, establishing a healthy sleep routine includes a regular sleep schedule and avoidance of alcohol, caffeine, nicotine, and excessive exercise prior to bedtime (See Box 6-4). In addition, blue light from phone and computer screens can adversely affect the production of melatonin. The quantity of sleep also is important (Box 6-5).

Box 6-4. Sleep Hygiene for Optimal Sleep

- Keep a consistent sleep routine and schedule
- Keep bedroom for sleeping (no TV, work, eating, screens)
- Keep room dark and cool
- Limit noise distractions
- Limit time in bed if not sleepy
- Keep naps to less than 30 minutes and before 3:00 pm
- Avoid caffeine, alcohol, smoking, heavy foods close to bedtime
- Avoid excessive fluid intake close to bedtime
- Try to reserve adequate time to wind down before bedtime
- Do not bring problems to bed with you; process prior to bedtime; make a "to do" list; keep a pad by bedside
- Consider mindfulness tools such as breath exercises
- If you cannot fall asleep, avoid clock watching and get out of bed until you are sleepy enough to return
- Do not look at the clock if you wake up at night

Box 6-5. Recommended Optimal Amount of Sleep by Age[83,86]

- Ages 6–12 years: 9–12 hours
- Ages 13–18 years: 8–10 hours
- Adults: ≥ 7 hours

Healthy People 2030[87] reports a deficit in good sleep and recommends that secondary schools have a start time of 8:30 am or later:

- 25.4% of youth in grades 9–12 get sufficient sleep (2017 data)
- 72.3% of adults ≥ 18 years received sufficient sleep (2020 data)

Obstructive Sleep Apnea

Another cause of poor sleep is obstructive sleep apnea (OSA), which is a reduced supply of air during sleep noted by hypopnea (partial collapse) and apnea (full collapse) of the airway. OSA increases the risk of cardiovascular disease and stroke.[88] Symptoms are often reported as loud snoring and daytime sleepiness. The prevalence has been reported to be lower in women (3%–23%) than in men (9%–49%).[89] In contact sports, the prevalence of OSA was reported to be 30%.[90] OSA has been described as more typical in older obese men. When studied in the National Football League, there were some trends relating to linemen being more affected, as well as those who had retired.[88] Studies have shown that up to 1 in 5 individuals diagnosed with OSA have normal body habitus, and their OSA is more difficult to treat.[89] Emerging evidence suggests that muscle development in the neck may be an important risk factor for OSA, along with neck size, not merely obesity. In addition to screening for optimal sleep, it is important to be attentive to OSA.

Assessing Sleep Quality and Quantity

Screening for and encouraging optimal sleep is vital to the overall health of anyone and, in particular, active individuals. The "gold standard" to assess sleep is polysomnography (PSG), which measures brain activity, heart rate (electrocardiogram), eye movements, muscle activity, blood oxygen levels, and breathing patterns. PSG is performed in a laboratory where the individual is monitored overnight. Sleep duration, sleep latency, sleep interruptions, and sleep quality in terms of time spent in each stage and in transitions between stages are also measured. The downside of PSG is that it is done in a laboratory, is expensive, and is intrusive for the person being studied, and that may affect the normal sleep pattern.

Newer technologies in many wearable devices use photoplethysmography, which may measure heart rate, oxygen saturation, and heart rate variability (sleep stages), and actigraphy (measurement of sleep-wake cycles), which measures vibration, movement, and acceleration. These wearable devices also use proprietary algorithms to improve the assessment of the stages of sleep. A study reviewing 53 wearable devices reported the average sleep-wake accuracy as 87.2%, the average 3-stage (wake, REM, NREM) accuracy as 69.7%, and average accuracy for all 4 stages (wake, light, deep, REM) as 65%.[91] Advancement and refinement of algorithms are making many wearable devices more effective, but cost is still an issue.

Several validated screening tools use questionnaires for sleep disorders. Two have been validated for an athlete population, and both tools are recommended by the NCAA and IOC: the Athlete Sleep Screening Questionnaire and the Athlete Sleep Behavior Questionnaire.[21,25,29]

MENTAL HEALTH AND ABUSE

When considering mental health disorders, it is important to take into account the possible role of abuse, as they commonly coexist. Mental health disorders can lead to abusive behaviors or set the stage for the individual to be the target of abuse from others. Alternatively, being the victim of abusive behaviors facilitates the development of certain mental health conditions. Thus, during any medical encounter with an individual, it is important to keep in mind how intertwined these conditions are. Refer to Chapter 9 for more information about abuse.

SUMMARY

Given the impact of mental health issues on active individuals and athletes, screening for mental health disorders is recommended. In this chapter, attention has been given to the most common mental health findings encountered in sport participation, and some reliable screening tools are offered. Frequent screening with the appropriate tools, having predetermined resources available for follow-up, and rendering treatment and intervention are emphasized. Also noted is the importance of destigmatizing mental health issues to allow for more comfortable conversations about these issues with individuals, their families, coaches, and communities.

It is also important to understand how so many common daily pressures can be a tipping point, moving from a more measured, normal response to one that is disproportionately affecting the individual. These instances may be the trigger leading to a mental health issue or crisis. The conditions discussed in this chapter can be observed independently, but they also may interact to compound an individual's response, impair coping ability, and lead to a crisis. Abusing substances can precipitate anxiety, depression, suicide, and other conditions. Exacerbation of stressors or abuse of alcohol can lead to interpersonal violence and abuse. Loss of a personal contact or family member can exacerbate a multitude of mental health issues, such as depression, suicide, and abuse of substances and alcohol. Time loss injuries and surgeries can lead to depressed mood or exacerbation of major depression and/or anxiety (as well as aggressive behavior or substance abuse).

Time loss injuries and surgeries can lead to depressed mood or exacerbation of major depression and/or anxiety (as well as aggressive behavior or substance abuse).

Clinicians working with athletes and other physically active individuals need to be aware of subtle changes in their moods and behaviors, looking for signs and symptoms of personal setbacks, whether they are physical, psychological, or social. Clinicians should encourage open dialogue about these issues, welcome communication, and break down barriers of access and stigma.

REFERENCES

1. Löwe B, Kroenke K, Gräfe K. Detecting and monitoring depression with a two-item questionnaire (PHQ-2). *J Psychosom Res.* 2005;58(2):163–171. PMID: 15820844
2. Lewinsohn PM, Rohde P, Seeley JR. Major depressive disorder in older adolescents: prevalence, risk factors, and clinical implications. *Clin Psychol Rev.* 1998;18(7):765–794. PMID: 9827321 doi: 10.1016/S0272-7358(98)00010-5
3. Kroenke K, Spitzer RL, Williams JB, Löwe B. An ultra-brief screening scale for anxiety and depression: the PHQ-4. *Psychosomatics.* 2009;50(6):613–621. PMID: 19996233 doi: 10.1176/appi.psy.50.6.613
4. Kroenke K, Spitzer RL, Williams JB. The PHQ-9: validity of a brief depression severity measure. *J Gen Intern Med.* 2001;16(9):606–613. PMID: 11556941 doi: 10.1046/j.1525-1497.2001.016009606.x
5. Smith PC, Schmidt SM, Allensworth-Davies D, Saitz R. Primary care validation of a single-question alcohol screening test. *J Gen Intern Med.* 2009;24(7):783–788. https://pmc.ncbi.nlm.nih.gov/articles/PMC2695521 PMID: 19247718 doi: 10.1007/s11606-009-0928-6
6. National Institute on Alcohol Abuse and Alcoholism. Screen and assess: use quick, effective methods. Updated May 8, 2025. https://www.niaaa.nih.gov/health-professionals-communities/core-resource-on-alcohol/screen-and-assess-use-quick-effective-methods
7. American Academy of Pediatrics. Screening for suicide risk in clinical practice. Updated February 22, 2023. https://www.aap.org/en/patient-care/blueprint-for-youth-suicide-prevention/strategies-for-clinical-settings-for-youth-suicide-prevention/screening-for-suicide-risk-in-clinical-practice/?srsltid=AfmBOoo4_HfevT7srvfrCZGNSI5aQZytt2Z21yaHSFMsx81CwQI_XPRa
8. Kellmann M, Günther K-D. *Recovery-Stress-Questionnaire for Athletes (RESTQ-S).* [Database record]. APA PsycTests; 2000. doi:10.1037/t55245-000
9. Grant CC, Van Rensburg DCJ, Collins R, Wood, PS, Du Toit PJ. The Profile of Mood State (POMS) questionnaire as an indicator of Overtraining Syndrome (OTS) in endurance athletes. *AJPHERD.* 2012;18(suppl 1). https://hdl.handle.net/10520/EJC119823
10. Mossman SA, Luft MJ, Schroeder HK, et al. The Generalized Anxiety Disorder 7-item scale in adolescents with generalized anxiety disorder: signal detection and validation. *Ann Clin Psychiatry.* 2017;29(4):227–234A. PMID: 29069107
11. Connor KM, Davidson JR, Churchill LE, Sherwood A, Foa E, Weisler RH. Psychometric properties of the Social Phobia Inventory (SPIN). New self-rating scale. *Br J Psychiatry.* 2000;176:379–386. PMID: 10827888 doi:10.1192/bjp.176.4.379
12. Adam GP, Caputo EL, Kanaan G, et al. Brief assessment tools for obsessive compulsive disorders in children: a systematic review. *Pediatrics.* 2025;155(3):e2024068993. PMID: 39639450 doi:10.1542/peds.2024-068993
13. Ouimette P, Wade M, Prins A, Schohn M. Identifying PTSD in primary care: comparison of the Primary Care-PTSD screen (PC-PTSD) and the General Health Questionnaire-12 (GHQ). *J Anxiety Disord.* 2008;22(2):337–343. PMID: 17383853
14. Pynoos RS, Weathers FW, Steinberg AM, et al. *Clinician-Administered PTSD Scale for DSM-5—Child/Adolescent Version.* 2015. National Center for PTSD. www.ptsd.va.gov
15. Levy SJL, Williams JF, et al; American Academy of Pediatrics Committee on Substance Use and Prevention. Substance use screening, brief intervention, and referral to treatment. *Pediatrics.* 2016;138(1):e20161211. PMID: 27325634 doi:10.1542/peds.2016-1211
16. DuPaul GJ, Power TJ, Anastopoulos AD, Reid R. *ADHD Rating Scale-5 for Children and Adolescents: Checklists, Norms, and Clinical Interpretation.* Guilford Press; 2016
17. Wolraich ML, Lambert W, Doffing MA, Bickman L, Simmons T, Worley K. Psychometric properties of the Vanderbilt ADHD Diagnostic Parent Rating Scale in a referred population. *J Pediatr Psychol.* 2003;28(8):559–567. PMID: 14602846
18. U.S. Preventive Services Task Force. Final Recommendation Statement: Intimate Partner Violence and Caregiver Abuse of Older or Vulnerable Adults: Screening. Updated June 24, 2025. Accessed March 10, 2026. https://www.uspreventiveservicestaskforce.org/uspstf/recommendation/intimate-partner-violence-and-abuse-of-elderly-and-vulnerable-adults-screening
19. Samuels C, James L, Lawson D, Meeuwisse W. The Athlete Sleep Screening Questionnaire: a new tool for assessing and managing sleep in elite athletes. *Br J Sports Med.* 2016;50(7):418–422. PMID: 26002952 doi:10.1136/bjsports-2014-094332

20. Bender AM, Lawson D, Werthner P, Samuels CH. The clinical validation of the Athlete Sleep Screening Questionnaire: an Instrument to identify athletes that need further sleep assessment. *Sports Med Open.* 2018;4(1):23. PMID: 29869021 doi:10.1186/s40798-018-0140-5
21. Driller MW, Mah CD, Halson SL. Development of the Athlete Sleep Behavior Questionnaire: a tool for identifying maladaptive sleep practices in elite athletes. *Sleep Sci.* 2018;11(1):37–44. PMID: 29796200
22. Reardon CL, Hainline B, Aron CM, et al. Mental health in elite athletes: International Olympic Committee consensus statement (2019). *Br J Sports Med.* 2019;53(11):667–699. PMID: 31097450
23. Chang CJ, Putukian M, Aerni G, et al. Mental health issues and psychological factors in athletes: detection, management, effect on performance, and prevention: American Medical Society for Sports Medicine position statement. *Clin J Sport Med.* 2020;30(2):e61–e87. PMID: 32000169
24. Van Slingerland KJ, Durand-Bush N, Bradley L, et al. Canadian Centre for Mental Health and Sport (CCMHS) position statement: principles of mental health in competitive and high-performance sport. *Clin J Sport Med.* 2019;29(3):173–180. PMID: 31033609
25. *Mental Health Best Practices: Understanding and Supporting Student-Athlete Mental Health.* An inter-association consensus document. NCAA. 2nd ed. Updated 2024. https://ncaaorg.s3.amazonaws.com/ssi/mental/SSI_MentalHealthBestPractices.pdf
26. Castaldelli-Maia JM, Gallinaro JGME, Falcão RS, et al. Mental health symptoms and disorders in elite athletes: a systematic review on cultural influencers and barriers to athletes seeking treatment. *Br J Sports Med.* 2019;53(11):707–721. PMID: 31092400 doi:10.1136/bjsports-2019-100710
27. Vella SA, Swann C, Bartterman M, et al. An intervention for mental health literacy and resilience in organized sports. *Med Sci Sports Exerc.* 2021;53(1):139–149. doi:10.1249/MSS.0000000000002433
28. U.S. Department of Health and Human Services, Office of the Surgeon General. Alcohol and cancer risk. Updated January 17, 2025. https://www.hhs.gov/surgeongeneral/priorities/alcohol-cancer/index.html
29. Gouttebarge V, Bindra A, Blauwet C, et al. International Olympic Committee (IOC) Sport Mental Health Assessment Tool 1 (SMHAT-1) and Sport Mental Health Recognition Tool 1 (SMHRT-1): towards better support of athletes' mental health. *Br J Sports Med.* 2021;55:30–37
30. Anderson T, Adams WM, Bartley JD, Brutus AL, Donaldson AT, Finnoff JT. Analysis of the Sport Mental Health Assessment Tool 1 (SMHAT-1) in Team USA athletes. *Br J Sports Med.* 2023;57(18):1187–1194. PMID: 37369554
31. Rice SM, Parker AG, Mawren D, et al. Preliminary psychometric validation of a brief screening tool for athlete mental health among male elite athletes: the Athlete Psychological Strain Questionnaire. *Int J Sport Exerc Psychol.* 2020;18(6):850–865
32. Rice S, Olive L, Gouttebarge V, et al. Mental health screening: severity and cut-off point sensitivity of the Athlete Psychological Strain Questionnaire in male and female elite athletes. *BMJ Open Sport Exerc Med.* 2020;6(1):e000712. PMID: 32231792
33. Mountjoy M, Edwards C, Cheung CP, Burr J, Gouttebarge V. Implementation of the International Olympic Committee Sport Mental Health Assessment Tool 1: screening for mental health symptoms in a Canadian multisport university program. *Clin J Sport Med.* 2023;33(1):5–12. PMID: 36599359
34. Yang J, Peek-Asa C, Corlette JD, Cheng G, Foster DT, Albright J. Prevalence of and risk factors associated with symptoms of depression in competitive collegiate student athletes. *Clin J Sport Med.* 2007;17(6):481–487. PMID: 17993792
35. Cadigan JM, Littlefield AK, Martens MP, Sher KJ. Transitions into and out of intercollegiate athletic involvement and risky drinking. *J Stud Alcohol Drugs.* 2013;74(1):21–29. PMID: 23200147 www.ncbi.nlm.nih.gov/pubmed/23200147
36. Hammond T, Gialloreto C, Kubas H, Hap Davis H IV. The prevalence of failure-based depression among elite athletes. *Clin J Sport Med.* 2013;23(4):273–277. PMID: 23528842
37. Daley MM, Reardon CL. Mental health in the youth athlete. *Clin Sports Med.* 2024;43(1):107–126. PMID: 37949505 doi:10.1016/j.csm.2023.06.003
38. Wolanin A, Hong E, Marks D, Panchoo K, Gross M. Prevalence of clinically elevated depressive symptoms in college athletes and differences by gender and sport. *Br J Sports Med.* 2016;50(3):167–171. PMID: 26782764
39. Radloff LS. The CES-D Scale: a self-report depression scale for research in the general population. *Appl Psychol Meas.* 1977;1:385–401
40. Lester D. Suicidal tendencies. In: Brown GT, ed. *Mind, Body and Sport: Understanding and Supporting Student-Athlete Mental Wellness.* National Collegiate Athletic Association; 2014:54–56

41. Rao AL, Asif IM, Drezner JA, Toresdahl BG, Harmon KG. Suicide in National Collegiate Athletic Association (NCAA) athletes: a 9-year analysis of the NCAA resolutions database. *Sports Health.* 2015;7(5):452–457. PMID: 26502423 doi:10.1177/1941738115587675
42. American Psychiatry Association. Suicide prevention. February 2023. https://www.psychiatry.org/patients-families/suicide-prevention
43. Whelan BM, Kliethermes SA, Schloredt KA, Rao A, Harmon KG, Petek BJ. Suicide in National Collegiate Athletic Association athletes: a 20-year analysis. *Br J Sports Med.* 2024;58(10):531–537. PMID: 38575202
44. Drum DJ, Denmark AB. Campus suicide prevention: bridging paradigms and forging partnerships. *Harv Rev Psychiatry.* 2012;20(4):209–221. PMID: 22894730
45. Suicide Prevention Resource Center. Learning center. Accessed December 30, 2025. https://sprc.org/settings/colleges-and-universities/#:~:text=Promote%20social%20networks%20and%20connectedness,when%20a%20suicide%20death%20occurs
46. Brenner JS, Watson A; American Academy of Pediatrics Council on Sports Medicine and Fitness. Overuse injuries, overtraining, and burnout in young athletes. *Pediatrics.* 2024;153(2):e2023065129. PMID: 38247370 doi:10.1542/peds.2023-065129
47. Stellingwerff T, Heikura IA, Meeusen R, et al. Overtraining syndrome (OTS) and Relative Energy Deficiency in Sport (RED-S): shared pathways, symptoms and complexities. *Sports Med.* 2021;51(11):2251–2280. PMID: 34181189 doi:10.1007/s40279-021-01491-0
48. Solomon ML, Weiss Kelly AK. Approach to the underperforming athlete. *Pediatr Ann.* 2016;45(3):e91–e96. PMID: 27031317 doi:10.3928/00904481-20160210-02
49. Morgan WP, Brown DR, Raglin JS, O'Connor PJ, Ellickson KA. Psychological monitoring of overtraining and staleness. *Br J Sports Med.* 1987;21(3):107–114. PMID: 3676635 doi:10.1136/bjsm.21.3.107
50. Mountjoy M, Ackerman KE, Bailey DM, et al. 2023 International Olympic Committee's (IOC) consensus statement on Relative Energy Deficiency in Sport (REDs). *Br J Sports Med.* 2023;57(17):1073–1097. PMID: 37752011 doi:10.1136/bjsports-2023-106994
51. Carrard J, Rigort A-C, Appenzeller-Herzog C, et al. Diagnosing overtraining syndrome: a scoping review. *Sports Health.* 2022;14(5):665–673. PMID: 34496702 doi:10.1177/19417381211044739
52. Schorb A, Niebauer J, Aichhorn W, Schiepek G, Scherr J, Claussen M. Overtraining from a sports psychiatry perspective. *Dtsch Z Sportmed.* 2021;72(6):271–279. doi:10.5960/dzsm.2021.496
53. Schall K, Tafflet M, Nassif H, et al. Psychological balance in high level athletes: gender-based differences and sport-specific patterns. PLoS One. 2011;6(5):e19007. doi:10.1371/journal.pone.0019007
54. American Psychiatric Association. *Diagnostic and Statistical Manual of Mental Disorders. Fifth Edition. Text Revision. DSM-5-TR.* American Psychiatric Association Publishing; 2022
55. Rice SM, Gwyther K, Santesteban-Echarri O, et al. Determinants of anxiety in elite athletes: a systematic review and meta-analysis. *Br J Sports Med.* 2019;53(11):722–730. PMID: 31097452
56. Pal S, Kalra S, Awsthi S. Influence of stress and anxiety on sports injuries in athletes. *J Clin Diagn Res.* 2021;15(4):YE01–YE05. https://www.jcdr.net/articles/PDF/14702/45973_CE%5bRa1%5d_F%5bSK%5d_PF1(AG_SL)_PFA(KM)_PB(AG_KM)_PN(KM).pdf
57. Schaal K, Tafflet M, Nassif H, et al. Psychological balance in high level athletes: gender-based differences and sport-specific patterns. *PLoS One.* 2011;6(5):e19007. PMID: 21573222 doi: 10.1371/journal.pone.0019007
58. Nixdorf I, Frank R, Beckmann J. Comparison of athletes' proneness to depressive symptoms in individual and team sports: research on psychological mediators in junior elite athletes. *Front Psychol.* 2016;7:893. PMID: 27378988
59. Powell DH. Treating individuals with debilitating performance anxiety: an introduction. *J Clin Psychol.* 2004;60(8):801–808. PMID: 15241808
60. Leray E, Camara A, Drapier D, et al. Prevalence, characteristics and comorbidities of anxiety disorders in France: results from the "Mental Health in General Population" survey (MHGP). *Eur Psychiatry.* 2011;26(6):339–345. PMID: 20430592 doi: 10.1016/j.eurpsy.2009.12.001
61. Reardon CL, Gorczynski P, Hainline B, Hitchcock M, Rice S. Anxiety disorders in athletes. *Clin Sports Med.* 2024;43(1):33–52. PMID: 37949513
62. Patel DR, Omar H, Terry M. Sport-related performance anxiety in young female athletes. *J Pediatr Adolesc Gynecol.* 2010;23(6):325–335. PMID: 20869282
63. Rocha VVS, Osó rio FdL. Associations between competitive anxiety, athlete characteristics and sport context: evidence from a systematic review and meta-analysis. *Arch Clin Psychiatry.* 2018;45(3):67–74
64. Grove JR, Eklund RC, Heard NP. Coping with performance slumps: factor analysis of the Ways of Coping in Sport Scale. *Aust J Sci Med Sport.* 1997;29(4):99–105. PMID: 9428990

65. Hofmann SG, Gómez AF. Mindfulness-based interventions for anxiety and depression. *Psychiatr Clin North Am.* 2017;40(4):739–749. PMID: 29080597
66. Brenner JS. Mindfulness for young athletes. *Sports Health.* 2024;16(2):300–302. PMID: 37936388 doi:10.1177/19417381231209219
67. Reardon CL, Creado S. Psychiatric medication preferences of sports psychiatrists. *Phys Sportsmed.* 2016;44(4):397–402. PMID: 27463033
68. Chang C, Putukia M, Aerni G, et al. American Medical Society for Sports Medicine Position: mental health issues and psychological factors in athletes: detection, management, effect on performance, and prevention—Executive Summary. 2020;30(2):91–95
69. Greydanus DE, Calles J, Patel DR. *Pediatric and Adolescent Psychopharmacology.* Cambridge University Press; 2008:61–76
70. World Anti-Doping Agency. World Anti-Doping Code International Standard Prohibited List 2026. https://www.wada-ama.org/sites/default/files/2025-09/2026list_en_final_clean_september_2025.pdf
71. Goodman WK, Grice DE, Lapidus KAB, Coffey BJ. Obsessive-compulsive disorder. *Psychiatr Clin North Am.* 2014;37(3):257–267. PMID: 25150561
72. Walitza S, Melfsen S, Jans T, Zellmann H, Wewetzer C, Warnke A. Obsessive-compulsive disorder in children and adolescents. *Dtsch Arztebl Int.* 2011;108(11):173–179. PMID: 21475565 doi: 10.3238/arztebl.2011.0173
73. Carney T, Myers B. Effectiveness of early interventions for substance-using adolescents: findings from a systematic review and meta-analysis. *Subst Abuse Treat Prev Policy.* 2012;7:25. PMID: 22697269 doi:10.1186/1747-597X-7-25
74. National Collegiate Athletic Association. Current findings on student-athlete substance use: NCAA Student-Athlete Health and Wellness Study. 2024. https://ncaaorg.s3.amazonaws.com/research/wellness/Jan2024RES_HW-SubstanceUseRelease.pdf
75. QuickStats: Percentage of children and adolescents aged 5–17 years who had ever received a diagnosis of attention-deficit/hyperactivity disorder, by urbanization level and age group—National Health Interview Survey, United States, 2020–2022. *MMWR Morb Mortal Wkly Rep.* 2024;73(5):116. PMID: 38329910 doi:10.15585/mmwr.mm7305a6
76. Han DH, McDuff D, Thompson D, Hitchcock ME, Reardon CL, Hainline B. Attention-deficit/hyperactivity disorder in elite athletes: a narrative review. *Br J Sports Med.* 2019;53(12):741–745. PMID: 31097459
77. Pujalte GGA, Narducci DM, Smith M, et al. Athletes with attention-deficit/hyperactivity disorder: position statement of the American Medical Society for Sports Medicine. *Clin J Sport Med.* 2023;33(3):195–208. doi:10.1097/JSM.0000000000001152
78. Zhong Y, Chen Y, Su X, et al. Global, regional and national burdens of bipolar disorders in adolescents and young adults: a trend analysis from 1990 to 2019. *Gen Psychiatr.* 2024;37(1):e101255. PMID: 38390238
79. Currie A, McAllister-Williams RH. Bipolar and psychotic disorders. In: Reardon CL, ed. *Mental Health Care for Elite Athletes.* Springer; 2022. doi:10.1007/978-3-031-08364-8_12
80. Kussman A, Choo HJ. Mental health and disordered eating in athletes. *Clin Sports Med.* 2024;43(1):71–91. PMID: 37949515 doi:10.1016/j.csm.2023.07.001
81. Martinsen M, Bahr R, Børresen R, Holme I, Pensgaard AM, Sundgot-Borgen J. Preventing eating disorders among young elite athletes: a randomized controlled trial. *Med Sci Sports Exerc.* 2014;46(3):435–447. PMID: 24549033
82. Thompson A, Petrie T, Tackett B, Balcom K, Watkins CE. Eating disorder diagnosis and the female athlete: a longitudinal analysis from college sport to retirement. *J Sci Med Sport.* 2021;24(6):531–535. PMID: 33423947
83. Watson NF, Badr MS, Belenky G, et al; Consensus Conference Panel. Joint consensus statement of the American Academy of Sleep Medicine and Sleep Research Society on the recommended amount of sleep for a healthy adult: methodology and discussion. *J Clin Sleep Med.* 2015;11(8):931–952. PMID: 26235159 doi:10.5664/jcsm.4950
84. Wojnar M, Ilgen MA, Wojnar J, McCammon RJ, Valenstein M, Brower KJ. Sleep problems and suicidality in the National Comorbidity Survey Replication. *J Psychiatr Res.* 2009;43(5):526–531. PMID: 18778837 doi:10.1016/j.jpsychires.2008.07.006
85. Drew M, Vlahovich N, Hughes D, et al. Prevalence of illness, poor mental health and sleep quality and low energy availability prior to the 2016 Summer Olympic Games. *Br J Sports Med.* 2018;52(1):47–53. PMID: 29056598

86. Paruthi S, Brooks LJ, D'Ambrosio C, et al. Recommended amount of sleep for pediatric populations: a consensus statement of the American Academy of Sleep Medicine. *J Clin Sleep Med.* 2016;12(6):785–786. PMID: 27250809
87. Healthy People 2030. Sleep health objectives. US Department of Health and Human Services. Accessed December 30, 2025. https://odphp.health.gov/healthypeople/objectives-and-data/browse-objectives/sleep
88. Rogers AJ, Xia K, Soe K, et al. Obstructive sleep apnea among players in the National Football League: a scoping review. *J Sleep Disord Ther.* 2017;6(5):278. PMID: 29984115 doi:10.4172/2167-0277.1000278
89. Gray EL, McKenzie DK, Eckert DJ. Obstructive sleep apnea without obesity is common and difficult to treat: evidence for a distinct pathophysiological phenotype. *J Clin Sleep Med.* 2017;13(1):81–88. PMID: 27655455
90. Howarth NE, White AJ, Pearce AJ, et al. Obstructive Sleep Apnea (OSA) and contact sports: a systematic review and meta-analysis. *Sleep Epidemiol.* 2022;2:100036. doi:10.1016/j.sleepe.2022.100036
91. Birrer V, Elgendi M, Lambercy O, Menon C. Evaluating reliability in wearable devices for sleep staging. *NPJ Digit Med.* 2024;7(1):74. PMID: 38499793 doi:10.1038/s41746-024-01016-9

CHAPTER 7

Individuals With Disabilities

Among nonelderly people with disabilities, 25% reported they had difficulty finding a health care professional who understood their disability. Many training and continuing education programs for health care professionals are now focusing on training them to understand disabilities.[1]

The goals of this chapter are to:

- Ensure our professional realm is open to all.
- Demystify caring for individuals with disabilities (IWDs).
- Educate health care providers about how to encourage a lifelong healthy lifestyle for IWDs, which includes participation in physical activity and adaptations needed for such.

Definitions

- *Adaptive sport* refers to any sport modified for IWDs.
- *Para sport* is under the adaptive sport umbrella and refers to sport sponsored by the International Paralympic Committee (IPC) in the Paralympic games. Para athletes are those who participate in Para sport.
- *Unified Sport* refers to a program with Special Olympics that includes participants with and without intellectual disability playing on the same team.

The American Academy of Pediatrics (AAP) book *Bright Futures: Guidelines for Health Supervision of Infants, Children, and Adolescents, 4th edition,* contains a section devoted to promoting physical activity for those with a disability. It includes recommendations for the health care provider to work with IWDs and their families to facilitate engagement in enjoyable activities.[2]

In 1990, the Americans with Disabilities Act (ADA) was passed by the US Congress to protect people with disabilities and stated that disability rights are civil rights. The ADA guarantees that people with disabilities have the same opportunities as everyone else without discrimination.[3] According to 2023 census data, there are over 44.7 million people (13.6%) with disabilities in the United States, which includes those with hearing, vision, cognitive, walking, self-care, or independent living difficulties. Disabilities are present in 6.5% of 5 to 17 year olds, 8.6% of 18 to 34 year olds, and 12.6% of people older than 35 years.[4] The codification of the ADA expanded opportunities for participation in sport and activities for people with a disability.

In the United States, the percentage of public school students who receive special education or related services has increased in recent years. The latest data from 2022 show that 7.3 million students received special education services, 15% of total enrollment, which was an increase from 13% the decade prior.[5] According to the National Federation of State

High School Associations survey data from 2022 to 2023, there were over 8 million participants in high school sports, an increase over previous years. Sixteen states reported adapted sports for boys, and 14 states reported adapted sports for both girls and boys, representing 691,280 (8.6%) of the 8,062,302 total participants. Additionally, there were 70,006 boys and girls in 16 Unified Sports supported by Special Olympics in 2024–2025 according to the National Federation of State High School Associations.[6] In addition, 21 states, as noted on their state high school athletic association website, offered programming for athletes with disabilities. Of these 21 states, 14 only offered programs for athletes with intellectual disabilities, and the majority of these were only provided as Unified Sports.

Special Olympics in North America has more than a half million athletes participating in 32 sports and is dedicated to empowering individuals with intellectual disabilities through its programs.[7] Worldwide, nearly 5.5 million participants (and Unified Sport teammates) representing 176 nations participated in the 2023 Summer World Games in Berlin, Germany.[8]

The International Paralympic Committee (IPC) (https://www.paralympic.org) hosts the Paralympic Games every 4 years at the site of the Olympic summer and winter games. Representation has increased rapidly from the original 16 wheelchair athletes (14 male and 2 female) at the Stoke Mandeville games in 1948 to 4,456 athletes from 170 nations competing in 22 sports and 549 medal events at the Paris Paralympic Games in 2024.[9]

In the United States, there are multiple opportunities for recreational and competitive participation for IWDs, including local programs, organized school programs, adaptive collegiate athletics, Special Olympics, World Deaf games, and Move United (https://moveunitedsport.org). Health care providers must be informed of these opportunities as well as the unique needs of participants. This chapter provides some of this background.

BENEFITS OF SPORTS AND ACTIVITY FOR INDIVIDUALS WITH DISABILITIES

As with individuals without disabilities, the short-term and long-term benefits of exercise to reverse a sedentary lifestyle have been shown to help IWDs feel better, function better, sleep better, and ward off cardiometabolic disease and cancers.[10] (See Table 7-1.) Physical activity and sport participation is even more important for IWDs given that 16% to 62% of those with disabilities are less likely than those without a disability to meet the guidelines established for healthy physical activity.[11] Use of tobacco products is greater in adolescents with disabilities, which compounds the negative impact on their physical health and financial well-being. Thus, the preparticipation evaluation (PPE) provides an opportunity to screen for risky behaviors.[12] Adolescents with a disability have lower levels of fitness, reduced rates of participation, and a higher prevalence of overweight and obesity compared with their peers without disabilities. Furthermore, adults with disabilities are more likely to have obesity, heart disease, stroke, diabetes, or cancer than adults without disabilities.[13] Therefore, the health care provider needs to emphasize screening for these risk factors.

When IWDs participate in activities and sports, there is improved mental health, development of social skills, and disease prevention. There are known benefits of exercise, including aerobic and anaerobic fitness, strength training, and functional/adaptive skills, for IWDs.[11] (See Box 7-1.)

Table 7-1. Benefits of Exercise for Individuals With Disability

Disability	Benefit
Cardiometabolic	
Stroke survivors	Reduced blood pressure and lower cholesterol levels
Spinal cord injury (SCI)	Improved waist circumference and insulin sensitivity
Para athletes in general	Improved peak cardiac output, respiratory function
Strength Training	
Wheelchair athletes	Improved upper body strength measures compared with nonathletes (with or without disability)
SCI	Reduced pain, improved lean muscle mass, and improved lipid profiles
Neurological (cerebral palsy, Parkinson)	Enhanced neurological and structural adaptations for improved muscular strength
Functional and Adaptive Skills	
Limb deficiency, visual and intellectual disability	Coordination, balance, and mobility are improved with aerobic and anaerobic exercise
Intellectual disability	The ability to learn and adaptive skills (communication skills, personal care, and ability to follow rules and routines) are improved with participation in sport

Derived from Fagher K, DeLuca S, Derman W, Blauwet C. Optimising health equity through para sport. *Br J Sports Med.* 2023;57(3):131–132. doi:10.1136/bjsports-2022-106229

Box 7-1. Benefits, Barriers, and Considerations for Participation in Sports by Individuals With Disabilities

Benefits of Participation

- Improved wellness
- Increased community integration
- Improved muscle strength
- Improved fundamental movement skills
- Enhanced psychosocial well-being
- Increased cardiorespiratory fitness
- Decreased morbidity (eg, pressure ulcers, infections, overweight and obesity)
- Improved bone health
- Improved motor coordination
- Improved attention and focus
- Decreased maladaptive behaviors

(*continued*)

Box 7-1. Benefits, Barriers, and Considerations for Participation in Sports by Individuals With Disabilities *(continued)*

Barriers to Participation
- False belief: no programs for this population
- False belief: participation is unsafe or too risky
- False belief: rules of sports too hard to learn or cannot be adapted to accommodate IWD
- Low physical literacy
- Lack of transportation to and from activities
- Lack of needed supervision or expertise
- Extra cost and time commitment

Facilitators to Participation
- Preparticipation evaluations to maximize safety with appropriate accommodations
- Organized sports that are focused on fun over competition
- Clinicians, physical education teachers, and coaches who create physical activity prescriptions and recognize individual needs
- Adaptations such as longer rest periods, lower coach-to-athlete ratios, copious positive feedback, and close monitoring for symptoms of fatigue or injury

Reproduced from Carbone PS, Smith PJ, Lewis C, et al; AAP Council on Children with Disabilities, Council on Sports Medicine and Fitness. Promoting the participation of children and adolescents with disabilities in sports, recreation, and physical activity. *Pediatrics*. 2021;148(6):e2021054664. doi:10.1542/peds.2021-054664

There are also established benefits for IWDs who engage in sport compared with those who do not. Athletes with paraplegia have fewer pressure ulcers and infections and a lower likelihood of hospitalization. Also, athletes with limb deficiencies have improved proprioception and increased proficiency using their prosthetic device.[14]

We know there is a problem persuading more IWDs to exercise and participate in activities, and we know the benefits of being active. However, many real barriers remain in accomplishing this goal. USA Soccer identified the following barriers to sport and exercise for those with disabilities[15]:

- Some young athletes with a disability may start in a youth recreation league with kids their own age without a disability. However, typically around puberty, many of these athletes do not continue to compete at the same level and, without any other competitive leagues to join, drop out of sport completely.
- Adaptive equipment for athletes with a disability can be costly or difficult to find.
- Public school interscholastic athletic programs exclusively for youth with disabilities are scarce.
- Athlete role models for athletes with disability are not as widely popularized in the US media.
- Physicians are less likely to counsel IWDs about the importance of exercise.
- Access to coaches and fitness experts who are skilled at advising an athlete with a disability can be difficult to obtain.

There are many barriers to participation in activities for those with disabilities that are far beyond the functional disability. Examples include negative self-perception and self-esteem; social barriers such as negative stereotypes, implicit biases, and unrealistic expectations for competition outcomes versus having fun; few to no opportunities at school or in the community; and cost of obtaining and maintaining adaptive equipment and prosthetics. Finally, there is a financial burden related to transportation, physical access, and equipment.[16]

The Special Olympics Healthy Athletes initiative offers free health screening and health education to Special Olympics athletes to improve the health care of those with intellectual disabilities. This initiative also trains health care professionals to treat people with intellectual disabilities.[17]

DISABILITIES DEFINED

Disabilities are defined for sport participation according to classification systems that attempt to allow for fair competition among all participants. These classification systems focus on the functional impact on the person's ability to participate in a particular sport due to a participant's eligible impairment secondary to their medical condition.

There is a distinction between an eligible disability and a health condition that is not considered an eligible disability, such as a condition that causes pain, fatigue, psychological conditions (eg, posttraumatic stress disorder), or hypermobility such as Ehlers-Danlos syndrome. The IPC recognizes 10 impairment types for eligibility for Para sport. The following is a summary of those definitions.[18]

- **Visual impairment** includes reduced vision or absent vision due to abnormalities of the eyes, visual pathways, and/or visual cortex, which can affect central or peripheral vision.
- **Intellectual impairment** is a restriction in intellectual functioning and adaptive behavior that affects conceptual, social, and practical adaptive skills needed for everyday life and must be present before the age of 18 years. Intellectual impairment includes cognitive and developmental conditions (autism spectrum is included).
- **Physical impairment**
  - **Impaired muscle power** reduces or eliminates the ability to voluntarily contract muscles to move or generate a force. Examples include spinal cord injury (SCI), muscular dystrophy, postpolio syndrome, and spina bifida.
  - **Impaired passive range of motion** involves a restriction or lack of passive movement in 1 or more joint(s). Examples include arthrogryposis, chronic joint immobilization, and trauma.
  - **Hypertonia** is an increase in muscle tension and reduced ability of a muscle to stretch owing to pathology involving the central nervous system. Examples include cerebral palsy, traumatic brain injury, and stroke.
  - **Ataxia** is an uncoordinated movement due to damage to the central nervous system. Examples include cerebral palsy, traumatic brain injury, stroke, and multiple sclerosis.
  - **Athetosis** involves continued slow involuntary movements. Examples include cerebral palsy, traumatic brain injury, and stroke.
  - **Limb difference** is a total or partial absence of bones or joints, such as from trauma, illness, or congenital limb difference.
  - **Leg length differences** are unequal lengths of the right and left legs. Examples include disturbance of limb growth that is developmental or results from trauma.

— **Short stature** is a reduced length in bones of upper limbs, lower limbs, and/or trunk. Examples include achondroplasia, growth hormone dysfunction, and osteogenesis imperfecta.

Hearing loss is not a recognized disability for Para sport by the IPC (see section on Governing Associations for IWD Sports). In deaf sports, all participants' needs are met and all participants have full access to communication. Deaf sport organizations provide opportunities for athletes with hearing loss to compete among their peers at recreational, amateur, or master levels. Deaf athletes benefit from adaptations that are specific to their needs, such as the use of a light flashing system instead of starting guns or buzzers and having officials use hand signals and flags instead of whistles. Full access to communication is also a critical factor in the success of any athlete.[19]

It is important to note that the formal definitions of disability for organized sport participation are stressed here. Health care providers should be advocating for opportunities for participation in activities for any IWD. The ADA definition of disability is a legal definition, not a medical definition, and encompasses many more disabilities than those of sporting organizations. For example, some learning disabilities and medical conditions affecting the cardiopulmonary system and metabolic system are not eligible disabilities for organized sport organizations. All IWDs should be encouraged to safely be active and participate in activities and sport. Health care providers should advocate for and facilitate this participation.

GOVERNING ASSOCIATIONS FOR IWD SPORTS

Most sport organizations for IWDs have governing bodies with oversight that serve to encourage, organize, and provide safe and fun opportunities for participants. Many organizations serve this purpose, from organizing the Paralympics to creating sporting opportunities such as Unified Sport, which partners people with and without intellectual disabilities on the same team. These organizations also serve as the governing body for official classification of IWDs for sport competition (see section on Classification of Individuals With Disabilities for Sport).

The first organized competition for IWDs occurred in 1948 at the Stoke Mandeville Games—coinciding with the 1948 London Olympics—and led to the creation of the International Sport Organization for the Disabled (ISOD) in 1960. The following is a general description of how these events progressed to the current oversight of sports for IWDs.

- ISOD expanded participation to individuals with vision impairment, amputees, individuals with cerebral palsy, and paraplegics. Initial membership included 16 countries.
- In 1982, the International Olympic Committee established the International Coordination Committee (ICC) of World Sport Organizations for the Disabled as a single governing body representing ISOD, Cerebral Palsy International Sports and Recreation Association (CPISRA), International Blind Sports Federation (IBSA), and International Stoke Mandeville Games Federation.
- These organizations were joined by the International Committee of Sport for the Deaf (ICSD) and the International Sports Federations for Persons with an Intellectual Disability in 1986.
- In 1989, the IPC replaced the ICC to oversee the Paralympic games in partnership with the International Olympic Committee.[20]

- Appendix A provides a listing of the sports currently offered by the oversight organizations: IPC, Special Olympics, Deaflympics, and the visually impaired sports (Virtus).
- The IPC recognizes 3 international organizations for sports for the disabled:
  - —IBSA for football, goalball, and judo
  - —Virtus, International Sports Federation for athletes with intellectual impairment (eg, autism, Down syndrome)
  - —World Ability Sport combined the International Wheelchair & Amputee Sports Federation and CPISRA[21]

Also, in the United States, Move United oversees opportunities for adaptive sports including the Wounded Warfighters to provide sports for severely wounded warriors.[22]

Special Olympics is a distinct entity that is a global sports movement to end discrimination against people with intellectual disabilities. Special Olympics supports 32 sports and over 50,000 competitions with more than 4 million athletes worldwide. It is open to all people with intellectual disabilities older than 8 years. Special Olympics does not use a classification system, but rather relies on "divisioning," which allows competition based on similar age, gender, and grouping within 15% of like performance levels between participants to encourage safe and fun participation.[23] Special Olympics also advocates for Unified Sport, which allows participants with and without intellectual disability to compete on the same teams. Unified Sport is popular in US high schools.

Since 1924, the ICSD has overseen the Deaflympics and is recognized by the IOC as an international federation with Olympic standing. However, the ICSD is not involved with the IPC. Advocates for deaf sports note that all needs are met and participants do not consider themselves to have a disability; rather, they have hearing loss. There are 2 recognized avenues for those with hearing loss to compete: the Olympics as they are or the Deaflympics, which has adaptations that are specific to their needs.[24]

CLASSIFICATION OF INDIVIDUALS WITH DISABILITIES FOR SPORTS

For the health care provider, working with an IWD is an opportunity to encourage activity and athletic participation and to more deeply explore their gifts and limitations to help them become or stay active. The PPE for IWDs has many similarities to the standard PPE outlined in this book; however, there are variances that should be addressed with a person with a disability. The PPE should serve as an opportunity to educate the IWD on strategies to prevent injury and illness with their training and competition. For example, for an individual with a prosthesis, part of the PPE should include evaluation of the prosthesis and fit, as well as preventive measures to prevent skin problems at the prosthesis-skin interface. A skilled physiatrist and/or prosthetist should be part of the evaluation and treatment team. IWDs who engage in organized competitions often need to be cleared for sport and classified according to their disability. Classification systems are overseen by the sport's governing body. Many are highly detailed and include a functional assessment of the athlete participating in their sport. But there are certain common frameworks with which the health care provider should be familiar.

Most national and international governing bodies use similar classification forms. All require an in-depth review of the individual's medical history, type of disability, the impact of the disability on their activities of daily living and sport, as well as any specific accommodations needed for participation. Most classification systems rely on the most significant disability if more than one is present (an athlete cannot participate in more than one sport classification). Keep in mind that a similar disability type can involve significant variation in function. For example, there can be many different functional outcomes for a disability to the same spinal cord level or the precise location of an amputation (eg, above-the-knee vs below-the-knee). Also, an impairment must be severe enough to impact the individual's sport performance; this is referred to as the "Minimum Impairment Criteria," which must be met for an athlete to compete in that sport. See Appendix B at the end of this chapter for links to several National Governing Bodies' screening clearance forms. It is important to note some unique applications.

The process starts with an Athlete Evaluation, which documents if the athlete has an eligible impairment for the sport. If so, does it meet the Minimum Impairment Criteria for that sport (see the 10 disabilities defined earlier)?

- Classifiers can be medical or technical, as determined by the rules of each sport and organization.
- *Medical* classifiers should be certified health professionals in a field relevant to the impairment (eg, medical doctor, physical therapist).
- *Technical* classifiers must have extensive background in and knowledge of impairments and activity limitations associated with the sport (eg, coaches, former athletes, individuals with a degree in physical education, biomechanics, or kinesiology).

Technical and medical classifiers are grouped together to form eligibility assessment committees to determine an athlete's sport class.[25]

- If one would like to become a classifier for the US Olympic & Paralympic Committee (USOPC), see https://www.usopc.org/become-a-parlaympic-classifier.
- For Paralympic sports managed by other organizations and federations, individuals should check their National Governing Bodies' websites.
- Note that Paralympic classifiers must be trained and certified domestically. After gaining experience as a classifier, they may apply to be an international classifier.

Special Olympics requires additional mention. Anyone older than 8 years with an intellectual disability is eligible for participation. For all local events, athletes must have completed a health history form by the time of registration; for regional/international events, a medical clearance form (in Appendix B) must be completed by a medical professional within 12 months of the games.[26]

SPECIAL HEALTH CONSIDERATIONS FOR THE PPE

The PPE for an athlete with a disability should be similar to that for an individual without disabilities, but extra attention should address the unique needs pertaining to the specific disability. The health care professional should be aware of common problems associated with different disabilities and be able to identify and help manage conditions that may compromise athletes' safety. Just as important, the health care professional should encourage physical activity and provide support as needed. As with a PPE for individuals without disabilities, it is important to perform the evaluation for IWDs at least 6 weeks prior to the deadline to coordinate consultations with specialists (eg, physiatrist, neurologists, cardiologist, orthotists, and prosthetists).

In addition to the usual recommendations for screening during a PPE, there are specific areas to focus on for IWDs. (See Table 7-2 and Table 7-3.)

Table 7-2. Issues in IWDs Associated With Organ Systems

Common Organ Systems With Associated Issues in IWDs	Common Signs/Symptoms or Issues to Screen
Cardiovascular	• Heart disease: electrocardiogram, echocardiograph • Hypertension
Dermatologic	• Abrasions • Blisters • Lacerations • Pressure ulcers • Rashes
Musculoskeletal	• Atlantoaxial instability signs • Decreased flexibility +/- contractures • Limited range of motion • Muscle strength: imbalance, decreased • Pelvic dysfunction due to limb deficiency or length discrepancies, impact of prosthetic devices • Shoulder: rotator cuff tendinitis, impingement • Torticollis
Neurological	• Ataxia • Atlantoaxial instability signs • Baclofen pump malfunction • Clonus • Hyperreflexia • Impaired hand-eye coordination • Inadequate motor control • Inadequate coordination and balance • Peripheral neuropathies (sensory dysfunction, muscle weakness) • Seizure • Shunt malfunction • Spasticity • Spinal cord syrinx • Tethered spinal cord • Upper motor neuron and posterior column involvement • Withdrawal or overdose from medications
Ocular	• Abnormalities in ocular appearance • Decreased visual acuity • Ocular health • Strabismus
Urological	• Bladder control • Catheterization required • Recurrent urinary tract infections

Derived from Slocum C, Blauwet CA, Allen JBA. Sports medicine considerations for the paralympic athlete. *Curr Phys Med Rehabil Rep.* 2015;3:25–35.

Table 7-3. Musculoskeletal Conditions Associated With Individual Disabilities

Disability	Condition	Injuries	Comments
Central neurological injury	Cerebral palsy Stroke TBI	Decreased range of motion and spasticity can lead to muscle strains and overuse injuries Premature osteoporosis and osteopenia	Because of reduced weight-bearing load, patients with SCI may experience premature osteoporosis and osteopenia below the level of the injury Oral antispasticity medications are not banned from competition but may alter sport classification
Limb difference	Amputation	Injuries to ligaments and tendons (both limbs residual and prosthetic) Overuse to contralateral limb, including osteoarthritis Skin breakdown	The prosthetic interface with residual limb poses potential problems
Wheelchair	Lower-extremity amputations, neuromuscular disorders SCI Spina bifida	Overuse/repetitive use (subacromial impingement) Carpal tunnel syndrome Ulnar nerve entrapment (wrist and/or elbow)	Important to evaluate the wheelchair for performance: seat position and height, conditioning of athlete, rear wheel camber and size, hand-rim configurations, material and construction of chair
Vison impaired	—	Injuries to lower extremities (tendinopathies, spasm, strains) Injuries to head, concussion: football Swimming: overuse to upper extremities and upper limbs	Often accompanied by sighted guides, use of blindfolds, and/or spotter goalkeepers

Abbreviations: SCI, spinal cord injury; TBI, traumatic brain injury.

Derived from Slocum C, Blauwet CA, Allen JBA. Sports medicine considerations for the Paralympic athlete. *Curr Phys Med Rehabil Rep.* 2015;3:25–35.

Ocular function. There is a high prevalence of vision abnormalities among Special Olympics athletes. A study at the 1995 International Summer Games revealed that almost one-third of the athletes had ocular problems.[27] The most common problems identified were poor visual acuity, refractive errors, astigmatism, and strabismus.

Cardiovascular system. Congenital heart disease is present in as many as 50% of children with Down syndrome who participate in sports, although most of these conditions are present at birth and should be screened for at that time.[28] In a study of Paralympic athletes, 12% had structural cardiovascular abnormalities and major tachyarrhythmias versus 1% to 2% in Olympic athletes who did not have a disability.[29] Most of these abnormalities were suggested by history and confirmed by electrocardiography and echocardiography. Also, a disproportionate number of Para athletes had systemic hypertension, which may require more frequent screening and observation. Medical eligibility decisions should take into consideration cardiac risk, and the clinician should provide precautions for safe sport participation.

Neurological function. Since many athletes with physical impairments may also have some form of neurological deficit, a complete neurological evaluation should be performed.

Peripheral nerve entrapment syndromes of the upper extremities are common in athletes who use wheelchairs. Two of the most common entrapment syndromes are carpal tunnel syndrome and ulnar neuropathy at the wrist (Guyon canal syndrome). The examiner should look for signs of muscle atrophy and weakness in the hand, test for sensory deficits associated with a specific nerve distribution, and perform provocative tests for nerve impairment, such as Tinel sign over the median nerve in the wrist or ulnar nerve in the elbow.

Individuals with **autism spectrum disorder** often have motor clumsiness and apraxia, placing them at increased risk for injuries when participating in sports.[30]

People with **cerebral palsy** frequently have difficulties with motor control, hand-eye coordination, and balance that can increase injury risk and affect their participation in certain sports. Evaluating these functions will reveal whether sports that require catching, throwing, and controlling equipment such as floor hockey sticks, rackets, and bats may be difficult for the athlete. Accommodation should be considered for athletes with functional deficits that may pose a risk to the athlete or their competitors.

Athletes with **multiple sclerosis** have varying degrees of disability. The health care provider should check for ataxia, muscle weakness, fatigue, spasticity, and sensory dysfunction.

Approximately 15% of children with Down syndrome have **atlantoaxial instability (AAI)**, although most are asymptomatic.[31] A very small number of these children develop signs and symptoms of cervical myelopathy. The neurological manifestations of symptomatic AAI include easy fatigue, abnormal gait, incoordination and clumsiness, sensory deficits, spasticity, hyperreflexia, clonus, and other upper motor neuron and posterior column signs and symptoms. Other people at increased risk for AAI include those who have rheumatoid arthritis, achondroplastic dwarfism (most common type of skeletal dysplasia), and Klippel-Feil syndrome (abnormal fusion of 2 cervical vertebrae).[32] Children with skeletal dysplasia often have associated cervical spine instability with the danger of spinal cord compression.[33] General screening must include a history and physical examination with a focus on the neurological assessment. Three key questions address AAI,[34] and if the answers are all "no," further assessment and restrictions are generally not needed: (1) Does the person show evidence of progressive myopathy? (2) Does the person have poor head/neck muscular control? and (3) Does the person's neck flexion allow the chin to rest on their chest?

Autonomic dysreflexia (AD) is an acute, potentially life-threatening syndrome of excessive, unregulated sympathetic output that can occur in people with SCIs at or above the sixth thoracic (T6) spinal cord level.[35] AD can occur in up to 90% of high thoracic or cervical SCI.[36] This condition may occur spontaneously or may be self-induced by an athlete ("boosting") (see next paragraph) to improve performance.[37,38] Spontaneous autonomic dysreflexia can be triggered by any irritant below the level of cord injury, including irritation or distention of the bladder wall, a urinary tract infection (UTI), and blocked catheter or overfilled collection bag; distended or irritated bowel, constipation or impaction, and hemorrhoids or anal infections; other infections; sunburn; pressure ulcers; ingrown toenails; and even menstrual cramps. Signs and symptoms of autonomic dysreflexia include excessively high blood pressure, bradycardia, pounding headache, blurred vision, sweating and flushing of the skin above the level of the spinal injury, and pale, cool clammy skin and piloerection (goose bumps) below the level of the SCI. Treatment initially includes sitting the individual upright and identifying the offending stimulus. Nifedipine is commonly used.

Boosting is an intentional self-induced AD to attempt to improve athletic performance (eg, overdistending the bladder [clamped catheter], sitting on sharp objects, overly tightening leg straps). The IPC bans boosting and has implemented a screening protocol for competition.[36]

Thermoregulation in people with SCIs can be impaired because of skeletal muscle paralysis (impaired shivering and reduced ability to produce heat) and a loss of autonomic nervous system control (impaired sweating and vasodilation to dissipate heat).[39] Impaired autonomic function can lead to decreased sweating and improper feedback from levels below the injury that are insensate. Some patients with cerebral palsy have hypothalamic dysfunction adversely affecting thermoregulation. Additionally, medications used for pain and bladder dysfunction can interfere with the normal sweating response. Also, athletes who have a history of heat illness are at greater risk of developing the condition again. Athletes with impaired thermoregulation should take extra precautions when training and competing in cold and hot conditions.[36]

Urogenital system. Examinations should involve the same evaluation as that for individuals who do not have a disability (see Chapter 5E). It is also important to examine any external devices used for bladder drainage. IWDs with SCI are predisposed to UTIs because of catheter use, incomplete voiding, and/or elevated intravesicular pressures. Further, symptoms of a UTI often present more subtly, with an increase in spasticity, fatigue, and fever. Often, individuals with SCI may be very aware of their genitourinary tract and have a sense of an impending UTI. Treatment for UTIs in those with SCI often consists of a 10- to 14-day course of antibiotics to adequately treat the infection and avoid partial treatment leading to resistance.

Bowel system. Attention to bowel symptoms is important. For some IWDs, dealing with incontinence may limit participation, and difficulty adequately evacuating bowel may adversely affect their competition.[36]

Dermatologic function. Athletes who use wheelchairs are especially prone to skin injuries. The upper extremities should be examined for abrasions and blisters caused by friction, shear, or irritation from repeated contact with the wheelchair push rim. Skin wounds can also result from contact with other chairs, wheelchair brakes, or sharp edges of the wheelchair.

The skin over the sacrum and ischial tuberosities should be inspected for pressure ulcers. Athletes using wheelchairs have elevated skin pressures in these regions for prolonged periods during training and competition, and if using wheelchairs for mobility, during normal daily activity. Sports wheelchairs are designed so that the athlete's knees are at a higher level than the buttocks, a position that leads to even more pressure over the sacrum and ischial tuberosities.[36] During sports participation, the combination of skin pressure, shear, and moisture increases the risk of pressure ulcers. An athlete using a wheelchair who has a pressure ulcer should be followed up closely to ensure healing of the wound. If wound healing is delayed or worsened by participation, medical eligibility should be rescinded until the skin is improving. The seat cushion should also be evaluated and modified to decrease skin pressures, improve skin healing, and reduce the risk of further skin trauma.

Prosthetic devices can cause skin trauma; thus, the prosthesis contact site should be inspected for abrasions, blisters, rashes, or pressure ulcers. The prosthesis should be evaluated for proper fit and reevaluated periodically to decrease the risk of future problems. Pressure ulcers may preclude full participation in sports until the condition is resolved or the prosthetic device is properly reconditioned and fitted to the athlete. In a skeletally immature individual, overgrowth of the stump can be a problem, leading to breakdown of the overlying skin and soft tissues.[40]

Musculoskeletal system. The musculoskeletal examination of an individual who uses a wheelchair should include evaluation of the stability, flexibility, and strength of commonly injured sites (eg, shoulder, hand, and wrist) and the trunk.[14]

Individuals with lower-limb amputation and prostheses require a full assessment of the lower back, pelvis, and lower extremities, and those with upper-limb amputation and prosthetic devices require a full assessment of the upper back, shoulder girdle, and upper extremities. Abnormal forces and motions placed onto the upper and lower extremities by prosthetic devices during sports activities commonly result in injury to these areas.

Athletes with musculoskeletal manifestations of AAI may develop either limited range of motion of the neck or torticollis (head tilt) (see Special Olympics below for discussion of screening for AAI). People with Down syndrome are often hypermobile with ligamentous laxity, and participating in sports increases the incidence of hip and knee injuries.[28] Examination may reveal signs of instability, coordination problems, or sensory deficits, or upper motor neuron findings and weakness. Exercise performance may be negatively affected by skeletal characteristics such as short stature and short limbs.[41]

As many as 78% of people with SCIs who use wheelchairs report experiencing shoulder pain at some time. Shoulder pain is more commonly reported by people using wheelchairs who are not involved in sports compared with athletes who use wheelchairs.[42]

Athletes with cerebral palsy have decreased strength, decreased musculotendinous flexibility (often with contractures), and muscle strength imbalances, especially of the lower extremities. These conditions vary in severity from mild and nearly imperceptible to very severe and requiring wheelchair use.[43] Overuse injuries, strains, and sprains are common, especially at the hips, knees, ankles, and feet. The PPE should include a thorough examination of these regions.

Functional assessment. An individualized functional assessment of all athletes with physical disabilities should be part of the PPE. An athlete's overall mobility—including during sport-specific tasks—while using prosthetic, orthotic, assistive, or adaptive devices should be evaluated by a provider with the necessary skills. A physical therapist or physiatrist with expertise in the area can perform this portion of the assessment.

Diagnostic studies. Diagnostic studies should be ordered based on the individual's medical history and physical examination findings that could put them at higher risk if competing. Refer to the section on Special Olympics for discussion of screening for AAI.

PREPARTICIPATION EVALUATION

Attention to the specific medical conditions that may be unique to IWDs results in the need for a more detailed and thorough PPE. It is important to establish a baseline of health at this examination, which is most important for assessing future injury or complications.[44] As noted earlier, this examination can be extremely useful for identifying areas in which early intervention can help optimize lifestyle and sporting activity. Providers may want to focus more attention on the following areas. See Appendix B at the end of this chapter for PPE forms and links.

Expanded Health History

- Define and document the individual's disability and impairments (note they may already have been formally classified).
- List competitive sports in which the individual participates.
- Date of the diagnosis
- The specific diagnosis (eg, SCI at what level; amputee, indicate the affected limb[s])
- Note any change in the individual's condition over time, and explain.
- Are there any other medical conditions?
- Treatments for their condition
- Surgical procedures
- Previous injuries
- Medications (note, for athletes competing in Paralympics, ensure compliance with the World Anti-Doping Agency and document any need for a Therapeutic Use Exemption)
- An additional 10 questions specific to IWDs have been recommended (see Table 7-4).
- Musculoskeletal questions are presented in Table 7-5, and limits to functional capacity are shown in Table 7-6.
- See Table 7-7 for musculoskeletal conditions associated with specific functional impairments.

Table 7-4. Special Health History Questions for IWDs

Further Medical Review	Yes	No
I. Have you ever had abnormal bowel or bladder control?		
II. Have you had problems with recurrent urinary tract infections?		
III. Are you concerned about recent bladder disturbances, including pain or bleeding?		
IV. Do you limit or carefully control what you eat or drink?		
V. Have you had pulmonary function tests? (if so, please specify the reason)		
VI. Do you have a history of recurrent skin wounds or pressure sores?		
VII. Have you been hospitalized for issues surrounding skin breakdown?		
VIII. Have you ever had unusual blood clotting, such as prolonged bleeding, deep vein thrombosis, or a pulmonary embolism?		
IX. Do you have any vision problems such as reduced vision in one or both eyes including legal blindness, need for glasses, eye crossing or drifting, and/or a history of eye surgery?		
X. For participant with SCI: Do you have a condition called autonomic dysreflexia?		

Adapted from Hawkeswood JP, O'Connor R, Anton H, Finlayson H. The preparticipation evaluation for athletes with disability. *Int J Sports Phys Ther.* 2014;9(1):103–115. PMC3924614

Table 7-5. Special Musculoskeletal History Questions for IWDs

Musculoskeletal History	Yes	No
a. Have you ever been told you have osteoporosis/osteopenia or low bone density?		
b. Have you ever had a stress fracture or a broken bone from a low-impact trauma?		
c. Have you ever taken prednisone for greater than a one week period?		
d. Do you currently have any metal in your body as a result of a bone surgery?		

Reproduced from Hawkeswood JP, O'Connor R, Anton H, Finlayson H. The preparticipation evaluation for athletes with disability. *Int J Sports Phys Ther.* 2014;9(1):103–115. PMC3924614

Table 7-6. Functional Review

Please circle major categories of limitation or difficulty due to the diagnosis.			
Mobility	**Independent**	**Cane/Walker**	**Wheelchair**
Transfers	Independent	Sliding board	Assist
Hygiene	Independent	Independent with modifications	Assist
Dressing upper body	Independent	Independent with modifications	Assist
Dressing lower body	Independent	Independent with modifications	Assist
Eating/drinking	Independent	Independent with modifications	Assist
Bowel care	Normal function	Modified routine (specify):	Assist
Bladder care	Normal function	Modified routine (specify):	Assist

Reproduced from Hawkeswood JP, O'Connor R, Anton H, Finlayson H. The preparticipation evaluation for athletes with disability. *Int J Sports Phys Ther.* 2014;9(1):103–115. PMC3924614

Table 7-7. Musculoskeletal Conditions Associated With Functional Impairments

Function	Common Conditions	Common Musculoskeletal Injuries	Comments
Primarily mobilizes via wheelchair	SCI, spina bifida, lower-extremity amputations, neuromuscular disorders	Overuse/repetitive use (subacromial impingement), carpal tunnel syndrome, ulnar nerve entrapment (wrist and/or elbow), skin breakdown	• Important to evaluate the wheelchair for performance: seat position and height, conditioning of athlete, rear wheel camber and size, hand-rim configurations, material and construction of chair • Evaluate ADLs and home environment/setup as this can increase the risk of overuse.
Primarily ambulates with prosthesis for mobility	Amputation/limb difference	Injuries to ligaments and tendons (both limbs residual and prosthetic); overuse to contralateral limb, including osteoarthritis; bony overgrowth in skeletally immature athletes; skin breakdown	• The prosthetic interface with residual limb poses potential problems.

Table 7-7. Musculoskeletal Conditions Associated With Functional Impairments (*continued*)

Function	Common Conditions	Common Musculoskeletal Injuries	Comments
All modes of mobility	Stroke, TBI, cerebral palsy, SCI	Decreased range of motion and spasticity can lead to muscle strains and overuse injuries; premature osteoporosis and osteopenia (especially in IWDs who have decreased ambulation/weight-bearing)	• Because of reduced weight-bearing load, patients with SCI may experience premature osteoporosis and osteopenia below the level of the injury. • Most oral antispasticity medications are not banned from competition (check each medication with antidoping databases) but may alter sport classification.
Vison impaired	—	Injuries to lower extremities (tendinopathies, spasm, strains); injuries to head, concussion–football; contusions or fractures due to impact into objects/other people they didn't see or impaired proprioception	• Ask athlete what their preferred assistance methods are (eg, sighted guide, cane, mobile apps, other methods). • Some sports require blindfolds, blacked-out goggles, and/or spotter goalkeepers.

Abbreviations: ADL, activities of daily living; IWD, individual with disability; SCI, spinal cord injury; TBI, traumatic brain injury.

Review of Any Adaptive Equipment

- Wheelchair: For activities of daily living and for performance. Review the seat position and height, rear wheel camber and size, any hand-rim configurations, the material and construction of the chair, and the overall condition.
- Prosthesis: Review what the individual uses for activities of daily living and for performance. Have there been any problems with fit (skin, pain, injury) or use, or any recent changes? Does the individual have a prosthetist/orthotist?

CONCUSSION IN IWDS

One should consider additional baseline testing to facilitate evaluation and treatment for concussion. Following current recommendations for evaluating concussion (eg, SCAT6) is helpful but not validated or appropriate for many athletes with a disability who have a sport-related concussion (see Table 7-8). As of the time of this book's publication, a working group known as the Para SCAT6-WC initiative intends "to develop a modified SCAT6 for athletes who use WCs as their primary means of mobility and then validate and establish the reliability and clinical utility of that tool." This offers the prospect of helpful evidence-based guidelines to improve the assessment and management of concussion in the Para sport population.[45]

Table 7-8. Examples of Issues Applying Current Concussion Evaluation Guidelines to IWDs

Condition	Issue With Evaluation
Limb difference	• Balance • Gait
Visual impairment	• May be unable to report vision issues (double vision, may not present with a "blank stare"
Intellectual impairment	• May have difficulty following commands or reporting symptoms • Neurocognitive testing • Reliability and repeatability of testing may suffer
Neuromuscular impairment	• Strength • Gait • Balance • Reflexes
Spinal cord injury	• Balance • Gait
Comorbid	• Many conditions overlap

Several key points are important for the evaluation and treatment of concussion in IWDs.[46]

- Perform a PPE and review any disabilities noted.
- Execute an evaluation tailored to the athlete with a disability to document a true baseline for function, symptoms (they may be described differently), balance, gait, and neurocognitive function.
- Engage a caregiver or another individual who is familiar with the IWD as part of the baseline evaluation (and concussion evaluation) to assist in tailoring the exam to the individual.

- If the athlete is concussed, a person medically familiar with the IWD should be part of the decision-making process for treatment and return to sport.
- For those with SCI, consider an alternative balance testing system, both for the baseline evaluation and for postconcussion: the Wheelchair Error Scoring System (WESS),[47] a proposed balance testing system for wheelchair athletes using 6 conditions tested (3 each with eyes open and closed). See Appendix C at the end of this chapter for a detailed explanation.

SPECIAL OLYMPICS

Under the umbrella of Special Olympics, many athletes may have a range of conditions that lead to qualification for participation. These include syndromes such as Apert, Down, fetal alcohol, fragile X, Prader-Willi, phenylketonuria, Williams, and cerebral palsy. Other health problems can coexist with these syndromes (see Box 7-2), and the health care provider should be aware of them.[48]

Box 7-2. Other Health Problems Seen With Special Olympic Participants

- AAI (atlantoaxial instability)
- Abnormal facies
- Dental problems
- Developmental disorders
- Diabetes
- Gait abnormalities
- Hearing and speech problems
- Hypertension
- Mood disorders, attention-deficit/hyperactivity disorder
- Obesity
- Seizure disorder
- Short stature
- Vision problems
- Skin (hypopigmentation, eczema, looseness)
- Congenital defects of extremities (webbing, fusion, undeveloped)
- Cardiac abnormalities (supravalvular aortic stenosis, mitral valve prolapse, ventricular septal defect)
- Musculoskeletal issues (tight muscles and joints, contractures, myoclonus, spasticity, joint laxity, scoliosis, postural problems

Atlantoaxial instability (AAI) deserves special attention. Any individual with Down syndrome needs to be screened for AAI, instability between C1 and C2 in the neck that can occur in up to 15% of individuals. Those with symptomatic AAI may have symptoms of fatigue, gait abnormalities, neck pain, limited neck range of motion, alterations in their coordination, spasticity, hyperreflexia, and clonus. If the answer to any of the following 3 questions is "yes," further assessment is required by a physician: (1) Does the individual show evidence of progressive myopathy, (2) Does the individual have poor head/neck control, and (3) Does the individual's neck flexion allow the chin to rest on their chest? Further, anyone diagnosed with AAI is restricted from participation until (1) the individual has been examined (including full flexion and extension radiographic views of the C-spine including C1-C2) and noted not to have AAI; and (2) the examining physician must notify the athlete and parents/guardians of the diagnosis, and they will be required to obtain written certifications from 2 physicians on Special Olympic forms, with acknowledgement of risks signed by an adult athlete or their parent/guardian if a minor.[49]

If the answer to any of the following 3 questions are "yes," further assessment is required by a physician: (1) Does the individual show evidence of progressive myopathy? (2) Does the individual have poor head/neck control? and (3) Does the individual's neck flexion allow the chin to rest on their chest? Further, anyone diagnosed with AAI is restricted from participation until (1) the individual has been examined (including full flexion and extension radiographic views of the C-spine including C1-C2) and noted not to have AAI; and (2) the examining physician must notify the athlete and parents/guardians of the diagnosis, and they will be required to obtain written certifications from 2 physicians on Special Olympic forms, with acknowledgement of risks signed by an adult athlete or their parent/guardian if a minor.

If further assessment is required, the following sports are restricted until the individual is cleared:

- Butterfly stroke and diving starts in swimming
- Diving
- Pentathlon
- High jump
- Equestrian sports
- Artistic gymnastics
- Football
- Alpine skiing
- Any warm-up exercise placing undue stress on the head and neck[50]

CONCLUSION

As health care professionals who evaluate and prepare individuals to be active and compete in sport and play, we are the gatekeepers for these opportunities. With a small amount of preparation, as well as additional knowledge and time, we can be the beacons of inclusion for IWDs. We have an opportunity to ensure our offices and examination rooms are welcoming to all individuals, especially those with disabilities. We have an additional opportunity to work within our practices, communities, and beyond to advocate for equity in participation for all people. Lastly, there remain tremendous gaps in research and data to support IWDs, even in terms of establishing adequate prosthetic services in all communities. We hope this chapter provides the framework for all health care providers to become advocates for all patients, especially those with disabilities.

REFERENCES

1. Office of the Surgeon General (US), Office on Disability (US). *The Surgeon General's Call to Action to Improve the Health and Wellness of Persons with Disabilities.* Office of the Surgeon General; 2005. III, health and wellness for persons with disabilities today. https://www.ncbi.nlm.nih.gov/books/NBK44662/
2. Hagan JF, Shaw JS, Duncan PM, eds. *Bright Futures: Guidelines for Health Supervision of Infants, Children, and Adolescents.* 4th ed. American Academy of Pediatrics; 2017
3. U.S. Department of Justice, Civil Rights Division. ADA.gov. https://www.ada.gov
4. United States Census Bureau. Disability characteristics. Accessed April 1, 2026. https://data.census.gov/table?q=S1810
5. Leppert R, Schaeffer K. 8 facts about Americans with disabilities. Pew Research Center. Updated July 24, 2023. Accessed April 1, 2026. https://www.pewresearch.org/short-reads/2023/07/24/8-facts-about-americans-with-disabilities/
6. NFHS. Flag Football helps drive high school athletics participation numbers to all-time high. *Athletic Business.* August 20, 2025. Accessed April 1, 2026. https://www.athleticbusiness.com/operations/governing-bodies/article/15753420/nfhs-participation-numbers-for-hs-athletics-hit-alltime-high-in-202425
7. Special Olympics. North America Region. Accessed April 1, 2026. https://www.specialolympics.org/regions/north-america
8. Special Olympics. 2024 Annual Report. Accessed April 1, 2026. https://www.specialolympics.org/about/reports/annual-report
9. International Paralympic Committee. Paris 2024 Paralympic Games. Accessed April 1, 2026. https://www.paralympic.org/paris-2024/
10. Centers for Disease Control and Prevention. Benefits of physical activity. Updated December 4, 2025. Accessed April 1, 2026. https://www.cdc.gov/physical-activity-basics/benefits/index.html
11. Fagher K, DeLuca S, Derman W, Blauwet C. Optimising health equity through para sport. *Br J Sports Med.* 2023;57(3):131–132. PMID: 36137733
12. Wells MB. Tobacco use in adolescents with disabilities: a literature review. *Subst Abuse.* 2023;17:11782218231179599. PMID: 37426876 doi: 10.1177/11782218231179599
13. Centers for Disease Control and Prevention. Disability and Health Data System (DHDS). Updated May 29, 2019. https://dhds.cdc.gov
14. Lape EC, Katz JN, Losina E, Kerman HM, Gedman MA, Blauwet CA. Participant-reported benefits of involvement in an adaptive sports program: a qualitative study. *PM R.* 2018;10(5):507–515. PMID: 29111464
15. U.S. Soccer Federation. Soccer for athletes with a disability. Accessed April 1, 2026. http://www.recognize-torecover.org/soccer-for-athletes-with-a-disability#disability-soccer
16. Carbone PS, Smith PJ, Lewis C, LeBlanc C; AAP Council on Children with Disabilities, Council on Sports Medicine and Fitness Promoting the participation of children and adolescents with disabilities in sports, recreation, and physical activity. *Pediatrics.* 2021;148(6):e2021054664. PMID: 34851421
17. Special Olympics. Healthy Athletes. Accessed April 1, 2026. https://www.specialolympics.org/what-we-do/inclusive-health/healthy-athletes?locale=en
18. International Paralympic Committee. International Standard for Eligible Impairments. September 2016. Accessed September 2024. https://www.paralympic.org/sites/default/files/2024-04/International%20Standard%20for%20Eligible%20Impairments_2016.pdf
19. Jordan J. The World Games for the Deaf and the Paralympic Games. International Committee of Sports for the Deaf. Accessed April 1, 2026. https://www.ciss.org/the-world-games-for-the-deaf-and-the-paralympic-games
20. International Paralympic Committee. Paralympics history. Accessed April 1, 2026. https://www.paralympic.org/ipc/history
21. United States Olympic and Paralympic Committee. Paralympic Sport Development. Accessed April 1, 2026. https://www.usopc.org/paralympic-sport-development
22. Move United. Accessed April 1, 2026. https://moveunitedsport.org
23. Special Olympics. Accessed April 1, 2026. https://www.specialolympics.org
24. International Committee of Sports for the Deaf. About the ICSD. Accessed April 1, 2026. https://www.ciss.org/icsd
25. International Paralympic Committee. Paralympic Classification. Accessed April 1, 2026. https://www.paralympic.org/classification
26. Special Olympics. Athlete Medical Form—Health History. Updated April 2021. Accessed April 1, 2026. https://media.specialolympics.org/resources/leading-a-program/registration-forms/SOI-Medical-Form-US-Programs-April-2021-English.pdf

27. Block SS, Beckerman SA, Berman PE. Vision profile of the athletes of the 1995 Special Olympics World Summer Games. *J Am Optom Assoc.* 1997;68(11):699–708. PMID: 9409105
28. Winell J, Burke SW. Sports participation of children with Down syndrome. *Orthop Clin North Am.* 2003;34(3):439–443. PMID: 12974493 doi: 10.1016/S0030-5898(03)00010-5
29. Pelliccia A, Quattrini FM, Squeo MR, et al. Cardiovascular diseases in Paralympic athletes. *Br J Sports Med.* 2016;50(17):1075–1080. PMID: 27231335 doi: 10.1136/bjsports-2015-095867
30. Ramirez M, Yang J, Bourque L, et al. Sports injuries to high school athletes with disabilities. *Pediatrics.* 2009;123(2):690–696. PMID: 19171639 doi: 10.1542/peds.2008-0603
31. Klenck C, Gebke K. Practical management: common medical problems in disabled athletes. *Clin J Sport Med.* 2007;17(1):55–60. PMID: 17304008 doi: 10.1097/JSM.0b013e3180302587
32. McKay SD, Al-Omari A, Tomlinson LA, Dormans JP. Review of cervical spine anomalies in genetic syndromes. *Spine (Phila Pa 1976).* 2012;37(5):E269–E277. PMID: 22045003
33. Svensson O, Aaro S. Cervical instability in skeletal dysplasia. Report of 6 surgically fused cases. *Acta Orthop Scand.* 1988;59(1):66–70. PMID: 3354325. doi: 10.3109/17453678809149348
34. Faculty of Sport and Exercise Medicine. Sport pre-participation screening for asymptomatic atlanto-axial instability (AAI) in Down syndrome (DS) patients. BJSM Blog. June 22, 2017. Accessed April 1, 2026. https://blogs.bmj.com/bjsm/2017/06/22/sport-pre-participation-screening-asymptomatic-atlanto-axial-instability-aai-syndrome-ds-patients.
35. Blackmer J. Rehabilitation medicine: 1. Autonomic dysreflexia. *CMAJ.* 2003;169(9):931–935. PMID: 14581313
36. Slocum C, Blauwet CA, Allen JBA. Sports medicine considerations for the paralympic athlete. *Curr Phys Med Rehabil Rep.* 2015;3:25–35
37. Chapter 4.2- Position statement on autonomic dysreflexia and boosting. In: International Paralympic Committee Handbook. International Paralympic Committee; 2016:4.21–4.23
38. Blauwet CA, Benjamin-Laing H, Stomphorst J, Van de Vliet P, Pit-Grosheide P, Willick SE. Testing for boosting at the Paralympic games: policies, results and future directions. *Br J Sports Med.* 2013;47(13):832–837. PMID: 23681503 doi: 10.1136/bjsports-2012-092103
39. Price MJ, Campbell IG. Effects of spinal cord lesion level upon thermoregulation during exercise in the heat. *Med Sci Sports Exerc.* 2003;35(7):1100–1107. PMID: 12840629 doi: 10.1249/01.MSS.0000074655.76321.D7
40. Patel DR, Greydanus DE. The pediatric athlete with disabilities. *Pediatr Clin North Am.* 2002;49(4):803–827. PMID: 12296534 doi: 10.1016/S0031-3955(02)00020-2
41. American College of Sports Medicine. Intellectual disability and Down syndrome: special considerations for individuals with Down syndrome. In: *ACSM's Guidelines for Exercise Testing and Prescription.* 10th ed. Wolters Kluwer; 2017:333
42. Fullerton HD, Borckardt JJ, Alfano AP. Shoulder pain: a comparison of wheelchair athletes and nonathletic wheelchair users. *Med Sci Sports Exerc.* 2003;35(12):1958–1961. PMID: 14652488 doi: 10.1249/01.MSS.0000099082.54522.55
43. Runciman P, Derman W. The athlete with cerebral palsy. *Aspetar Sport Med J.* 2018;7:142–147
44. Pinheiro L, Verhagen E, Ocarino J, et al. Periodic health evaluation in Para athletes: a position statement based on expert consensus. *BMJ Open Sport Exerc Med.* 2024;10(4):e001946. PMID: 39411023
45. Post EG, Anderson T, Triplett AN, et al. Advancing concussion assessment for para sport athletes through the Para SCAT6 initiative. *Br J Sports Med.* 2026;60(7):500-502. PMID: 41667157 doi:10.1136/bjsports-2025-110566
46. Weiler R, Blauwet C, Clarke D, et al. Concussion in para sport: the first position statement of the Concussion in Para Sport (CIPS) Group. *Br J Sports Med.* 2021;55(21):1187–1195. PMID: 33837003 doi: 10.1136/bjsports-2020-103696
47. Moran RN, Broglio SP, Francioni KK, Sosnoff JJ. Exploring baseline concussion-assessment performance in adapted wheelchair sport athletes. *J Athl Train.* 2020;55(8):856–862. PMID: 32607535
48. Special Olympics. Other Intellectual Disabilities. Accessed April 1, 2026. https://www.specialolympics.org/about/intellectual-disabilities/other-intellectual-disabilities
49. Special Olympics. Article 1: Sports Rules. Accessed April 1, 2026. https://media.specialolympics.org/resources/sports-essentials/general/Sports-Rules-Article-1-2017.pdf
50. Special Olympics. Coaching Guide: Basics of Special Olympics. Accessed April 1, 2026. https://media.specialolympics.org/soi/files/sports/Essentials/English/Basics_of_Special_Olympics.pdf

APPENDIX A: ORGANIZATIONS AND SPORTS OFFERED

International Paralympic Sports

The Paralympic Movement currently includes 28 sports, each run by its own international federation that follows International Paralympic Committee (IPC) standards:

Summer Sports

- Para archery
- Para athletics
- Para badminton
- Blind football
- Boccia
- Para canoe
- Para cycling
- Para equestrian
- Goalball
- Para judo
- Para powerlifting
- Para rowing
- Shooting Para sport
- Sitting volleyball
- Para swimming
- Para table tennis
- Para taekwondo
- Para triathlon
- Wheelchair basketball
- Wheelchair fencing
- Wheelchair rugby
- Wheelchair tennis

Winter Sports

- Para alpine skiing
- Para biathlon
- Para cross-country skiing
- Para ice hockey
- Para snowboard
- Wheelchair curling

Further, the IPC recognizes other Para sports run by international federations that are not currently eligible to be IPC members:

- Arm wrestling (WAF)
- Bobsleigh (IBSF)
- Bowling (IBF)
- Climbing (IFSC)
- CP football (IFCPF)

- Flying disc (WFDF)
- Golf (IGF)
- Handball (IHF)
- Hockey (FIH)
- Karate (WKF)
- Modern pentathlon (UIPM)
- Powerchair football (FIPFA)
- Sailing (WS)
- Surfing (ISA)

Special Olympic Sports

Here are the sports currently included in Special Olympics:

Summer Sports

- Aquatics (open water and swimming)
- Athletics (track & field)
- Badminton
- Basketball
- Bocce
- Bowling
- Competitive cheer
- Cricket
- Cycling
- Dance sport
- Equestrian sports
- Floor ball
- Floor hockey
- Football (soccer)
- Golf
- Kayaking
- Motor Activity Training Program
- Netball
- Powerlifting
- Gymnastics (artistic, rhythmic)
- Handball
- Judo
- Roller skating
- Sailing
- Softball
- Swimming
- Table tennis
- Tennis
- Triathlon
- Volleyball

Winter Sports

- Alpine skiing
- Cross-country skiing
- Figure skating
- Short-track speed skating
- Snowboarding
- Snowshoeing

Deaflympic Sports

Here are the sports currently included in the Deaflympics:

Summer Sports

- Athletics
- Badminton
- Basketball
- Beach volleyball
- Bowling
- Cycling Road
- Football (soccer)
- Futsal
- Golf
- Handball
- Judo
- Karate
- Mountain bike
- Orienteering
- Shooting
- Swimming
- Table tennis
- Taekwondo
- Tennis
- Volleyball
- Wrestling freestyle
- Wrestling Greco-Roman

Winter Sports

- Alpine skiing
- Chess
- Cross-country
- Curling

Visually Impaired Sports

Sports for Visually Impaired Currently Included in the International Blind Sports Federation

- Chess
- Ninepin bowling
- Tenpin bowling
- Showdown
- Torball

Visually Impaired Sports Part of IPC

- Athletics
- Cycling
- Equestrian
- Blind football (soccer)
- Goalball
- Judo
- Rowing
- Shooting
- Skiing (Alpine and Nordic)
- Swimming
- Triathlon

Virtus (Intellectually Impaired) Sports

- Athletics
- Basketball
- Cricket
- Cycling
- Equestrian
- Football/futsal
- Judo
- Rowing
- Skiing
- Table tennis
- Tennis

Promoting these sports:

- Golf
- Karate
- Para-hockey
- Sailing
- Taekwondo

APPENDIX B: FORMS AND LINKS

- International Committee of Sport for the Deaf (ICSD): https://www.ciss.org
- International Paralympic Committee: https://www.paralympic.org
- Move United: https://moveunitedsport.org
- Special Olympics: https://www.specialolympics.org
- Virtus: https://www.virtus.sport

Forms

- Special Olympics medical release form: https://media.specialolympics.org/resources/leading-a-program/registration-forms/SOI-Medical-Form-US-Programs-April-2021-English.pdf
- Athletes Without Limits (US member of Virtus, intellectual impairment): https://www.athleteswithoutlimits.org/eligibility
- World Ability Sport, World Para Dance Sport form: https://worldabilitysport.org/wp-content/uploads/2024/02/2024-WPDS-Medical-Diagnostics-Form.pdf
- Parasport Classification Guide: https://lexi.global
- World Paralympic Medical Diagnostic Form: https://www.paralympic.org/sites/default/files/document/180508150843738_2017_11+Medical+Diagnostic+Form+for+ALL+Athletes+with+Physical+Impairment_Athletics_0.pdf

APPENDIX C: SCREENING, TESTING, AND MANAGING CONCUSSION IN INDIVIDUALS WITH A DISABILITY

Adaptive and Para athletes sustain sport-related concussions. However, there is a gap in the validated approach to evaluating and managing an IWD with suspected concussion compared to the norms that have been published for concussion evaluation and management in individuals without a disability. Therefore, being cognizant of the differences and having a planned approach to managing IWDs with concussion is essential.

One should consider additional baseline testing for IWDs to facilitate evaluation and treatment for concussion. Using current recommendations for evaluating concussion (eg, SCAT 6) may be helpful but is not validated or appropriate for many athletes with a disability who are suspected of having a sport-related concussion.[a]

Examples of Issues Applying Current Concussion Evaluation Guidelines to IWDs

Condition	Issue With Evaluation
Limb difference	• Balance • Gait
Visual impairment	• May be unable to report vision issues (double vision, may not present with a "blank stare") • Neurocognitive tests and reaction times • Glasgow Coma Scale may have limited "eye response"
Intellectual impairment	• May have difficulty following commands or reporting symptoms • Neurocognitive testing • Reliability and repeatability of testing may suffer
Neuromuscular impairment	• Strength • Gait • Balance • Reflexes
Spinal cord issue	• Balance • Gait
Comorbid	• Many conditions overlap

Several key points are important for the evaluation and treatment of concussion in IWDs.[b]

- Use a PPE and review any disabilities noted.
- Execute a concussion baseline evaluation tailored to the athlete with a disability to document a true baseline for function, symptoms (they may be described differently), balance, gait, and neurocognitive function.
- Engage a caregiver or someone who is familiar with the IWD (eg, coach, teammate) as part of the baseline evaluation (and after suspected concussion evaluation) to assist in tailoring the examination to the individual.
- If the IWD is concussed, a person medically familiar with the individual should be part of the decision-making process for treatment and return to sport.
- Consider implementing an alternative reaction time test (although not yet validated).[c]
- For those with spinal cord injury, consider using an alternative balance testing system for both the baseline and post-concussion evaluation: the WESS (Wheelchair Error Scoring System).[d]

WESS (Wheelchair Error Scoring System)[d]

Six conditions are tested, 3 each with eyes open and eyes closed. Each is tested for 20 seconds. Record the error(s) for each 20-second test (see Figure 7-1).

- Seated on a firm surface, hands on hips, legs dangle over the edge of the surface
- Seated on a balance disc, hands on hips, legs dangle over the edge of the surface
- In a standard wheelchair (no front or posterior coasters), perform a wheelie on the 2 main back wheels

Error Scoring

- Lifting hands off hips
- Moving trunk into > 30° of flexion or abduction
- Coming out of the wheelie task
- Changing grip during the wheelie task
- Lifting hands off the wheels during the wheelie task
- Remaining out of position for more than 5 seconds
- For eyes-closed testing, opening of the eyes

Note: One point is added for each error during the 20-second tests. A maximum of 10 errors are counted for any single testing condition.

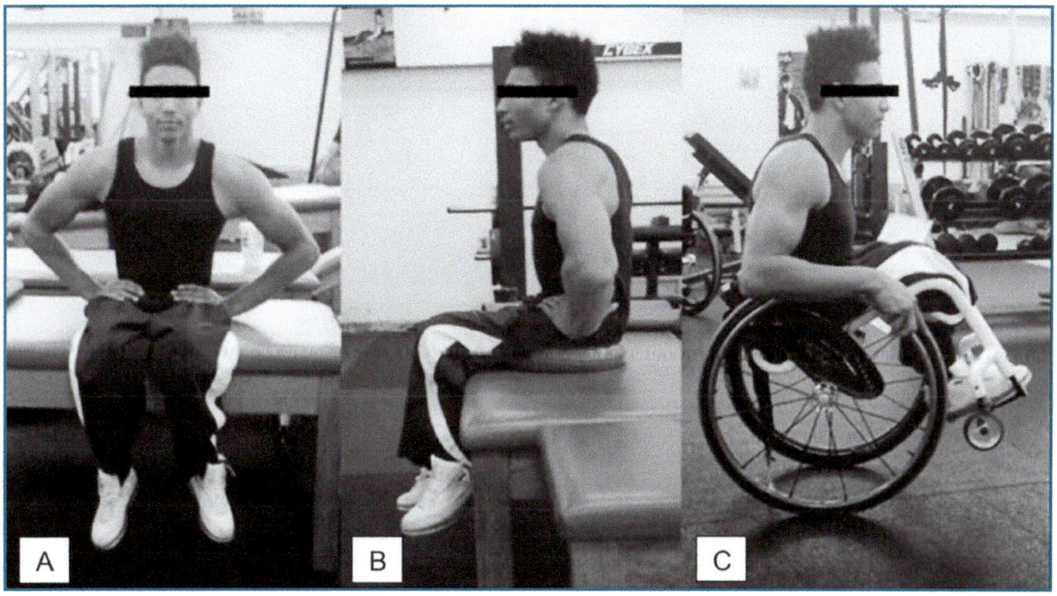

Figure 7-1. Positioning and stances on the Wheelchair Error Scoring System

A, seated on firm surface; B, seated on balance disk (unstable surface); C, wheelie.

Reproduced from Moran RN, Broglio SP, Francioni KK, et al. Exploring baseline concussion-assessment performance in adapted wheelchair sport athletes. *J Athl Train.* 2020;55(8):856–862.

REFERENCES

Consider reading the following resources to better plan for managing concussion in IWDs.

a. Lee K, Harper MW, Uihlein MJ, McCrea M. *Concussion Management for Wheelchair Athletes.* Springer; 2021. doi:10.1007/978-3-030-83004-5

b. Weiler R, Blauwet C, Clarke D, et al. Concussion in para sport: the first position statement of the Concussion in Para Sport (CIPS) Group. *Br J Sports Med.* 2021;55(21):1187–1195. PMID: 33837003 doi:10.1136/bjsports-2020-103696

c. Eckner JT, Whitacre RD, Kirsch NL, Richardson JK. Evaluating a clinical measure of reaction time: an observational study. *Percept Mot Skills.* 2009;108(3):717–720. PMID: 19725308 doi:10.2466/pms.108.3.717–720

d. Moran RN, Broglio SP, Francioni KK, Sosnoff JJ. Exploring baseline concussion-assessment performance in adapted wheelchair sport athletes. *J Athl Train.* 2020;55(8):856–862. PMID: 32607535

CHAPTER 8

Gender-Diverse Individuals

A transgender person has a gender identity that is different from their sex assigned at birth, whereas *cisgender* is a term often used to describe a person whose gender identity is in concordance with their sex assigned at birth. The term *gender-diverse* includes transgender, nonbinary, and gender nonconforming individuals. Gender-diverse individuals of all ages are less physically active and less likely to participate in organized sports than their cisgender peers.[1,2] The preparticipation evaluation (PPE) serves as an opportunity to engage people of all genders with their providers in routine preventive health care, encourage regular physical activity, and determine medical clearance for sport. The PPE process is the same for all individuals, regardless of their gender. The designation of sex and gender and the determination of competition status based on either sex or gender has become a topic of scrutiny for transgender participants. The determination of eligibility for male versus female categories of sport is governed by state law and sports governing bodies. The role of the health care provider is to determine medical clearance for sports and to provide quality care that is free from discrimination or bias and supports the health care needs of all individuals regardless of gender.

Determination of eligibility for male versus female categories of sport is based on law/policy, while medical clearance is based on the PPE assessment.

The World Health Organization (WHO) has distinguished the meanings of sex and gender to prevent their interchangeable use in society and in the medical community.[3] The WHO confines sex to the biological and physiological characteristics that define male and female. Gender refers to the socially constructed roles, behaviors, activities, and attributes that society considers culturally appropriate for men, women, and people of other gender categories. The fundamental concepts of sex and gender extend beyond the traditional male and female biological designations assigned at birth. While there are exceptions based on certain medical conditions, biological sex is primarily defined by the human genotype and usually leads to the development of internal and external genitalia, chromosomes, hormone levels, and secondary sex characteristics. Gender is a complex concept that represents psychosocial self-perceptions, social constructs, and cultural expectations including attitudes regarding men and women[4] and encompasses a broad range of gender identity categories. Gender identity may be a fluid concept for some individuals that changes over time during psychological and/or physiological development. Self-awareness is a determining factor that also influences one's perception, recognition, and expression of gender identity.[5] Similarly to other aspects of one's personality, individuals may have varying degrees of comfort when expressing gender identity within different personal, professional, athletic, and public personas. Societal norms, cultural conditions, and institutional policies also affect the degree to which gender-diverse individuals may express or conceal their gender identity.[6]

Sex: Biological and physiological characteristics that define male and female
Gender: Socially constructed roles, behaviors, activities, and attributes that society considers culturally appropriate

It is important for providers to know that a patient's sexual orientation and gender identity are considered protected personal/health information under federal privacy laws.[7]

Depression, suicidality, nonsuicidal self-injuries, and other mental and emotional health concerns are more common in gender-diverse people compared with cisgender populations.[8] LGBTQ+ youth experience elevated rates of suicide attempts, illicit substance use, and sexual risk behaviors compared with cisgender, heterosexual youth.[9] Minority stress theory likely explains the increased rates of mental health disparities experienced by gender-diverse people.[10]

The 2022 US Transgender Survey found that 44% of participants reported psychological distress within the previous 30 days.[11] Of those who sought medical care, nearly one-half reported negative experiences because of gender identity, including refusal of care, labeled undesired gender, and receipt of harmful language or rough touch or abuse.[11] Transgender individuals who describe their health care providers as less inclusive have reported lower general health scores.[12] Transgender athletes also experience barriers to seeking care owing to the lack of clinician education, lack of a safe and supportive environment, and lack of supportive team or local environment.[13] By addressing these barriers, health care professionals can improve access to and delivery of care for gender-diverse individuals.[14]

It is important for providers to know that a patient's sexual orientation and gender identity are considered protected personal/health information under federal privacy laws.

Measures that build trust and emphasize safety for gender-diverse individuals strengthen the provider–patient relationship and access to care.[13] Improved mental health outcomes such as lower depressive symptoms, suicidal ideation, and suicidal behaviors among transgender youth have been associated with increased use of one's chosen name in multiple contexts, including in the health care setting.[15] As such, providers' willingness to learn and use language that positively impacts gender-diverse individuals can improve their health outcomes. LGBTQ+ educational programs, policy statements, and professional conferences that focus on inclusivity and recognize intentional and unintentional biases increase knowledge and broaden acceptance of diverse backgrounds among members of the health care team.[1] Formal training that emphasizes safety and fosters an interest in improving care for LGBTQ+ populations may assist those who feel unequipped to support and care for LGBTQ+ individuals and their families.

Environments can also be constructed with language and terminology that is respectful and culturally responsive to support privacy and promote safety. Use of "Safe Zone" posters, pins, and signs placed in highly visible locations delivers a broad message to patients, visitors, and staff. Forms that include antidiscrimination policies and gender-inclusive language convey support for all who read, complete, and review the information. The use of preferred pronouns and chosen names within all forms of communication and documentation assists providers and staff in supporting a health care setting that is welcoming and free from bias. Preferred pronouns and names may be obtained directly from the individual, either verbally in a private setting or by providing additional space on forms so that the information can be included in the medical history and consent documents.[1,13] Pronouns may be gender specific and/or gender neutral. Examples of preferred pronouns include he/him/his, she/her/hers, and they/them/theirs. Some individuals may prefer a mix of pronouns (eg, he/they). It is important for these preferred pronouns and names to be used consistently by all providers and staff in both oral and written communication to foster trust and improve respect within the health care setting. As with cisgender individuals, confidentiality remains essential to the provider–patient relationship. Like all health care information and medical decision-making, conversations regarding gender identity are protected and private. Permission to disclose gender-specific information should be obtained as individuals may not be comfortable reporting their gender identity to all family, friends, coworkers, and members of the sports team and staff. Clarification of the individual's wishes is important to maintain trust and convey sensitivity. Medical forms should remain secure to avoid inappropriate disclosure.

Examples of preferred pronouns include he/him/his, she/her/hers, and they/them/theirs.

Recommendations to Support Gender-Diverse Individuals

- **Be empowering and inclusive through advocating respect, equity, safety, and privacy.**
- **Inform and involve individuals in decision-making to promote health and well-being.**
- **Use preferred names and pronouns verbally and in documentation.**
- **Complete training about the specific health care needs of gender-diverse individuals.**

Suggested Resources Available to Health Care Providers

- **Thegenderbook.com**
- **AAP Policy Statement: Ensuring comprehensive care and support for transgender and gender-diverse children and adolescents[5]: https://doi.org/10.1542/peds.2018-2162**
- **National Athletic Trainers' Association (NATA) LGBTQ+: https://www.nata.org/professional-interests/more/lgbtq-formerly-inclusion/lgbtq-resources**

POLICIES ON GENDER-DIVERSE INDIVIDUALS PARTICIPATING IN ORGANIZED SPORTS

Sports competitions have traditionally been divided by sex, but as more transgender individuals partake at different levels of organized sports, participation across sex divisions challenges these traditional constructs. Transgender individuals may face barriers when engaging in organized sport.[2] Exclusion from sport on the basis of gender identity contributes to social isolation and limits personal and social development, physical fitness, networking opportunities, and team building.[16] It is important for health care providers to encourage physical activity and sport participation for all individuals regardless of gender while being aware of the needs that are specific to transgender and gender-diverse individuals. Providers who maintain current knowledge of legal issues and policy changes pertinent to LGBTQ+ participation are better prepared to understand and address any resultant psychosocial impact on these individuals.

High School Policy

Policy regarding transgender competition is continually evolving at all levels of sport. At the high school level, the National Federation of State High School Associations recommends school administrators follow statutes and policies set at the state and community levels. Thus, state high school athletic associations have developed individual policies, which vary from state to state. Some state laws and policies ban transgender students from participating in sports consistent with their gender identity. Such policies can limit access to activities that are beneficial to physical and mental health. The controversial legal culture surrounding transgender youth and the lack of unified messaging among organizations have a profound impact on the mental health of the LGBTQ+ youth, as messaging may be internalized to negatively impact self-worth, self-perception, self-regard, and personal agency.[6] Health care providers can play an important role in evaluating and supporting the mental health of gender-diverse individuals. The provider needs to keep abreast of changing policies, encourage participation in physical activities, and offer support to the adolescent transgender individual.

National Collegiate Athletic Association Policy

The National Collegiate Athletic Association (NCAA) policy on transgender athlete participation can be found at https://www.ncaa.org/sports/2022/1/27/transgender-participation-policy.aspx.

The rules apply to all practices and competitions in NCAA sports where participants are separated by gender throughout the regular season, conference championships, the postseason, scrimmages, and exhibitions. Schools remain responsible for certifying student-athlete eligibility for practice and competition.[17] The policy also notes that schools fall under the jurisdiction of local, state, and federal legislation.

International Olympic Committee Policy

Eligibility for elite-level athletes is set by the International Olympic Committee (IOC) or a given sport's governing body. In 2026, the IOC modified its consensus frameworks regarding transgender athletes. The IOC policy can be found at https://stillmed.olympics.com/media/Documents/International-Olympic-Committee/EB/policy/policy-on-the-protection-of-the-female-category-english.pdf.

HORMONE GUIDELINES

For individuals receiving hormone therapy, the World Anti-Doping Agency (WADA) and the US Anti-Doping Agency (USADA) provide testosterone-dosing guidelines[18] to maintain fairness. These guidelines may be found at:

- WADA Guidelines for Therapeutic Use Exemption (TUE): https://www.wada-ama.org/en/resources/world-anti-doping-program/guidelines-international-standard-therapeutic-use-exemptions[18]
- USADA TUE Application: https://www.usada.org/athletes/testing/tue/apply/

Individuals with specific medical conditions, including those unique to transgender participants, must review and comply with the USADA checklist and WADA guidelines to maintain eligibility for sport. The TUE process allows for review of the medical needs and therapies of the individual while also considering fairness of competition and the rights of all athletes who participate. For the TUE, documentation and administration of the medications and supplements must include dose, route, and frequency in accordance with hormone replacement guidelines, and should be completed by the health care provider who is prescribing the hormone replacement therapy. This process is not unique to transgender individuals as it also pertains to cisgender males who require testosterone replacement therapy postorchiectomy.

RESOURCES

A helpful resource for the care of transgender and gender-diverse people designed to address issues for children, adolescents, young adults, adults, and older adults is the Gender Affirmative Lifespan Approach, with approaches to care aimed at countering the internalization of stigma and improving mental health outcomes (www.sexualhealth.umn.edu/ncgsh/gala).

REFERENCES

1. Rogers SM, Crossway AK, Aronson PA. Creating a LGBTQ+ inclusive culture in the athletic training facility. *Clin Pract Athl Train.* 2018;1(1):11–14
2. Jones BA, Arcelus J, Bouman WP, Haycraft E. Sport and transgender people: a systematic review of the literature relating to sport participation and competitive sport policies. *Sports Med.* 2017;47(4):701–716. PMID: 27699698 doi:10.1007/s40279-016-0621-y
3. World Health Organization (WHO). Gender and health. Accessed March 9, 2026. http://www.who.int/health-topics/gender#tab=tab_1
4. Bassett AJ, Ahlmen A, Rosendorf JM, Romeo AA, Erickson BJ, Bishop ME. The biology of sex and sport. *JBJS Rev.* 2020;8(3):e0140. PMID: 32224635
5. Rafferty J, et al; American Academy of Pediatrics Committee on Psychosocial Aspects of Child and Family Health, Committee on Adolescence; Section on Lesbian, Gay, Bisexual and Transgender Health and Wellness. Ensuring comprehensive care and support for transgender and gender-diverse children and adolescents. AAP Policy Statement. *Pediatrics.* 2018;142(4):e20182162. doi:10.1542/peds.2018-2162
6. Ramos N, Burgess A, Ollen E. The current status of sociopolitical and legal issues faced by lesbian, gay, bisexual, transgender, queer and questioning youth. *Adolesc Psychiatry (Hilversum).* 2022;12(3):180–195. PMID: 37064428
7. US Department of Health and Human Services, Office for Civil Rights. Protecting the Rights of Lesbian, Gay, Bisexual, Transgender, Queer, and Intersex (LGBTQI+) People. Updated February 18, 2025. Accessed March 9, 2026. https://www.hhs.gov/ocr/lgbtqi/index.html

8. James SE, Herman JL, Durso LE, Heng-Lehtinen R. *Early Insights: A Report of the 2022 U.S. Transgender Survey.* National Center for Transgender Equality; 2024. https://transequality.org/sites/default/files/2024-02/2022%20USTS%20Early%20Insights%20Report_FINAL.pdf
9. Kann L, Olsen EO, McManus T, et al. Sexual identity, sex of sexual contacts, and health-related behaviors among students in grades 9-12–United States and selected sites. *MMWR Surveill Summ.* 2016;65(9):1–202. PMID: 27513843
10. Marra J, Christensen D, Harper JM, et al. Medical Care of Transgender Athletes and Policy Implications: ACSM Contemporary Issue Statement. *Med Sci Sports Exerc.* 2026;58(3):606–618. doi:10.1249/TJX.0000000000000336
11. Rastogi A, Menard L, Miller GH, et al. Health and wellbeing: a report of the 2022 U.S. Trangender Survey. Advocates for Transgender Equality. June 2025. Accessed March 9, 2026. https://ustranssurvey.org/download-reports/
12. Seelman KL, Colón-Diaz MJP, LeCroix RH, Xavier-Brier M, Kattari L. Transgender noninclusive healthcare and delaying care because of fear: connections to general health and mental health among transgender adults. *Transgend Health.* 2017;2(1):17–28. PMID: 28861545
13. Munson EE, Ensign KA. Transgender athletes' experiences with health care in the athletic training setting. *J Athl Train.* 2021;56(1):101–111. PMID: 33259593
14. Coleman E, Bockting W, Botzer M, et al. Standards of care for the health of transsexual, transgender, and gender-nonconforming people, version 7. *Int J Transgenderism.* 2012;13(4):165–232. doi:10.1080/15532739.2011.700873
15. Russell ST, Pollitt AM, Li G, Grossman AH. Chosen name use is linked to reduced depressive symptoms, suicidal ideation, and suicidal behavior among transgender youth. *J Adolesc Health.* 2018;63(4):503–505. PMID: 29609917
16. Hargie OD, Mitchell DH, Somerville IJ. 'People have a knack of making you feel excluded if they catch you on your difference': transgender experiences of exclusion in sport. *Int Rev Sociol Sport.* 2017;52(2):223–239. doi:10.1177/1012690215583283
17. Office of Inclusion. NCAA inclusion of transgender student-athletes. National Collegiate Athletic Association; May 2024. Participation policy for transgender student-athletes. Updated February 6, 2025. Accessed March 17, 2026. https://www.ncaa.org/sports/2022/1/27/transgender-participation-policy.aspx
18. World Anti-Doping Agency (WADA). TUE Physician Guidelines-Transgender Athletes. 2022. https://www.wada-ama.org/en/resources/therapeutic-use-exemption/tue-physician-guidelines-transgender-athletes

CHAPTER 9

Preventing and Addressing Abuse and Sexual Violence

HISTORY FORM QUESTION

1. *Has anyone ever touched you in a way or pressured you to engage in any physical or sexual acts that made you uncomfortable?*

SECONDARY QUESTIONS

- In sport, have you ever felt bullied, harassed, threatened, neglected, or placed into situations in which your health may have been at risk?
- Have you ever been humiliated, emotionally abused, or made to feel uncomfortable by your teammates, coaches, or athletic staff?
- Have you ever been afraid for your safety when attending a practice, competition, or meeting with an athletic staff member?

KEY POINTS

- Abuse can, and does, present in a variety of forms (Table 9-1).
- Sports have historically brandished a culture normalizing certain forms of maltreatment and dissuading reporting, which perpetuates the abuse.
- It is essential that all medical professionals be educated regarding the various forms abuse may take, screen during preparticipation evaluations (PPEs) and routine medical encounters, and understand next steps in protecting each individual.
- There is zero tolerance for abuse in any form.

COMMON FORMS OF ABUSE

Table 9-1. Forms of Abuse

Form of Abuse	Definition, Regardless of Age	Example
Psychological abuse	Deliberate, prolonged, repeated noncontact deleterious language and nonphysical actions that involve more than just an individual's emotions. This form of abuse is used to weaken, damage, coerce, or frighten a person and is the root of all forms of abuse.	A coach regularly critically compares a player to other teammates with the ultimate goal of motivation.
Sexual abuse	Any and all acts sexual in nature, where consent is not—or *cannot* be—given or in which consent is coerced. According to the International Olympic Committee (IOC), a minor is not able to provide consent.[1]	An adult assistant coach texts an athlete who is a minor flirty messages and shirtless photos.
Physical abuse	Nonaccidental trauma or injury caused by contact with an individual's person. May also consist of physical actions intended to coerce, discipline, or harm an individual that do not necessarily result in visible or medical injury.	More senior players on a team repeatedly slap a junior player's helmet every time they make a mistake.
Bullying/harassment	Unwanted, harmful, repetitive antagonistic behaviors directed toward an individual in the setting of an actual or perceived imbalance of power. Harassment involves similar offensive actions specifically targeted at a protected class of individuals (disability, age, sex, race, color, nationality, or religion).	Bullying: Teammates taunting a basketball athlete for regularly missing free throws Harassment: A few teammates imitate a player's accent every time she speaks, laughing and telling her to learn how to speak "right."
Neglect	Failure of parents or caregivers (including coaches and staff) to provide medical care, meet a child's psychological or developmental needs, and/or failure to protect against danger.	An individual returns after taking a few days off for a viral illness. During the first practice back, the coach refuses to let her rest or come out of drills after an episode of emesis.

Participation in sports promotes health, unifies people with similar interests, and creates a culture of teamwork, discipline, respect, and personal achievement. Athletic culture supports well-being, yet can serve as a breeding ground for harmful behaviors, including abuse and sexual violence—an increasingly pressing issue that has gained significant attention in recent years. Data indicate that these behaviors are pervasive, yet difficult to identify because of biopsychosocial complexities. More than ever, this underscores the unique and crucial position that any medical professional working in the sporting world and performing PPEs plays in the identification, management, and prevention of all forms of maltreatment.

The prevalence of abuse in sport is difficult to gauge owing to a multitude of factors including lack of recognition, taboo nature of the topic, and fear surrounding reporting. Data are scant, and the available information is difficult to interpret because of the widely varying definitions and study designs.[2] Prevalence rates have been reported as high as 3 out of 4 athletes up to 16 years old,[3] whereas the *NCAA myPlaybook Survey,* collecting data from 2021 to 2022, reported that 1 in 10 athletes experienced at least one type of interpersonal violence during their college sports career.[4] As many as 45% of youth athletes experience some form of abuse throughout their career.[2,5] Rates of interpersonal violence have also been reported to be higher at more elite levels of competition.[3,6]

There are several aspects of the sports environment that increase the risk for abuse. These include unequal power dynamics between coaches or staff and participants.[7] The presence of a hierarchy; demands on time for training, travel, and competition; distance from home environments; and situations that may expose participants to being isolated with a potential abuser in a vehicle, home, or hotel room are factors that increase opportunities for abuse to occur. The pervasive nature of social media and potential access to communication is a newer consideration that is being explored. Research indicates that athletes, particularly women, youth, elite-level participants, and marginalized groups such as individuals who identify as LGBTQ+ or people with disabilities, are disproportionately affected.[3,6,8–12] Contrary to previous suggestion, there are no data to support the degree of physical contact in the sport or the amount of clothing worn as sporting attire as risk factors.[13]

Violence in sport can take on many forms, making it extremely difficult to identify. The culture of sport touts resilience as a desirable feature, leading to an environment in which the athlete may be pushed too far physically, mentally, or sexually. It is important for health care providers to stay informed about the different forms of abuse in sports.

DEFINING VIOLENCE IN SPORT

The World Health Organization defines child maltreatment in sport as all forms of physical, emotional, or sexual abuse; neglect; and negligent treatment.[14] Strong evidence shows that physical, sexual, and psychological abuse are highly correlated, and it is important to acknowledge that psychological abuse is present at the core of all forms of child maltreatment.

Defining forms of maltreatment improves the understanding and identification of the various forms to which individuals of all ages may be exposed to and/or the recipient of, including unwanted actions, words, and attention. Individuals participate in sports and activities during various stages of growth, maturation, and psychological development. Children are inherently vulnerable to adult pressures in sport at all stages of growth and maturation. They are particularly at risk for abuse because of their dependence on adults for care, protection, and supervision during development. Abusers in positions of power coerce, manipulate, and/or dominate youth athletes. In addition to individuals in positions of power, peers and teammates may be perpetrators. Furthermore, abuse or maltreatment can be perpetrated through electronic communication, such as social media platforms that provide direct access. There is a need to clearly define appropriate, inappropriate, and violent behaviors in sport to improve the ability to categorize forms of child maltreatment that occur in sport.

GROOMING WITHIN SPORT

Hierarchical relationships, such as those that exist between coaches or staff and participants, increase the risk for abuse because of the power structure and the dependent nature of the relationship. Relationships of abuse often lack proper boundaries, which allows unhealthy interactions to be introduced, established, and maintained. The process of grooming describes a perpetrator's intentional coercion to create dependence and build trust while exploiting boundaries of acceptable behavior (Table 9-2). The growth and continuation of manipulative interactions allows the perpetrator to slowly violate emotional, physical, and sexual boundaries and renders the athlete powerless to seek help.

It is important to recognize that the grooming process may not simply occur between a perpetrator and athlete alone, but also with parents, staff, other trusted adults, as well as the larger organization itself. Over time, these manipulative individuals gain the respect and trust of others, including the organization. Insidious patterns of behaviors ensue in which the offender skirts existing policies or practices that were created to protect the athlete. This tacit endorsement by other trusted figures including the organization further disempowers the individual being groomed. Four stages of grooming illustrate the intent the perpetrator disguises as coaching to facilitate the normalization and tolerance of unhealthy behaviors.[15–17]

(1) Targeting the victim

(2) Building trust and friendship

(3) Developing isolation and building loyalty

(4) Building and securing secrecy

Table 9-2. The Four Stages of the Grooming Process

1. Targeting the victim	The individual is targeted through unique invitations, special training sessions, or individual attention. Commonly, the perpetrator identifies the presence of vulnerable qualities such as lack of strong peer or parental relationships, financial or physical dependence, and/or the desire of specific skill training, which are exploited.
2. Building trust and friendship	The perpetrator provides gifts or rewards for specific acts or behaviors to support an exclusive relationship reliant on the perpetrator. Conditions directed by the perpetrator are dependent on the individual's increased cooperation, emotional reliance, and affection, which is often confused as consent.
3. Developing isolation and building loyalty	The perpetrator restricts time, meeting, and communication with other relationships, friends, and groups while strengthening the individual's commitment to the abuser.
4. Building and securing secrecy	The perpetrator delivers statements of guilt or demands to preserve anonymity, preventing reports of abuse. The abuser threatens consequences that destroy the opportunities and eliminate privileges to preserve the entrapment and command the individual's cooperation.

FORMS OF DELIVERY OF ABUSE

Abuse may be delivered either directly or indirectly. Direct acts or words of abuse are clearly unacceptable behaviors that deliver harm to the individual. Indirect abuse occurs when an individual witnesses the abuse of others. Both forms of delivery may bring immediate and long-term detriment to the recipients. Relationships among those who witness abuse are also affected when abuse continues and is not reported.

FORMS OF ABUSE

Psychological Abuse

Psychological abuse targets the identity of the individual, their beliefs and systems of value. This involves more than just the individual's emotions; it presents as a pattern of deliberate, prolonged, repeated noncontact behavior that is at the root of all forms of abuse. It serves as the foundation on which other abusive relationships are fostered. A pattern of verbal and nonverbal psychological communication is delivered to the athlete, who slowly loses value of self.

One of the only large-scale studies of over 6,000 youth-athlete respondents on this topic identified the prevalence of psychological abuse to be as high as 75%.[3] Athletes reported that coaches performed behaviors to belittle, humiliate, reject, isolate, and threaten.

Case Example

A basketball player who experiences a stress fracture is called obese by the coach, who falsely states this is the reason she developed the injury.

Sexual Abuse

Sexual abuse includes all acts that are sexual in nature, where consent is not or cannot be given or in which consent is coerced. Any unwanted touch, comments, coercion, or other sexual acts are sexual abuse regardless of age. The International Olympic Committee Statement on Youth Athletic Development[1] states that minors are not able to provide consent. Forms of sexual abuse may include sexual discrimination, sexual harassment, and physical acts of abuse. Although identification labels are provided, it is important to note one form may develop into another, or multiple forms may coexist in a culture of maltreatment and exploitation. Suggestive activities include voyeurism, exhibitionism, masturbation, and pornography. Sexual discrimination is the unfavorable and unfair behavior directed toward an individual based on their sex. Harassment is any unwanted attention such as through jokes, comments, verbal or written threats, invitations, and innuendos. Acts of sexual abuse present as forced physical contact. All sexual acts performed with manipulation are acts of abuse.

Sexual abuse may be perpetrated in any sport and at any level; however, a greater prevalence has been reported at the more elite levels. On the one hand, this may be due to an increased comfort with reporting the abuse. Alternatively, this may represent a higher rate of abuse, which has previously been attributed to the nature of elite sports in which talent is identified earlier in life, when individuals are more susceptible to abuse. This, too, may simply be a result of the increased time spent with coaches, including travel. It may also represent systemic failures by large organizations to protect the participants.

Case Example

A physically inappropriate and unwanted rubdown is delivered by an assistant coach to an athlete in the locker room after practice.

Physical Abuse

Physical abuse is nonaccidental trauma or injury caused by contact with an individual's person. Common examples include hitting, biting, beating, kicking, and other physical activities that deliver harm. Activity that is mandated but is inappropriate for age, or that is demanded in poor environmental conditions, can also be identified as physical abuse. Examples include practicing in excessive heat or in conditions with limited access to water or cooling.

It is important to note that activities of physical abuse also encompass psychological abuse. Examples to consider involve the perpetrator blurring the lines of acceptable behavior to obtain participation by the individual. Individuals who are coerced into using substances to enhance physique or achieve desired effects are targets of physical abuse with psychological involvement. This may present as an athlete pressured to use performance-enhancing substances to reduce weight or gain muscle, or forced to restrict calories to achieve a desired appearance or body weight. Similarly, those bullied to consume alcohol during team parties/celebrations or elsewhere—both minors and those of legal drinking age—are subject to this abuse.

As mentioned earlier, excessive training despite exhaustion or injury can also be considered physical abuse.[18] The concept of "exercise as punishment" is considered corporal punishment, an action found to be unethical and harmful to the individual, with recommendations that it be abolished across school systems.[18] A coach may punish the athlete for poor performance or use enhanced training strategy to coax them to participate through the pain and possibly to the point of collapse. Preventing an athlete from meeting basic biological needs such as cooling, hydration, nutrition, and bathroom breaks poses risks to the individual. An injured athlete may feel pressured to return to sport without proper medical evaluation. Similarly, the individual may feel pressured to resume activity prior to recovery despite environmental or biological conditions. In these circumstances, physical and psychological abuse coexist as the health of the individual is invalidated, and the injury is dismissed by the perpetrator.

Case Example

The adolescent marathon runner is pressured to practice in humid temperatures without access to frequent hydration stops.

Bullying/Harassment

Abuse commonly presents in the form of bullying or harassment. Bullying is defined as unwanted, harmful, repetitive, antagonistic behaviors directed toward an individual in the setting of an actual or a perceived imbalance of power. The perpetrator gains enjoyment at the persecution of the abused. Harassment involves similar aggressive and offensive actions specifically targeted at a protected class of individuals (disability, age, sex, race, color, nationality, or religion), thus constituting discrimination. Bullying and harassment can take on differing forms including physical, psychological, or social bullying and can be delivered in direct open actions or by indirect methods such as exclusion.

Case Example
A high school lacrosse team captain nicknames a teammate who he has never liked "Runt" owing to his smaller stature. This name clearly distresses the individual, yet several teammates laugh each time it is said, and the nickname sticks.

Neglect

Neglect is defined as the failure of parents or caregivers (including coaches and staff) to provide medical care, meet the child's psychological or developmental needs, and/or protect against danger. The physical impact of neglect may cause greater risk to the developing youth athlete as a result of their distinct physical, psychological, and cognitive vulnerabilities.

Forms of neglect may accompany other abuses. For example, neglect may overlap with physical abuse when preventable overtraining injuries result from disregarding recovery guidelines. Neglect can also coexist with psychological abuse. Athletes who are purposely excluded from practices, competition, or social gatherings are isolated from teammates and peers.

Case Example
An athlete who does not drive is denied transportation to appropriate medical care to treat a severe ankle sprain, coupled with the coach belittling the injury by stating, "Just walk it off like every other boo-boo you have."

Negative Bystander Effect

The negative bystander effect is a contributing issue to the various abuses. This occurs when a person besides the perpetrator and abusee witnesses maltreatment but does not intervene.[19] The bystander effect has historically been noted as widespread in sporting environments.

SAFEGUARDING THE INDIVIDUAL

It is well established that early intervention can mitigate ongoing victimization and adverse long-term outcomes.[20] Once identified, these problems need to be addressed. While the presence of a single form of violence can lead to posttraumatic stress disorder, depression, anxiety, social isolation, eating disorders, self-harm, and suicide attempts, it is important to understand that multiple exposures potentiate this effect.[9,21–23] The safeguarding of an individual is at the core of a physician's responsibility, and specifically the team physician's obligation to the athlete.[6,24–26] Table 9-3 lists signs and symptoms that may present as a result of abuse. When caring for individuals reporting more than 1 of these symptoms, consider screening for abuse.

Table 9-3. Signs and Symptoms That Warrant Screening for Abuse

Physical Health	Mental Health	Sport Related
Bruising pattern inconsistent with sport	Anxiety	Absenteeism
Chronic musculoskeletal pain	Depression	Conflict with teammates
Dysmenorrhea	Eating disorder	Decline in performance
Headaches	Mood swings	Difficulty concentrating
Fatigue	Self-harm behavior/suicidality	Early fatiguing
Gastrointestinal complaints	Sleep disturbances	Injury/recurrent injuries
Pelvic pain	Substance use/misuse	Retirement/dropout
Sexually transmitted infections		
Unwanted pregnancy/abortion		

Many challenges exist in reporting these concerns to authorities. Recent data suggest that hesitation to report sexual violence stems from worries that the individual will not be believed or supported.[27] There is a fear of negative reactions by others such as doubt, blame, and insensitive treatment. The possibility of unwanted consequences such as changed relationships and career interference has been documented.

The legal system, too, has been cited as daunting to survivors because of unwanted police or court involvement or because of a mistrust in the process in which disclosure will not result in further action. A concern that confidentiality is not guaranteed is yet another fear.[28]

The actual disclosure experience can deliver beneficial or harmful effects to the survivor. Positive outcomes include enhanced psychological and physical health. Alternatively, others experience feelings of desolation and isolation upon reporting.[28,29] Trust and communication are the crux of patient care, setting the foundation for disclosure. Normalizing conversations and providing an open atmosphere can make it easier for individuals to report. Providing various opportunities or methods to disclose is recommended.[27] Securing a safe and quiet clinic environment can help place the individual more at ease. Addressing confidentiality limits early in the encounter is important so that the individual understands what may require mandatory reporting. During the encounter, it is helpful for the health care professional to use a trauma-informed approach, offering a safe and caring atmosphere.[24] Aligning oneself with the survivor to create a "together we will do this" method to next steps can foster reassurance.

As it has been shown that others' responses to disclosure play a critical role in a survivor's recovery process, it is important to pay particular attention to appropriate ways to respond.[28] Individuals who experience sexual abuse pursue medical care more often than those who have not been victimized, albeit without necessarily revealing the abuse; thus, it is important to keep one's index of suspicion high.

Education programs such as SafeSport[24] or those offered by individual sporting organizations provide a variety of resources: learning modules geared toward different members of the sports entourage and a library of resources such as printable posters underscoring athlete rights for an environment free from abuse and misconduct.

Upon hearing the history, the provider's next step is to consider the health needs of the survivor by encompassing physical as well as psychological support. Emergency conditions such as bodily trauma (eg, lacerations, fractures) require expeditious attention. In cases of sexual assault, access to an official and properly conducted sexual assault forensic examination by a trained professional is time sensitive, ideally completed within 72 hours, particularly if there is interest in pregnancy prevention. If outside this time window, this examination is still recommended. Questions regarding details of the assault will guide the head-to-toe examination, which may consist of a full-body examination including external and internal assessments of the mouth, vagina, and/or anus. Body areas may be swabbed and samples of blood, urine, and hair obtained.[30] Screening for sexually transmitted infections and postexposure prophylaxis may also be addressed. Psychological services involving acute crisis support and future therapy/counseling referrals are crucial.

There are legal considerations regarding disclosures. Laws require mandatory reporting of suspected abuse, neglect, or exploitation of a minor or vulnerable (eg, disabled) adult. If the provider learns information and/or identifies reasonable suspicion of child abuse including sexual abuse, as a mandated reporter they must immediately report concerns to law enforcement, child protective services, and any additional agency mandated by the sporting organization, state law, or federal law. For example, National Governing Bodies require reporting to the US Center for SafeSport.[24] Specific information regarding each state's regulations is available through the *Rape, Abuse and Incest National Network* (RAINN) State Law Database.[30] Mandatory reporting is also applied by Title IX and the Clery Act in the college and university setting. Title IX requires educational institutions to have clear policies and procedures in place to address and prevent sexual discrimination and harassment.[31] Every institution is required to have a designated Title IX coordinator to serve as the responsible authority. Such coordinators act on behalf of the institution and receive complaints, allegations, and grievances via website, electronic mail, or written notice or in person. Mandatory reporting to the medical licensing board applies if another health care professional is suspected of perpetrating sexual violence.

When filing a report, it is important to include the name, title, and contact information of the survivor and perpetrator; information disclosed regarding the abuse; and the reporting professional's name, title, and contact information. This report should be purely objective in nature, providing only facts and observations.[24]

When filing a report, it is important to include the name, title, and contact information of the survivor and perpetrator; information disclosed regarding the abuse; and the reporting professional's name, title, and contact information. This report should be purely objective in nature, providing only facts and observations.

PREVENTION

The PPE functions on a prevention framework. This is also the recommended approach to addressing interpersonal and sexual violence in sport. Individuals should be able to participate in sports without emotional, physical, or sexual abuse or misconduct.[24] Because a PPE may be the single point of contact between a health care provider and a participant over the course of up to 2 years, it is important to use the opportunity to screen for potential interpersonal and sexual violence.

The PPE provides an opportunity for physicians to screen all participants to determine whether they are currently, or have in the past, experienced interpersonal violence, including psychological abuse, sexual abuse or misconduct, physical abuse, or neglect. Creating a safe disclosure atmosphere and environment is paramount to participants' feeling comfortable reporting episodes of interpersonal or sexual violence.

Screening works best when it is repetitive. The individual can be encouraged to respond to a history questionnaire prior to their appointment, then be given the opportunity to disclose any history of sexual or interpersonal violence during a face-to-face encounter.

Anticipating disclosures during the PPE and having written policies or strategies in place for circumstances in which a disclosure is made allows for equitable and timely assessments and recommendations.[6,31–33] This includes an established multidisciplinary support system that will provide complex comprehensive care in such cases. These services help protect and empower survivors, while lessening chances of repeat abuse. They provide a network of care and support moving forward, with the goal of favorable mental health and a productive life inclusive of sports.[6,28]

Best clinical practice includes respect for patient privacy for any undressing and dressing. For every sensitive examination, it is important to provide an explanation of the examination and purpose, implement proper draping to minimize exposure, and provide a chaperone.[9,34,35]

Developing an emergency action plan (EAP) for disclosures of interpersonal or sexual violence helps delineate the process for contacting individuals or agencies that may need to be notified based on the disclosure.[36]

Developing an emergency action plan for disclosures of interpersonal or sexual violence helps delineate the process for contacting individuals or agencies that may need to be notified based on the disclosure.

Health care professionals performing PPEs are encouraged to receive training in how to observe for signs or symptoms of interpersonal or sexual violence among participants, as well as abusive behaviors, including grooming, among other individuals in positions of authority.

Ensuring participant safety in sport requires a culture shift. Creating a climate of empowerment can potentially be protective and enacted on many levels.[7] There is an opportunity to educate participants, families, and other staff and health care providers in interventions to shift widespread bystander behavior. Various organizations are creating bystander intervention training programs to assist with both abuse identification and intervention measures.[19,24] It is important that access to resources, including how to report episodes of abuse, is readily available. Creating these relationships with local partners will further foster the healing environment.

The message is zero tolerance. All members of the sports medicine team and primary care providers need to advocate for participation in all sports and activities free from abuse of any kind.

SCREENING TOOLS

- **The Violence Towards Athletes Questionnaire (VTAQ)** is a tool designed for athletes aged 14 to 17 years to identify interpersonal violence including coach derived.[37]
- Components of the IOC's **Sport Mental Health Assessment Tool 1 (SMHAT-1).**[38] This tool addresses various aspects of mental health and well-being:
  - — Athlete Psychological Strain Questionnaire (APSQ)—general well-being
  - — General Anxiety Disorder-7 (GAD-7)—anxiety
  - — Patient Health Questionnaire-9 (PHQ-9)—depression
  - — Brief Eating Disorder in Athletes Questionnaire (BEDA-Q)—disordered eating patterns

RESOURCES

- 988 Lifeline: https://988lifeline.org
- National Collegiate Athletic Association (NCAA) Sexual Violence Prevention Tool Kit: https://www.ncaa.org/sports/2016/9/28/sexual-violence-prevention-tool-kit.aspx
- National Sexual Assault Hotline: 1-800-656-4673
- National Sexual Violence Resource Center: https://www.nsvrc.org
- RAINN (Rape, Abuse and Incest National Network): http://www.Rainn.org
- U.S. Center for SafeSport: http://uscenterforsafesport.org

REFERENCES

1. Bergeron MF, Mountjoy M, Armstrong N, et al. International Olympic Committee consensus statement on youth athletic development. *Br J Sports Med.* 2015;49(13):843–851. PMID: 26084524
2. Vertommen T, Parent S. Measuring the prevalence of interpersonal violence against children in sport. In: *Routledge Handbook of Athlete Welfare.* Routledge; 2020:385–395
3. Stafford A, Alexander K, Fry D. 'There was something that wasn't right because that was the only place I ever got treated like that': children and young people's experiences of emotional harm in sport. *Childhood.* 2013;22(1):121–137. doi:10.1177/0907568213505625
4. Zogg CK, Runquist EB III, Amick M, et al. Experiences of interpersonal violence in sport and perceived coaching style among college athletes. *JAMA Netw Open.* 2024;7(1):e2350248. PMID: 38227316
5. ChildHelp. Accessed June 2025. https://www.childhelp.org/
6. Mountjoy M, Brackenridge C, Arrington M, et al. International Olympic Committee consensus statement: harassment and abuse (non-accidental violence) in sport. *Br J Sports Med.* 2016;50(17):1019–1029. PMID: 27118273
7. Ohlert J, Schmitz H, Schäfer-Pels A, Allroggen M. An empowering climate as a protective factor against sexual violence in sport? *Soc Sci.* 2022;11(8):330. doi:10.3390/socsci11080330
8. Vertommen T, Schipper-van Veldhoven N, Wouters K, et al. Interpersonal violence against children in sport in the Netherlands and Belgium. *Child Abuse Negl.* 2016;51:223–236. PMID: 26516053
9. Joy EA, Herring SA, Nelson C, et al. Sexual violence in sport: expanding awareness and knowledge for sports medicine providers. *Curr Sports Med Rep.* 2021;20(10):531–539. PMID: 34622818
10. Denison E, Bevan N, Jeanes R. Reviewing evidence of LGBTQ+ discrimination and exclusion in sport. *Sport Manage Rev.* 2020;24(3):389–409. doi:10.1016/j.smr.2020.09.003

11. Denison E, Faulkner N, Jeanes R, Toole D. Relationships between attitudes and norms with homophobic language use in male team sports. *J Sci Med Sport.* 2021;24(5):499–504. PMID: 33279424
12. Tuakli-Wosornu YA, Sun Q, Gentry M, et al. Non-accidental harms ('abuse') in athletes with impairment ('para athletes'): a state-of-the-art review. *Br J Sports Med.* 2020;54(3):129–138. PMID: 31023860 doi:10.1136/bjsports-2018-099854
13. Fletcher S. Touching practice and physical education: deconstruction of a contemporary moral panic. *Sport Educ Soc.* 2013;18(5):694–709. doi:10.1080/13573322.2013.774272
14. World Health Organization (WHO). Child maltreatment. November 5, 2024. https://www.who.int/news-room/fact-sheets/detail/child-maltreatment
15. Marks S, Mountjoy M, Marcus M. Sexual harassment and abuse in sport: the role of the team doctor. *Br J Sports Med.* 2012;46(13):905–908. PMID: 22171340
16. Brackenridge CH. *Spoilsports: Understanding and Preventing Sexual Exploitation in Sport.* Routledge; 2001:35
17. Brackenridge C, Fasting K. The grooming process in sport: narratives of sexual harassment and abuse. *Auto/Biography.* 2005;13:33–52 doi:10.1191/0967550705ab016oa
18. Allison MA, Beers N, Peterson JW; COUNCIL ON SCHOOL HEALTH. Corporal punishment in schools. *Pediatrics.* 2023;152(3):e2023063284. PMID: 37599648 doi:10.1542/peds.2023-063284
19. Verhelle H, Vertommen T, Peters GY. Preventing sexual violence in sport: determinants of positive coach-bystander behavior. *Front Psychol.* 2022;13:862220. PMID: 35936332 doi:10.3389/fpsyg.2022.862220
20. Eisenberg ME, McMorris BJ, Gower AL, Chatterjee D. Bullying victimization and emotional distress: is there strength in numbers for vulnerable youth? *J Psychosom Res.* 2016;86:13–19. PMID: 27302541
21. Vertommen T, Kampen J, Schipper-van Veldhoven N, Uzieblo K, Van Den Eede F. Severe interpersonal violence against children in sport: associated mental health problems and quality of life in adulthood. *Child Abuse Negl.* 2018;76:459–468. PMID: 29253798
22. Ohlert J, Rau T, Allroggen M. Association between sexual violence experiences and well-being and risk for depression in elite athletes depends on the context of the incidents. *J Clin Sport Psychol.* 2019;13(2):311–329
23. Hamby S. Intimate partner and sexual violence research: scientific progress, scientific challenges, and gender. *Trauma Violence Abuse.* 2014;15(3):149–158. PMID: 24464246
24. U.S. Center for SafeSport. Accessed January 10, 2026. https://uscenterforsafesport.myabsorb.com/#/public-dashboard
25. Koontz JS, Mountjoy M, Abbott KE, et al. Sexual violence in sport: American Medical Society for Sports Medicine Position Statement. *Br J Sports Med.* 2021;55(3):132–134. PMID: 32554408
26. Herring SA, Putukian M, Leclere LE, et al. The Team Physician Consensus Statement 2024. *Med Sci Sports Exerc.* 2025;57(5):1067–1075
27. DeStefano S, Peterson E, Pham DC, et al. Screening college athletes for sexual violence: athletes' experiences and opinions on best practices. *Br J Sports Med.* 2024;58(22):1369–1375. doi:10.1136/bjsports-2023-107622
28. Halstead V, Williams JR, Gonzalez-Guarda R. Sexual violence in the college population: a systematic review of disclosure and campus resources and services. *J Clin Nurs.* 2017;26(15-16):2137–2153. PMID: 28102917
29. Mountjoy M, Vertommen T, Denhollander R, Kennedy S, Majoor R. Effective engagement of survivors of harassment and abuse in sport in athlete safeguarding initiatives: a review and a conceptual framework. *Br J Sports Med.* 2022;56(4):232–238. PMID: 35110362
30. RAINN. Explore the state law database. Accessed January 10, 2026. https://apps.rainn.org/policy/
31. Young J, Neil ER, Granger K, Walker SE, Chadburn JL, Eberman LE. Preparedness, confidence, and best practices in preventing, recognizing, managing mental health cases in NCAA institutions. *J Athl Train.* 2023;58(2):156–162. PMID: 33150415
32. World Players Association. *Supporting Player Associations to Address Abuse in Sport: Mapping Interest Capacity and Opportunities.* May 23, 2023. https://uniglobalunion.org/wp-content/uploads/CARE_Mapping_Report-2023.pdf
33. The Foundation for Global Sports Development. Empowering communities through movement, learning, and opportunity. Accessed January 10, 2026. https://globalsportsdevelopment.org/
34. Berhane A, Hackell JM, Wallace S; Committee on Practice and Ambulatory Medicine; Committee on Adolescence. Use of chaperones for the pediatric and adolescent encounter: policy statement. *Pediatrics.* 2025;155(6):e2025071810. PMID: 40383537 doi:10.1542/peds.2025-071810
35. American Medical Association. Code of Medical Ethics. Opinion 1.2.4. Use of chaperones. https://code-medical-ethics.ama-assn.org/ethics-opinions/use-chaperones

36. DeStefano S, Agnew M, Deccy S, et al. Developing a sexual assault emergency action plan: modified Delphi consensus recommendations from the American Medical Society for Sports Medicine. *Br J Sports Med.* 2026;60(5):326-339. PMID: 41771704 doi:10.1136/bjsports-2025-110966
37. Parent S, Fortier K, Vaillancourt-Morel M-P, et al. Development and initial factor validation of the Violence Toward Athletes Questionnaire (VTAQ) in a sample of young athletes. *Loisir et Société/Society and Leisure.* 2019;42(3):471–486. https://doi.org/10.1080/07053436.2019.1682262
38. Gouttebarge V, Bindra A, Blauwet C, et al. International Olympic Committee (IOC) Sport Mental Health Assessment Tool 1 (SMHAT-1) and Sport Mental Health Recognition Tool 1 (SMHRT-1): towards better support of athletes' mental health. *Br J Sports Med.* 2021;55(1):30–37. PMID: 32948518 doi:10.1136/bjsports-2020-102411

CHAPTER 10

Implementation in Practice

- **Purpose of PPE:** The preparticipation evaluation (PPE) serves as an entry point to health care for young athletes, aiming to identify medical risks, promote safe sports participation, and support overall health.
- **Effectiveness:** While their effectiveness as a screening tool is debated, PPEs provide opportunities for early detection of health issues.
- **Evaluator qualifications:** PPEs should be performed by physicians, nurse practitioners, and physician assistants, with appropriate training, particularly in the context of cardiovascular screening for athletes.
- **Timing:** The best timing for a PPE is at least 6 weeks before the sports season starts. Aligning the PPE with the annual health supervision visit optimizes care and can prevent delays.
- **Setting:** The PPE authoring societies recommend that PPEs be conducted within the medical home for comprehensive, long-term care.
- **Frequency and monitoring:** The PPE authoring societies recommend that youth and high school–aged individuals undergo a PPE every 1 to 2 years.
- **Electronic health record integration:** Integrating the PPE history, examination findings, and medical eligibility forms into electronic health records enhances continuity of care, streamlines the process, standardizes evaluations across providers, and facilitates research on sports-related health trends.
- **Challenges and accessibility:** Barriers such as the lack of an established medical provider, insurance limitations, and scheduling difficulties can hinder access to PPEs. While group-setting PPEs are discouraged, in situations where the individual lacks a medical home or health care insurance, a group-setting PPE may be their only access point for a PPE and hence sports participation.
- **Forms:** Having the individual and their parents or legal guardians complete the History Form together improves accuracy and completeness. Health care providers should review the Medical Eligibility form with them, highlighting any conditions or restrictions. Providing the Medical Eligibility form to the school or sports organization contributes to a safer environment for the individual by ensuring that key medical information is accessible to school personnel or other staff.
- **Chaperones:** Offering the presence of a chaperone during sensitive examinations is recommended, as is shared decision-making between the individual, parent or guardian, and provider on the use of chaperones.
- **Emergency action plans:** A mental health emergency action plan (EAP) can be developed for the medical home to address mental health crises and emergencies during the PPE.

With millions of young people participating in sports, the PPE can serve as an entry point into, or a periodic touchpoint with, the health care system. The primary goal of the PPE is to identify medical or physical conditions or concerns that may put individuals at increased risk of injury or health complications during physical activity or sports. Additionally, the PPE provides an opportunity to promote safe sports involvement and foster health and wellness among participants. Although its effectiveness as a screening tool remains contested, the PPE provides a touchpoint for preventive care and early detection of medical issues, which can have long-term health implications.

It is very important that health care providers completing the evaluation have training in identifying physical and medical conditions that may predispose to injury or illness (particularly cardiac and neurologic issues); sport/activity-specific requirements for safe participation (including an understanding of the physical requirements for various sports and activities); state-specific rules and laws related to participation in sports or activities; addressing mental health issues common in young people; and identifying individuals experiencing interpersonal or sexual violence. The PPE authoring societies recommend that only health care professionals with this appropriate training—physicians (medical doctors/doctors of osteopathic medicine), nurse practitioners, and physician assistants—perform PPEs to provide a more thorough assessment of an individual's health and safety. Chiropractors, for example, do not receive the comprehensive medical training required to conduct PPEs.

The PPE authoring societies recommend that the PPE be conducted at least 6 weeks before the start of a new activity or new season. This time frame allows adequate opportunity to address any issues identified during the evaluation prior to the first day of practice. While most individuals will be cleared to participate in their chosen activities, some will need further evaluation before being allowed to participate. Educating the participant and the parent or guardian on the importance of a timely evaluation will limit unnecessary delays in clearance and minimize the chance of missing practices or competitions. Rather than waiting until the weeks prior to the start of a sports season, incorporating the PPE into the annual health supervision visit may help alleviate the burden on health care providers of having PPEs clustered together during the short summer. Additionally, when the PPE is incorporated into the annual health supervision visit for all children and adolescents, even those not currently involved in sport, it will be complete if the individual chooses to participate in a sport anytime in the next 1 to 2 years.

The PPE authoring societies recommend that the PPE be conducted within the medical home, where the sport- or activity-specific portions can be integrated into the annual health supervision visit. This approach allows for a more comprehensive understanding of the individual's medical history and fosters the development of a long-term, trusting relationship with health care providers. These providers can offer guidance on safe sport practices, injury prevention, and overall health promotion. For participants with preexisting medical conditions, shared decision-making is crucial in ensuring their safety and well-being. The PPE presents an opportunity to develop or refine management plans to support medically reasonable participation in these activities. Additionally, incorporating the PPE into electronic health records can streamline the process, improve consistency among health care providers, and provide data for future research.

The PPE authoring societies recommend that PPEs not be performed in an urgent care center, a retail clinic, or another environment where continuity of care cannot be maintained. Similarly, group and station-based evaluations are discouraged because of significant limitations in the personalization and continuity of care, difficulty performing thorough or sensitive examinations, and difficulty obtaining delicate and critical history elements. However, in situations where the individual lacks a medical home or health care insurance, a group-setting PPE may serve as both their sole opportunity for sports participation and a gateway to establishing a medical home.

Some school districts require a sports physical to be completed after an arbitrary date. However, the PPE authoring societies' recommended timing for the PPE is every 1 to 2 years after the previous PPE and not after an arbitrary date. For a student who had a recent physical examination, being required to repeat it simply to meet a school requirement leads to redundancy, added financial burden, strain on the health care system, and stress for families.

If the PPE is performed every 2 years, an interim health update questionnaire is recommended in the year between full evaluations to monitor any new or emerging health conditions and help support ongoing fitness for participation throughout the year.

The American Academy of Pediatrics recommends offering a chaperone be present during sensitive exams and using shared decision-making between the patient, parent or guardian, and provider on the use of chaperones.[1] While patients can decline a chaperone, offering this as an option may make them feel more in control and empowered to advocate for themselves.

Health care providers are encouraged to develop a structured EAP for addressing acute and subacute mental health crises in the office setting. An effective EAP integrates community and emergency services, enabling a safe, systematic, and compassionate response.

CONCLUSION

The primary purpose of the PPE is to promote healthy and safe participation; it is not primarily intended to exclude individuals from participating in activities. The PPE offers a comprehensive assessment that extends beyond simply determining eligibility for participation. It serves as a valuable opportunity to address preventive care, identify high-risk behaviors, address mental health and substance use, assess for interpersonal or sexual violence, provide health education, and foster a relationship and build trust between the participant and the health care provider. Additionally, the PPE facilitates attention to the unique health care needs of individuals with disabilities, promoting inclusivity and equitable access to care. For many, the PPE, or the routine health supervision visit with sport-specific portions, is the individual's only touchpoint with the health care system. By taking a thorough, individualized approach, the health care provider can identify potential risks, offer guidance on injury prevention, and support individuals in achieving a healthy, active lifestyle.

Effective implementation of the PPE requires consistent adherence to evolving best practices and guidelines, while also acknowledging its inherent limitations. As research advances, particularly in areas like cardiovascular screening, mental health, and injury prevention, health care providers are encouraged to be proactive in staying informed. The PPE is more than just an evaluation; it is an opportunity to educate, advocate for safety, and champion a safe, active, and healthy lifestyle. By embracing this role, health care providers enhance the effectiveness of the PPE and significantly contribute to the overall well-being of every individual evaluated.

REFERENCE

1. Berhane A, Hackell JM, Wallace S; American Academy of Pediatrics Committee on Practice and Ambulatory Medicine; Committee on Adolescence. Use of chaperones for the pediatric and adolescent encounter: policy statement. *Pediatrics*. 2025;155(6):e2025071810. PMID: 40383537 doi:10.1542/peds.2025-071810

FORMS

This form should be placed into the individual's medical file and should *only* be shared with other health care professionals.
The Medical Eligibility Form is the only form that should be submitted to nonmedical personnel at a school or sports organization.

PREPARTICIPATION EVALUATION

HISTORY FORM

Note: Complete and sign this form (with your parents if younger than 18) before your appointment.

Name: ______________________ Date of birth: ________________ Date of examination: ___________________

Sports and Activities: ____

List past and current medical conditions (including mental health disorders such as ADHD, anxiety, depression).

____

Have you ever had surgery? If yes, list all past surgical procedures. ________________________________

____

Medicines and supplements: List all current prescriptions, over-the-counter medicines, vitamins, and supplements (herbal and nutritional).

____

Do you have any allergies? If yes, please list all your allergies (eg, medicines, pollens, food, stinging insects).

____

Sex assigned at birth (F, M, or intersex): ______ How do you identify your gender? (F, M, nonbinary, or another gender): ______

Patient Health Questionnaire Version 4 (PHQ-4)

Over the past 2 weeks, how often have you been bothered by any of the following problems? (Circle response)

	Not at all	Several days	Over half the days	Nearly every day
Feeling nervous, anxious, or on edge	0	1	2	3
Not being able to stop or control worrying	0	1	2	3
Little interest or pleasure in doing things	0	1	2	3
Feeling down, depressed, or hopeless	0	1	2	3

Over the past 2 weeks, have you had thoughts that you would be better off dead or hurting yourself in some way? (Circle response)

Not at all	Several days	Over half the days	Nearly every day
0	1	2	3

GENERAL QUESTIONS (Explain "Yes" answers at the end of this form. Circle questions if you don't know the answer.)	Yes	No
1. Do you have any concerns that you would like to discuss with your provider?		
2. Has a provider ever denied or restricted your participation in sports for any reason?		
3. Have you had any recent illness?		
HEART HEALTH QUESTIONS ABOUT YOU	**Yes**	**No**
4. Have you ever had pain, discomfort, or shortness of breath in your chest during exercise?		
5. Have you ever passed out or nearly passed out during or after exercise, or in response to sudden loud noises?		
6. Has a doctor ever told you that you have any heart problem, heart murmur, or high blood pressure?		
7. Has a doctor ever ordered a test for your heart (for example, electrocardiography [ECG/EKG] or echocardiography [ECHO])?		
8. Have you ever had a seizure?		

HEART HEALTH QUESTIONS ABOUT YOUR FAMILY	Unsure	Yes	No
9. Has any family member or relative died or had a disability from heart problems before age 50 or had an unexpected or sudden unexplained death (SUD) before age 50 (including drowning, unexplained car accident, or sudden infant death syndrome)?			
10. Does anyone in your family have hypertrophic cardiomyopathy (HCM), dilated cardiomyopathy, Marfan syndrome, arrhythmogenic cardiomyopathy (ACM), long QT syndrome (LQTS), Brugada syndrome, or catecholaminergic polymorphic ventricular tachycardia (CPVT) or have a pacemaker or an implanted defibrillator?			

BONE AND JOINT QUESTIONS	Yes	No
11. Have you ever had a fracture or an injury to a bone, muscle, ligament, joint, or tendon that caused you to miss a practice or game?		
12. Do you have a bone, muscle, ligament, or joint injury that currently bothers you?		

MEDICAL QUESTIONS		Yes	No
13. Have you ever had a hit or blow that caused confusion, prolonged headache, or memory problems or been diagnosed with a concussion?			
14. Have you ever had numbness, tingling, or weakness in your arms or legs, or been unable to move your arms or legs after being hit or falling?			
15. Are you missing a kidney, an eye, a testicle, spleen, or any other organ? Are any of these organs not functioning properly?			
16. Have you ever become ill while exercising in the heat?			
17. Do you or does someone in your family have sickle cell trait or disease?	Unsure		
18. Have you ever had or do you have any problems with your eyes or vision?			
19. Do you cough, wheeze, or have difficulty breathing during or after physical activity?			
20. Do you have groin or testicular pain or a bulge or lump in the groin area?			
21. Do you have any recurring skin rashes or rashes that come and go, including herpes or methicillin-resistant *Staphylococcus aureus* (MRSA)?			

MEDICAL QUESTIONS (*CONTINUED*)	Yes	No
22. Are you happy with your current weight?		
23. Do you feel pressured to lose or gain weight?		
24. Do you follow a specific diet plan?		
25. Has anyone ever touched you in a way or pressured you to engage in any physical or sexual acts that made you uncomfortable?		

MENSTRUAL QUESTIONS
26. How old were you when you had your first menstrual period?
27. When was your most recent menstrual period?
28. How many periods have you had in the past 12 months?

Explain "Yes" answers here.

____

____

____

____

____

____

____

____

____

____

____

____

I hereby state that, to the best of my knowledge, my answers to the questions on this form are complete and correct.

Signature of athlete: ____

Signature of parent or guardian: ____

Date: ____

This form should be placed into the individual's medical file and should *only* be shared with other health care professionals.
The Medical Eligibility Form is the only form that should be submitted to nonmedical personnel at a school or sports organization.

EVALUACIÓN PREVIA A LA PARTICIPACIÓN

FORMULARIO DE ANTECEDENTES

Nota: complete y firme este formulario (con sus padres, si es menor de 18 años) antes de su cita.

Nombre:_______________ Fecha de nacimiento:_______________ Fecha de examen:_______________

Deportes y actividades:_______________

Enumere las afecciones médicas pasadas y actuales (incluyendo trastornos de salud mental como TDAH, ansiedad o depresión).

____

¿Alguna vez le hicieron una cirugía? Si la respuesta es sí, haga una lista de todas las cirugías pasadas. _______________

____

Medicamentos y suplementos: Haga una lista de los medicamentos actualmente recetados, los de venta libre, las vitaminas y los suplementos (herbales y nutricionales).

____

¿Sufre de algún tipo de alergia? Si la respuesta es afirmativa, haga una lista de todas sus alergias (por ejemplo, a algún medicamento, al polen, a los alimentos, a las picaduras de insectos).

____

Sexo asignado al nacer (femenino, masculino o intersexual): ___ ¿Con qué género se identifica? (femenino, masculino, no binario u otro género): ___

Cuestionario de salud del paciente, versión 4 (PHQ-4)

Durante las últimas 2 semanas, ¿con qué frecuencia le han molestado los siguientes problemas? (Encierre en un círculo su respuesta)

	Ningún día	Varios días	Más de la mitad de los días	Casi todos los días
Sentirse nervioso, ansioso o inquieto	0	1	2	3
No poder dejar de preocuparse o controlar sus preocupaciones	0	1	2	3
Poco interés o placer por hacer cosas	0	1	2	3
Sentirse triste, deprimido o sin esperanza	0	1	2	3

Durante las últimas 2 semanas, ¿ha pensado que sería mejor estar muerto o hacerse daño de alguna manera? (Encierre en un círculo su respuesta)

Ningún día	Varios días	Más de la mitad de los días	Casi todos los días
0	1	2	3

PREGUNTAS GENERALES (Explique las respuestas "Sí" al final de este formulario. Encierre en un círculo las preguntas si no sabe la respuesta).	Sí	No
1. ¿Tiene alguna preocupación sobre la que le gustaría hablar con su proveedor de atención médica?		
2. ¿Algún proveedor de atención médica alguna vez le prohibió o restringió su participación en deportes por alguna razón?		
3. ¿Ha tenido alguna enfermedad reciente?		
PREGUNTAS SOBRE LA SALUD DEL CORAZÓN	**Sí**	**No**
4. ¿Alguna vez ha tenido dolor, molestias o falta de aire en el pecho durante el ejercicio?		
5. ¿Alguna vez se ha desmayado o casi se ha desmayado durante o después del ejercicio, o por ruidos fuertes repentinos?		
6. ¿Algún médico alguna vez le ha dicho que tiene un problema del corazón, un soplo cardíaco o presión arterial alta?		

PREGUNTAS SOBRE LA SALUD DEL CORAZÓN (*CONTINUACIÓN*)	Sí	No
7. ¿Algún médico alguna vez le indicó que se haga una prueba del corazón (por ejemplo, un electrocardiograma [ECG/EKG] o un ecocardiograma [ECHO])?		
8. ¿Alguna vez tuvo una convulsión?		

PREGUNTAS SOBRE LA SALUD DEL CORAZÓN DE SU FAMILIA	No estoy seguro	Sí	No
9. ¿Algún familiar o pariente murió o tuvo una discapacidad por problemas del corazón antes de los 50 años, o tuvo una muerte inesperada o repentina sin explicación antes de los 50 años (incluyendo ahogamiento, accidente automovilístico sin explicación o síndrome de muerte súbita del lactante)?			

PREGUNTAS SOBRE LA SALUD DEL CORAZÓN DE SU FAMILIA (*CONTINUACIÓN*)	No estoy seguro	Sí	No
10. ¿Alguien en su familia tiene miocardiopatía hipertrófica (HCM), miocardiopatía dilatada, síndrome de Marfan, miocardiopatía arritmogénica (ACM), síndrome de QT largo (LQTS), síndrome de Brugada o taquicardia ventricular catecolaminérgica polimórfica (CPVT), o tiene un marcapasos o un desfibrilador implantado?			

PREGUNTAS SOBRE LOS HUESOS Y LAS ARTICULACIONES	Sí	No
11. ¿Alguna vez tuvo una fractura o una lesión en un hueso, músculo, ligamento, articulación o tendón que le hizo faltar a una práctica o juego?		
12. ¿Tiene una lesión en un hueso, músculo, ligamento o articulación que actualmente le molesta?		
PREGUNTAS MÉDICAS	**Sí**	**No**
13. ¿Alguna vez recibió un golpe que le causó confusión, dolor de cabeza prolongado o problemas de memoria, o le diagnosticaron una conmoción cerebral?		
14. ¿Alguna vez tuvo entumecimiento, hormigueo o debilidad en los brazos o las piernas, o no ha podido mover los brazos o las piernas después de un golpe o una caída?		
15. ¿Le falta un riñón, un ojo, un testículo, el bazo o algún otro órgano? ¿Alguno de estos órganos no funciona correctamente?		
16. ¿Alguna vez se ha enfermado mientras hacía ejercicio en el calor?		
17. ¿Usted o alguien de su familia tiene enfermedad depranocítica o rasgos de células falciforme? — No estoy seguro: ☐		
18. ¿Alguna vez tuvo o tiene problemas con los ojos o la visión?		

PREGUNTAS MÉDICAS (*CONTINUACIÓN*)	Sí	No
19. ¿Tiene tos, sibilancias o dificultad para respirar durante o después de la actividad física?		
20. ¿Tiene dolor en la ingle o en los testículos, o un bulto o hinchazón en el área de la ingle?		
21. ¿Tiene sarpullidos frecuentes o sarpullidos que aparecen y desaparecen, incluyendo herpes o *Staphylococcus aureus resistente a la meticilina* (MRSA)?		
22. ¿Está conforme con su peso actual?		
23. ¿Siente presión por bajar o subir de peso?		
24. ¿Sigue un plan de alimentación específico?		
25. ¿Alguna vez alguien lo tocó de una manera que lo hizo sentir incómodo o lo presionó para participar en actos físicos o sexuales que lo hicieron sentir incómodo?		
PREGUNTAS MENSTRUALES		
26. ¿A qué edad tuvo su primera menstruación?		
27. ¿Cuándo fue su última menstruación?		
28. ¿Cuántas menstruaciones tuvo en los últimos 12 meses?		

Explique aquí las respuestas "Sí".

____

____

____

____

____

____

____

____

____

____

____

____

Por la presente, declaro que, a mi leal saber y entender, mis respuestas a las preguntas de este formulario son correctas e íntegras.

Firma del deportista o participante: ____

Firma de padre, madre o tutor: ____

Fecha: ______________________________

Spanish translation of Preparticipation Physical Evaluation Medical History form.

This form should be placed into the individual's medical file and should *only* be shared with other health care professionals. The Medical Eligibility Form is the only form that should be submitted to nonmedical personnel at a school or sports organization.

Disclaimer: Athletes who have a current Preparticipation Physical Evaluation (per state and local guidance) on file should not need to complete another examination.

PREPARTICIPATION EVALUATION

PHYSICAL EXAMINATION FORM

Name: ______________________________ Date of birth: ______________

PHYSICIAN REMINDERS

1. **Consider additional questions on more sensitive issues.**
   - Do you feel stressed out or under a lot of pressure?
   - Do you have enough food at home?
   - Do you ever worry about becoming homeless?
   - Do you feel safe at your home/residence, in your neighborhood, at school, and in sports/activities?
   - Have you ever tried cigarettes, e-cigarettes, chewing tobacco, snuff, or dip?
   - During the past 30 days, did you use chewing tobacco, snuff, or dip?
   - Do you drink alcohol or use any other drugs?
   - Do you wear a seat belt, use a helmet, and use condoms?
   - Have you ever taken anabolic steroids or used any other performance-enhancing supplement?
   - Have you ever taken any supplements to help you gain or lose weight or improve your performance?

EXAMINATION		
Height: Weight:		
BP: / Pulse: Vision: R 20/ L 20/ Corrected: ☐ Y ☐ N		
MEDICAL	**NORMAL**	**ABNORMAL FINDINGS**
Appearance • Marfan stigmata (kyphoscoliosis, high-arched palate, pectus excavatum, arachnodactyly, hyperlaxity, myopia)		
Eyes, ears, nose, and throat		
Lymph nodes		
Cardiovascular • Murmurs (auscultation standing, auscultation supine, and ± Valsalva maneuver) • Pulses (radial and femoral)		
Lungs		
Abdomen • Mass or enlarged liver/spleen • CVA tenderness		
Skin • Herpes simplex virus (HSV), *Staphylococcus aureus*, or tinea corporis		
Neurological		
MUSCULOSKELETAL	**NORMAL**	**ABNORMAL FINDINGS**
Neck		
Back		
Shoulder and arm		
Elbow and forearm		
Wrist, hand, and fingers		
Hip and thigh		
Knee		
Leg and ankle		
Foot and toes		
Functional • Consider single-leg squat test and/or box drop test		

Consider electrocardiography (ECG), echocardiography, referral to a cardiologist for abnormal cardiac history and/or examination findings.

Name of health care professional (print or type): ______________________ Date: __________

Address: ______________________________ Phone: ______________

Signature of health care professional: ______________________________, MD, DO, NP, or PA

This form should be placed into the individual's medical file and should *only* be shared with other health care professionals.
The Medical Eligibility Form is the only form that should be submitted to nonmedical personnel at a school or sports organization.

PREPARTICIPATION EVALUATION

SUPPLEMENT TO THE HISTORY FORM FOR INDIVIDUALS WITH DISABILITIES

Name: ______________________________ Date of birth: ______________

1. Type of disability:		
2. Cause of disability (traumatic, medical, genetic):		
3. Date of disability (age of onset):		
4. Specific diagnosis (for individuals with limb deficiencies and spinal cord injuries, please include the levels affected):		
5. Medical treatments (eg, medications, surgery, orthosis/prosthesis, medical devices, technical aids):		
6. Is your condition changing over time? If so, how?		
7. Classification (if available):		
8. List the activities you are participating in:		
	Yes	**No**
9. Do you limit or carefully control what you eat or drink?		
10. Have you had pulmonary function tests? (if yes, please state the reason)		
11. Have you ever had unusual blood clotting such as prolonged bleeding, deep vein thrombosis, or a pulmonary embolism?		
12. Do you have any visual problems such as decreased vision in one or both eyes, legal blindness, need for glasses, eye crossing or drifting, and/or history of eye surgery?		
13. Have you ever had abnormal bowel or bladder control?		
14. Do you have a history of recurrent skin wounds or pressure sores?		
15. Have you been hospitalized for issues related to skin breakdown?		
16. Have you ever been told you have osteoporosis, osteopenia, or low bone density?		
17. Have you had problems with recurrent urinary tract infections?		
18. Are you concerned about recent bladder disturbances, including pain or bleeding?		
19. Have you had a condition called "autonomic dysreflexia"?		

Explain "Yes" answers here.

____

____

____

____

____

____

Functional Review

Please circle any major category of limitation or difficulty for you because of your diagnosis:

Mobility:	Independent	Cane/walker	Wheelchair
Transfers:	Independent	Sliding board	Assist
Hygiene:	Independent	Independent with modifications	Assist
Dressing upper body:	Independent	Independent with modifications	Assist
Dressing lower body:	Independent	Independent with modifications	Assist
Eating, drinking:	Independent	Independent with modifications	Assist
Bowel care:	Normal function	Modified routine (specify below)	Assist
Bladder care:	Normal function	Modified routine (specify below)	Assist

Specify modified routine for bowel or bladder:

____

____

____

Adaptive/Prosthetic Equipment ***(nonsport)***

Item: __________________ Date obtained: ____________ Date last modified? ____________

Is this used for daily nonsporting activities? ________________________

Do you have any concerns about fit, performance, comfort, or safety? __________________

Have you had any associated pain, skin lesions, injuries, or other issues with this equipment?

____

____

____

Adaptive/Prosthetic Equipment ***(sport)***

Item: __________________ Date obtained: ____________ Date last modified? ____________

Is this used for your sporting activities? ________________________

Do you have any concerns about fit, performance, comfort, or safety? __________________

Have you had any associated pain, skin lesions, injuries, or other issues with this equipment?

____

____

I hereby state that, to the best of my knowledge, my answers to the questions on this form are complete and correct.

Signature of athlete: ______________________________

Signature of parent or guardian: ________________________

Date: ________________________

The Medical Eligibility Form is the only form that should be submitted to nonmedical personnel at a school or sports organization.

PREPARTICIPATION EVALUATION

MEDICAL ELIGIBILITY FORM

Name: ______________________________ Date of birth: ______________

SHARED EMERGENCY INFORMATION

Medical Conditions (Check all that apply)

☐ Anaphylaxis ☐ Asthma ☐ Cardiac Condition ☐ Concussion History ☐ Diabetes ☐ Heat Stroke/ Rhabdomyolysis

☐ Missing Organ ☐ POTS ☐ Seizures ☐ Sickle Cell Disease ☐ Sickle Cell Trait ☐ Stinger History

☐ Other (Specify): ______________________________

____

☐ Known triggers for conditions listed above (eg, exercise, weather): ______________

____

☐ Environmental & Food Allergies: ______________________________

____

Condition-Specific Activity Guidelines

☐ Emergency Medications (eg, inhaler, EpiPen): ______________________________

☐ Medications used before, during, or after activity (eg, inhaler before exercise, insulin): ______________

____

☐ Activity Modifications (eg, limit exertion, monitor symptoms, extra hydration breaks): ______________

____

☐ Other: ______________________________

For Evaluating Health Care Professional

☐ Medically eligible for all sports and activities without restriction

☐ Medically eligible for all sports and activities without restriction, with recommendations for further evaluation or treatment of: __________

____

☐ Medically eligible **AFTER** evaluation and clearance for: ______________________________

____

☐ Medically eligible for certain sports and activities (list the specific sports or type of sports): ______________

____

☐ Not medically eligible for any sports or activities

Recommendations: ______________________________

____

____

I have examined the student named on this form and completed the preparticipation physical evaluation. The athlete does not have apparent clinical contraindications to practice and can participate in the sport(s) as outlined on this form. A copy of the physical examination findings are on record in my office and can be made available to the school at the request of the parents. If conditions arise after the athlete has been cleared for participation, the physician may rescind the medical eligibility until the problem is resolved and the potential consequences are completely explained to the athlete (and parents or guardians).

Name of health care professional (print or type): ______________________ Date: ______________

Address: ______________________ Phone: ______________

Signature of health care professional: ______________________, MD, DO, NP, or PA

Legal Guardian Acknowledgment to Share With Individual's School or Sports Organizations

☐ I acknowledge that this form may contain protected medical information and authorize its sharing with the participant's school, coaches, and relevant personnel.

Legal guardian name (print or type): ______________________

Signature of legal guardian: ______________________ Date: ______________

Emergency contacts: ______________________

Index

Page numbers followed by an *f*, a *t*, or a *b* indicate a figure, a table, or a box, respectively.

A

B

E

F

G

H

I

J

K

L

M

N

O

P

R

S

T

U

V

W

Y